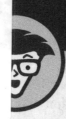

Depression

2nd Edition

by Laura L. Smith, PhD
Charles H. Elliott, PhD

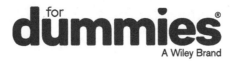

for
dummies®
A Wiley Brand

Depression For Dummies®, 2nd Edition

Published by: **John Wiley & Sons, Inc.**, 111 River Street, Hoboken, NJ 07030-5774, www.wiley.com

Copyright © 2021 by John Wiley & Sons, Inc., Hoboken, New Jersey

Published simultaneously in Canada

For general information on our other products and services, please contact our Customer Care Department within the U.S. at 877-762-2974, outside the U.S. at 317-572-3993, or fax 317-572-4002. For technical support, please visit https://hub.wiley.com/community/support/dummies.

Wiley publishes in a variety of print and electronic formats and by print-on-demand. Some material included with standard print versions of this book may not be included in e-books or in print-on-demand. If this book refers to media such as a CD or DVD that is not included in the version you purchased, you may download this material at http://booksupport.wiley.com. For more information about Wiley products, visit www.wiley.com.

Library of Congress Control Number: 2021932518

ISBN 978-1-119-76859-3 (pbk); ISBN 978-1-119-76860-9 (ebk); ISBN 978-1-119-76861-6 (ebk)

Manufactured in the United States of America

SKY10025322_030921

Contents at a Glance

Table of Contents

Introduction

Decadent luxuries, dazzling technology, and startling new knowledge flood the senses and excite the imagination. What was the domain of science fiction less than a generation ago is now commonplace in many living rooms. Today, cable companies beam recently released movies to inches-thick televisions that hang on walls. All you have to do is press a few buttons on your remote control and your home is a cinema. And, with a couple of words to your virtual assistant, you can order a pizza that arrives in time for the start of the movie.

In the field of healthcare, advancing knowledge of the immune system promises new cancer treatments that go to the source of the disease. Nanotechnology eventually will allow inconceivably small machines to clean out congested arteries like a plumber's snake. And the human genome project begins to solve the mysteries behind countless inherited diseases. Sure, the world still has plenty of problems, but solutions for many of them lie on the horizon.

Yet the World Health Organization paints a less optimistic picture. It estimates that on any given day, 264 million people worldwide suffer from depression. Over the course of a year, about 10 percent of the world's population suffer from an episode of depression. Depression rates continue to increase. And most experts believe that the increase is real — not just a result of more people seeking help.

Theories abound concerning the alarming increase in depression today. But regardless of the cause, this scourge robs its victims of happiness, joy, and the capacity to give and receive love.

The good news is that more weapons exist for defeating depression than ever before. Clinicians have devised new psychotherapies that have been verified as effective in treating depression and preventing relapse. Medications, methods of stimulating key nerve centers, and other psychotherapies continue to be refined and developed. The majority of people no longer need to suffer with long-standing, intractable depression.

About This Book

We have two primary goals in writing this book. First, we want you to understand the nature of depression. Understanding depression makes the idea of dealing with it less frightening. Second, we present what you're probably most interested in discovering — how to overcome your depression or help someone you love who has depression.

We leave no stone unturned in our quest to bring you every possible means for battling depression. We draw strategies for defeating depression from the fields of medicine and psychotherapy. We tell you about the arsenal of medications and other strategies that can combat depression. We show you how focusing on your overall health with exercise and nutrition can pay off. Plus, we extract elements from the psychotherapeutic approaches that have stood up to the tests of rigorous research and been verified as highly effective treatments for depression. These approaches include

>> Cognitive therapy

>> Acceptance and commitment therapy (ACT)

>> Behavior therapy

>> Interpersonal and relationship therapy

Then we go one step further. We turn to the field of *positive psychology* for ideas on navigating your way from feeling *good* again to feeling *even better*. We want you to make your life more joyful and more meaningful.

Depression For Dummies offers you the best advice available based on scientific research. We believe that, if you practice the techniques and strategies we provide in this book, you'll very likely feel better. For some people, this book may be a complete guide for defeating mild depression. Numerous studies show that self-help often works.

However, depression frequently needs more care and attention than you can receive through self-help. If your depression significantly hinders your ability to work or play, you need to get professional help. No book can completely replace therapy. Start by seeing your family doctor. If you're seeing a therapist or counselor, you may find that *Depression For Dummies* can help augment your therapy. Be sure to discuss that possibility with your therapist. Depression can be conquered, so please don't give up.

Foolish Assumptions

Who would want to read this book? We assume, perhaps foolishly, that you or someone you love suffers from depression. We also figure that you want to banish depression from your life. Finally, we imagine that you're curious about a variety of helpful strategies that can fit your lifestyle and personality. If these descriptions strike a chord, this book is for you.

On the other hand, you may be a professional who is looking for a good, easy-to-understand resource for your patients who suffer from depression. Readers over the years have told us that our *For Dummies* books on mental health issues have been helpful in both their recovery and their understanding of what they're dealing with in therapy.

Icons Used in This Book

Throughout this book, we use icons in the margins to quickly point out different types of information. Here are the icons you'll see and a few words about what they mean.

REMEMBER

As the name of this icon implies, we don't want you to forget the information that accompanies it.

TIP

This icon emphasizes pieces of practical information or bits of insight that you can put to work.

WARNING

This icon appears when you need to be careful or seek professional help.

TECHNICAL STUFF

This piece of art alerts you to information that you may find interesting, but not reading it won't put you at a disadvantage in the battle against depression.

Beyond the Book

There is a free Cheat Sheet available online. Go to www.dummies.com and type "Depression For Dummies Cheat Sheet" in the Search box. The cheat sheet gives you signs that you may be depressed, some depression dos and don'ts, as well resources to get professional help.

Where to Go from Here

Most books are written so that you have to start on page one and read straight through. But we wrote *Depression For Dummies* so that you can use the detailed Table of Contents to pick and choose what you want to read based on your individual interests. Don't worry too much about reading chapters and parts in any particular order. Read whatever chapters apply to your situation. However, we suggest that you at least skim Part 1 because it contains a variety of fascinating facts as well as important ideas for getting started.

In addition, the more severe your depression, the more we urge you to start with Chapter 5 and continue with Part 3. These chapters contain a variety of ways for overcoming the powerful inertia that keeps severely depressed people from taking actions. After you read those chapters, feel free to continue picking and choosing what topics you want to explore.

1

Discovering Depression and Preparing a Plan

Chapter **1**

Demystifying and Defeating Depression

Like solitary confinement, depression isolates those who experience it. Alone, fearful, and feeling powerless, sufferers withdraw. Hope, faith, relationships, work, play, and creative pursuits — the very paths to recovery — seem meaningless and inconceivable. A cruel, inhuman punishment, depression incarcerates the body, mind, and soul.

Though depression feels inescapable, we have a set of keys for unlocking the jail cell of depression that confines you or someone you care about. You may find that the first key you try works, but more often than not escape requires a combination of keys. We're here to help, and we have a ring of keys for you to try out. We also tell you how to choose a great locksmith (mental health professional) if you can't find the right key.

In this chapter, we clarify the difference between sadness and depression; they're not the same. Next, we show you how depression looks among various groups of people. We calculate the costs of depression in terms of health, productivity, and relationships. We tell you about the treatment options for depression. And finally, we offer a glimpse of life beyond depression.

Just Singing the Blues or Depressed?

Life delivers death, divorce, disaster, disease, disorder, disgrace, and distress. Inescapable and inevitable. Even if nothing else goes wrong, you're eventually going to die. Expecting to live a life absent of sharp episodes of sadness, despair, or grief is unrealistic. In fact, without times of sorrow, how would you truly appreciate life's blessings?

Yet, misfortunes and loss need not lead to depression. What's the difference? Sadness and grief lessen in intensity as time passes. (See Chapter 2 for more information about grief and types of depression.) Sadness and grief may seem fairly overwhelming when they occur. But time does eventually heal (unless the grief turns into depression over time).

REMEMBER

Unlike episodes of despair, depression involves deep feeling of guilt and loss of self-esteem. People suffering from depression feel hopeless, helpless, and unforgiving of themselves. Depression disrupts the body, often impacting sleep, appetite, concentration, energy, and sex. And depression profoundly diminishes the ability to love, laugh, work, and play.

Depression is a mood disorder in which a person feels profoundly sad, joyless, despondent, and unable to experience pleasure. Depression comes in various types that have somewhat different symptoms. We describe these categories of depression in Chapter 2, but all involve a low mood or diminished sense of pleasure.

The Varying Faces of Depression

Depression doesn't discriminate; it can affect anyone regardless of race, social class, or status. Typical symptoms of sadness, loss of energy and interests, low self-esteem, feelings of guilt, and changes in appetite and sleep appear in men, women, children, and the elderly. Such symptoms also manifest themselves across different cultures. However, a depressed preschooler may not exactly look the same as a depressed 80-year-old.

In Chapter 2, we dissect the various categories of depression. In this chapter, we show you how depression looks in different people at different life stages. The cases we present in this chapter, and throughout this book, don't represent real people. However, they're loosely based on the people we've worked with in our collective careers.

Young and depressed

Depression can be found among children of any age, from preschool through young adulthood. However, preschoolers have relatively low rates of depression. Depression increases throughout childhood and is most common in adolescence.

WARNING

The rates of depression in children are likely underreported because parents and professionals often fail to recognize the problem. Children rarely spontaneously report depression to others. Instead, they more typically remain unaware of their feelings, which manifest themselves through changes in their behavior, appetite, and sleep.

> **Mackenzie's** mom surprises her by bringing cupcakes to school on her eighth birthday. The teacher leads the class in singing "Happy Birthday," but Mackenzie barely smiles. After quickly devouring the two overloaded trays of cupcakes, the kids all race out to the playground for recess. Mackenzie trails behind.
>
> Mackenzie's teacher approaches her mother, "I'm concerned about Mackenzie. She seems quiet and less interested in her schoolwork. I often see her alone on the playground. She doesn't raise her hand in class like she used to, either. Is something wrong?"

When children are depressed, they lose interest in activities that they previously enjoyed. If you ask them if they're sad, they may not be able to connect their feelings with words. However, they will show various signs of depression, such as low energy, sleep problems, appetite changes, irritability, and low self-esteem.

KIDS, DEPRESSION, AND OBESITY

In a study reported in the journal *Pediatrics,* more than 9,000 teens participated in a study on the relationship between depression and obesity. The researchers gave the kids a questionnaire that measured depression and calculated their body mass index (BMI), a measure of obesity. They assessed the kids once again a year later. Kids who were obese and depressed at the first assessment tended to become more obese by the second assessment. Kids who were not obese at the first assessment, but were depressed, had double the risk of becoming obese a year later. Much remains to be discovered about exactly how depression may increase this risk of obesity; however, these findings underscore the importance of addressing depression when it occurs.

Watch children at play for subtle signs of depression. Depressed children may weave themes of death or loss into their play. All children's play includes such themes on occasion, but dark topics show up more often in kids who are depressed. You may need to observe kids over a period of time because their moods change. They may not look as continuously depressed as adults with depression. Their moods may fluctuate throughout the day. Consult a professional if you have any doubts.

Depression in seniors

Some people view old age as inherently depressing. They assume that upon reaching a certain age, quality of life deteriorates. In fact, there is some truth to these assumptions: Old age brings increases in illness and disability and losses of friends, family members, and social support. Therefore, *some* sadness is to be expected.

Nevertheless, depression is absolutely *not* an inevitable consequence of old age. Most symptoms of depression in the elderly mimic those of depression in anyone. However, the elderly are a little more likely to focus on aches and pains rather than feelings of despair. Furthermore, they commonly express regret and remorse about past events in their lives.

Depression interferes with memory. If you notice increased memory problems in grandpa or grandma, you could easily chalk the problem up to the worst-case scenario: Alzheimer's or dementia. However, such memory problems also occur as a result of depression.

And depression in the elderly increases the chances of death. Yet, if asked about depression, elders may scoff at the idea. Denying depression, the elder person may not get needed treatment.

Elderly men are at particularly high risk of suicide. Men older than 60 are more likely to take their own lives than any other combination of age and gender. If you have any doubts, check the possibility of depression with a doctor or mental health professional.

Real men don't get depressed, or do they?

Most studies show that men get depressed about half as frequently as women. But then again, men tend to cover up and hide their depression; they feel far more reluctant to talk about weaknesses and vulnerabilities than women do. Why?

Many men have been taught that admitting to any form of mental illness or emotional problem is unmanly. From early childhood experiences, these men learn to cover up negative feelings.

> **Scott** looks forward to retirement from his job as a marketing executive. He can't wait to start traveling and pursuing long-postponed hobbies. Three months after he retires, his wife of 20 years asks for a divorce. Shocked, yet showing little emotion, Scott tells his friends and family, "Life goes on."

> Scott starts drinking more heavily than usual. He pursues extreme sports. He pushes his abilities to the limit in rock climbing, hang gliding, and skiing in remote areas. Scott distances himself from family and friends. His normal, even temperament turns sour. Yet Scott denies the depression so evident to those who know him well.

REMEMBER

Rather than own up to disturbing feelings, men commonly turn to drugs or alcohol in an attempt to cope. Some depressed men express anger and irritation rather than sadness. Others report the physical signs of depression, such as lack of energy, poor sleep, altered appetite, and body aches, but adamantly deny feeling depressed. The cost of not expressing feelings and not getting help may account for the fourfold greater rate of suicide among depressed men than women.

Women and depression

Why do women around the world appear to suffer from depression about twice as often as men? Biological and reproductive factors may play a role. The rate of depression during pregnancy, after childbirth, and prior to menopause is higher than at any other time in women's lives.

However, cultural or social factors likely contribute to women's depression as well. For example, women who have been sexually or physically abused outnumber men with similar experiences, and such abuse increases the likelihood of depression. Furthermore, risk factors, such as low income, stress, and multiple responsibilities like juggling housework, childcare, and a career, occur more frequently among women than men.

> **Janine** gently lays her baby down in the crib. Finally, the baby has fallen asleep. Exhausted after a challenging day at work, she desperately longs to go to bed herself. But, laundry waits, the bills need to be paid, and the house is a disaster. Six months ago, her husband was called to active duty in the Army Reserves and life hasn't been the same since. Janine realizes her overwhelming fatigue and loss of appetite are due to depression setting in.

Depression and diversity

Everyone experiences depression in unique ways. Attempting to generalize about depression based merely on ethnicity or membership in a certain group can lead to misperceptions. But risk factors for depression include discrimination, social ostracism, poverty, and major losses (like loss of a job or loved one). And unfortunately all these risk factors occur more frequently among minorities. Being different may take the form of race, culture, physical challenge, or sexual orientation.

In addition to these risk factors, many groups face special obstacles when dealing with depression. For example, some ethnic populations have limited access to mental health care because of language differences, embarrassment, economic difficulties, and lack of nearby facilities. More resources designed at helping these groups access care are clearly needed.

Adversity and depression

People who undergo traumatic events (especially repeatedly) have an increased risk of depression. For example, the social isolation that came during the pandemic increased rates of depression and anxiety. Those who experience chronic financial difficulties can easily succumb to a sense of hopelessness and depression. Those who live in high-risk areas such as forests in western states and coastal areas vulnerable to extreme weather events such as hurricanes may also be susceptible to higher risks of depression.

Adding Up the Costs of Depression

Depression has existed since the beginning of humankind. But today depression is a worldwide epidemic. No one knows why for sure, but the risk of depression for those born after World War II has mushroomed.

Estimates vary considerably, but today depression appears to hover around 20 percent of all people over the course of a lifetime. Furthermore, in any given 12-month period, about 10 percent of the population experiences an episode of significant depression. And at this very moment, the World Health Organization estimates that 264 million people are suffering from depression throughout the world. That's an awful lot of people.

TIP

Guess what? Estimates on depression are only rough approximations. Because most people with depression fail to seek treatment and many folks with depression don't even realize they're depressed, reliable statistics are few and far between. Whatever the real figures are, huge numbers of people suffer from depression at some point in their lives. And depression has all kinds of costs associated with it.

Financial costs of depression

The World Health Organization (WHO) has created a statistic called the Global Burden of Disease (GBD) that puts a number on the worldwide economic cost of various diseases. Depression is now one of the top-five largest contributors to the GBD.

The financial cost of depression is staggering. In the United States alone, the American Psychiatric Association pegs the price tag of depression at $210.5 billion per year.

Where do these costs come from? Depressed people miss work more often and get less done when they do work. Parents of depressed kids may have to miss work to get their children to treatment appointments. Treatment also represents part of the total tab, but remember that alleviation of depression increases productivity, reduces absenteeism, and reduces medical costs.

Previewing personal costs of depression

Economic facts and figures do little to describe the human costs of depression. The profound suffering caused by depression affects both the sufferer and those who care. Words can't adequately describe these costs:

>> The anguish of a family suffering from the loss of a loved one to suicide

>> The excruciating pain experienced by someone with depression

>> The diminished quality of relationships suffered both by people with depression and those who care about them

>> The loss of purpose and sense of worth suffered by those with depression

>> The loss of joy

Detailing depression's physical toll

Depression's destruction radiates beyond personal and economic costs — depression damages the body. Scientists discover new information almost daily about the intricate relationship between mood and health. Today, we know that depression affects:

» **Your immune system.** Your body has a complex system for warding off infections and diseases. Various studies have shown that depression changes the way the immune system responds to attack. Depression depletes the immune system and makes people more susceptible to disease.

» **Your skeletal system.** Untreated depression increases your chances of getting osteoporosis, though it's unclear exactly how depression may lead to this problem.

» **Your heart.** The relationship between depression and cardiovascular health is powerful. Johns Hopkins University studied healthy doctors and found that among those people who developed depression, their risk of heart disease increased twofold. This risk is comparable to the risk posed by smoking.

Another study reported in the journal *Circulation* followed more than 4,000 elderly people who were initially free of heart disease. Researchers found that elderly persons with depression were 40 percent more likely to develop heart disease and 60 percent more likely to die. Intriguingly, they discovered that every increase in depression scores led to even greater increases in heart disease risk. This risk occurred above and beyond the risks posed by smoking, high cholesterol levels, and age.

» **Your mind.** Although depression can mimic dementia in terms of causing poor memory and concentration, depression also increases the risk for dementia. We're not sure why, but scientists have discovered that an area in the brain thought to govern memory is smaller in those with chronic depression.

If left untreated, depression can disrupt and possibly damage connections in your brain and may lead to the degeneration and death of brain cells.

» **Your experience of pain.** Of course depression inflicts emotional pain. However, depression also contributes to the experience of physical pain. Thus, if you have some type of chronic pain, such as arthritis or back pain, depression may increase the amount of pain you feel. Scientists aren't entirely sure how depression and pain interact, but the effect may be due to disruption of neurotransmitters involved in pain perception. As a matter of fact, many people with depression fail to realize they're depressed and only complain of a variety of physical symptoms such as pain.

Depression likely affects the entire way the body functions. For example, altered appetite may lead to obesity or malnourishment and serious weight loss. In addition, depression is associated with disrupted hormonal levels and various other subtle physiological changes. In a sense, depression harms your body, mind, and soul.

REMEMBER

Don't let yourself get depressed by all these frightening effects caused by depression. If you're depressed, you can feel better — and we spend the remainder of this book helping you to do so. Effective treatments currently exist and new ones are emerging.

Feeling Good Again

Depression is treatable. With good diagnosis and help, most folks can expect to recover. If you feel a loss of pleasure, reduced energy, a diminished sense of your worth, or unexplained aches and pains, you may be depressed. Please pursue help. See Chapter 5 for ideas on how to find the right help for you.

Many types of help exist for depression. This book is one of them and falls under the category of self-help. Self-help does work for many people. However, self-directed efforts are often not enough (although self-help often can supplement professional assistance). In the following sections, we briefly outline the different kinds of help that you may find useful.

REMEMBER

You don't have to choose only one option. You may need or want to combine a number of these strategies. For example, many people with depression have found the combination of medication and psychotherapy helpful. And combining more than one type of psychotherapy sometimes proves useful as well.

WARNING

If your depression doesn't start to lift or if you have severe symptoms such as thoughts of suicide, please seek professional assistance immediately.

Exploring cognitive therapy

Cognitive therapy is based on the premise that the way you think strongly influences the way you feel. Studies support the value of cognitive therapy above any other approach to the alleviation of depression. Dr. Aaron T. Beck, who developed cognitive therapy, discovered that depressed people

>> View themselves in distorted, overly negative ways

>> See the world in bleak, dark terms

>> Envision a future of continual gloom and doom

Depression causes people to believe that their dark views are completely accurate and correct. Cognitive therapy helps untangle twisted thinking. You can find out more about this approach in Part 2 of this book. We encourage you to give cognitive therapy a try. Research shows that cognitive therapy even protects you against future recurrences of depression. Skeptical? Try it anyway!

Trying behavior therapy

Another well-tested approach to the alleviation of depression is what's known as *behavior therapy*, which is based on the premise that changing behavior changes moods. The problem: When you're depressed, you don't feel like doing much of anything. So in Part 3 we help you figure out how to take small steps and overcome this mind hurdle using behavior-therapy based tools. In addition, we tell you how

>> Exercise can kick-start your battle with depression.

>> You can bring small pleasures back into your life.

>> Problem-solving strategies can improve coping.

Reinventing relationships

Depression sometimes follows the loss of a significant relationship and such losses often come in the form of death of a loved one or divorce. But depression can also come on the coattails of other types of relationship losses — like changing a way you relate to the world. For example, retirement requires you to give up (to lose) one role, that of an employee, and take on another. Major life changes or transitions sometimes lead to depression if you don't have a way of dealing with them. So in Chapter 15, we tell you how to handle loss and transitions.

Depression also often causes problems with important current relationships. In Chapter 16, we provide you with various ways of enhancing your relationships. The process of improving your relationships may decrease your depression as well.

Finding biological solutions

Perhaps you think the easiest approach to treating depression is found at the pharmacy or health food store. Simply pop the right potion and voilà, you're cured! If only getting better were so easy!

In Chapter 17, we review the pharmacological therapies. You'll find quite a few to choose from and we help you sort out the options. We also give you strategies for making the complicated decision as to whether antidepressant medication makes sense for you or if you'd prefer alternative approaches.

In Chapter 18, we discuss the so-called natural way of treating depression. We also bring you information about shock therapy and other not-so-common treatments for depression.

Feeling Better Than Good

After you've overcome your depression, you will likely feel much better. However, you'll want to sustain that improvement. Depression, like the common cold, has a nasty habit of returning. But you can do much to hold off or prevent future depression. We show you how to avoid future bouts in Chapter 19. Should you catch another round of depression, we also show you how to recover more quickly and keep the symptoms mild.

So, you feel better. You feel good. But guess what? You don't have to settle for good. We want you to feel better than good; perhaps better than you have ever felt in your life. That may sound too good to be true. However, in Chapter 21, we give you ways to add purpose and meaning to your life. In addition, we provide secret keys for unlocking your potential for happiness — those keys probably aren't what you would imagine them to be.

Celebrating Sadness

We begin this book with promises of relief from depression. However, no therapy, behavior, or pill provides a life free from sadness. We're glad that one doesn't exist. And if such a cure existed, we wouldn't take it.

Because without sadness, how could one feel happy? Who would write great plays or create emotionally powerful works of art or songs that sing to the depths of the soul? Human emotions serve a purpose. They distinguish us from computers and give life meaning.

Thus, we write this book wishing you a life of happiness interspersed with moments of pain. To have pain is to live.

Chapter **2**

Detecting Depression

D epression has a variety of symptoms, from subtle to obvious. Sometimes depression slowly and silently possesses the mind and soul, virtually shutting down day-to-day living. Other times, depression explodes, bursts through the door, and robs its victims of joy and pleasure. Some people are unaware that they have depression, although other people fully recognize depression's presence in their lives. Sometimes depression has no obvious signs, masquerading as a set of physical complaints like fatigue, poor sleep, changes in appetite, and even indigestion.

Depression is a disease of extremes. Its power can not only depress appetite but also create insatiable hunger. People with depression may find sleep distressingly evasive; others may find that fatigue is overwhelming, confining them to bed for days at a time. Depressed people sometimes pace frantically or collapse and hardly move. Depression can take root and endure for months or years. Other times it blows through like a series of afternoon thunderstorms.

In this chapter, we help you recognize whether you or someone you care about suffers from depression. We do so by categorizing the effects depression has on individuals. We outline the major types of depression and their symptoms. We explore the connections between disease and depression, and we look at the grief/depression link. We delve into the causes of this disorder. And finally, we tell you how you or a loved one can monitor and track your moods if you suspect that you may be battling depression.

Recognizing the Ravages of Depression

Everyone feels down from time to time. Stock market plunges, health problems, natural disasters, loss of a friend, pandemics, divorce, or failure to reach sales quotas — events like these can make anyone feel sad and upset for awhile. But depression is more than a normal reaction to unpleasant events and losses. Depression deepens and spreads well beyond sadness, disrupting both the mind and the body in serious, sometimes deadly ways.

Depression impacts every aspect of life. In fact, even though a number of types of depression exist (see "The Faces of Depression" later in this chapter), all types of depression affect people in four areas, although each individual may be affected in different ways. Depression disrupts

>> Thoughts

>> Behaviors

>> Relationships

>> The body

In the following sections, we touch on the ways that each form of depression affects individuals.

Dwelling on bleak thoughts

When you get depressed, your view of the world changes. The sun shines less brightly, the sky clouds over, people seem cold and distant, and the future looks dark. Your mind may fill with recurrent thoughts of worthlessness, self-loathing, and even death. Typically, depressed people complain of difficulty concentrating, remembering, and making decisions.

For **Ellen,** depression emerges about one year after her divorce. She finds herself thinking that she'll never find a good relationship. Ellen is quite attractive, although when she looks in the mirror, she only sees the beginning of wrinkles, a bad haircut, and an occasional blemish. She concludes that even if there are any good people left, they'll be repulsed by her awful looks. She feels tense. Her concentration is shot, and she starts to make careless errors at work. Her boss understands that she's been under stress lately, but Ellen sees her mistakes as proof of incompetence. Although she believes that she's in a job well below her skill level, she doesn't see herself as capable of doing anything better. She begins to wonder why she bothers to go to work every day.

TIP

Does your mind dwell on negative thoughts? If so, you may be suffering from depression. The following quiz in Table 2-1 gives you a sample of typical thoughts that go along with depression. Check the box preceding each thought that you often have.

TABLE 2-1

Depressed Thoughts Quiz

Check If Yes	Depressed Thought
	Things are getting worse and worse for me.
	I think I'm worthless.
	No one would miss me if I were dead.
	My memory is shot.
	I make too many mistakes.
	By and large, I think I'm a failure.
	I don't look forward to much of anything.
	I find it almost impossible to make decisions.
	The world would be a better place without me.
	Basically, I'm extremely pessimistic about things.
	I can't think of anything that sounds interesting or enjoyable.
	My life is full of regrets.
	I can't concentrate, and I forget what I read.
	I don't see my life getting better in the future.
	I'm deeply ashamed of myself.

Unlike many of the self-tests you may have seen in magazines or online, no specific score indicates depression here. All the items are typical of depressed thinking. However, merely checking one or two doesn't mean you're depressed. But, the more items you check, the greater the concern of possible depression. And if you check any of the items related to death or suicide, that's plenty of cause for concern.

TIP

Don't get too depressed about your depressive thinking. Depression is treatable. If you checked a lot of boxes in Table 2-1, we urge you to consider seeing your primary care provider for a depression screening and a possible referral for treatment.

If you're having serious suicidal thoughts, you need an immediate evaluation and treatment. If the thoughts include a plan that you believe you may actually carry out now or in the very near future, go to a hospital emergency room. They have trained personnel who can help. If you're not able to get yourself to an emergency room, call 911 for more rapid attention. The National Suicide Helpline is particularly useful and is staffed 24/7: Call 800-273-TALK (800-273-8255). For more information, but not for emergencies, see Chapter 10.

For more information about depressive thinking and what you can do about it, see Part 2.

Dragging your feet: Depressed behavior

Not everyone who's depressed behaves in the same way. Some people speed up and others slow down. Some folks sleep more than ever, while others complain of a dreadful lack of sleep.

> **Darryl** drags his body out of bed in the morning. Even after ten hours of sleep, he feels depleted of energy. He starts showing up at work late. He uses up his sick leave. He can't make himself go to the gym, an activity he used to enjoy. He reasons that he'll work out again when he gets the energy. His friends ask him what's going on, because he hasn't been spending much time with them. He says that he doesn't really know; he's just tired.

> **Cheryl,** on the other hand, is averaging about three and a half hours of sleep each night. She awakens at about 3 a.m. with racing thoughts. When she gets up, she feels a frantic pressure and can't seem to sit still. Irritable and cranky, she snaps at her friends and co-workers. Unable to sleep at night, she finds herself drinking too much. Sometimes she cries for no apparent reason.

Although everyone is different, certain behaviors tend to go along with depression. Do your actions and behaviors concern you? Depressed people tend to either feel like they're walking in wet cement or running full speed on a treadmill. The following quiz in Table 2-2 can give you an idea as to whether your actions indicate a problem. Check each item that applies.

All these items are typical of depressed behavior or, in some cases, a health problem. On a bad day, anyone might check off a single item. However, the more items you check, the more likely it is that something's wrong, especially if the problem exists for more than a couple of weeks.

TABLE 2-2

Depressed Behavior Quiz

Check If Yes	Depressed Behaviors
	I've been having unexplained crying spells.
	The few times I force myself to go out, I don't have much fun.
	I can't make myself exercise like I used to.
	I haven't been going out nearly as much as usual.
	I feel agitated and frantic, but can't get anything done.
	I've been missing a lot of work lately.
	I can't get myself to do much of anything, even important projects.
	I'm moving at a slower pace than I usually do, for no good reason.
	I haven't been doing things for fun like I usually do.
	Even when others are laughing, I don't join in.
	My home and workspace are more and more disorganized.
	I start projects but can't seem to finish them.
	I struggle to make myself get out of bed in the morning.

For more information about depressed behavior and what you can do about it, see Part 3.

Reflecting upon relationships and depression

Depression damages the way you relate to others. Withdrawal and avoidance are the most common responses to depression. Sometimes depressed people get irritable and critical with the very people they care most about.

> **Antonio** trips over a toy left on the living room floor and snaps at his wife Sylvia, "Can't you get the kids to pick up their damn toys for once?" Hurt and surprised by the attack, Sylvia apologizes. Antonio fails to acknowledge her apology and turns away. Sylvia quickly picks up the toy and wonders what's been happening to her marriage. Antonio hardly talks to her anymore, other than to complain or scold her about something trivial. She can't remember the last time they had sex. She worries that he may be having an affair.

TIP

Have you or perhaps someone you care about been responding differently in one or more of your relationships? Table 2-3 describes some of the ways in which depression affects relationships. Check the items that fit your situation.

TABLE 2-3

Depression and Relationships Quiz

Check If Yes	Depressed Behaviors
	I've been avoiding people, including friends and family, more lately.
	I can't share with others what I am feeling.
	I've been unusually irritable with others.
	I don't feel like being around anyone.
	I feel isolated and alone.
	I'm sure that no one understands or cares about me.
	I haven't felt like being physically intimate with anyone lately.
	I feel like I've been letting everyone down.
	I'm pretty sure that no one wants to be around me.
	Lately, I don't really care about whether others like me or not.
	Frankly, I don't care that much about other people right now.
	I'm not really being a good partner in my relationship.

REMEMBER

When you're depressed, you turn away from the very people who may have the most support to offer you. Either you feel that they don't care about you, or perhaps you can't muster up positive feelings for them. You may avoid others or find yourself irritated and crabby.

The more items you checked in the previous list, the more likely depression is affecting your relationships. For more information about how depression can affect your relationships and what you can do about it, see Part 4.

Feeling funky: The physical signs of depression

Depression typically includes at least a few physical symptoms. These symptoms include changes in appetite, sleep, and energy. However, for some people, the experience of depression *primarily* consists of physical symptoms and doesn't necessarily include as many other symptoms such as sadness, withdrawal from people, lack of interests, and missed work.

Many folks who experience depression primarily in physical terms are very unaware of their emotional life. Sometimes, that's because they were taught that feelings are unimportant. In other cases, their parents scolded them for crying or showing other appropriate feelings such as excitement or sadness.

When **Carl** was growing up, his father scolded him for crying. He said that big boys tough things out and that Carl should never show weakness. His father also jumped on him for showing too much excitement in anticipation of holidays or vacations. He said that men don't get emotional. Over time, Carl learned to keep his feelings to himself.

After five years of marriage, Carl's wife leaves him; she says that he's an unfeeling and uncaring man. In the ensuing six months, Carl finds his appetite diminished, and food no longer tastes good to him. His energy drains away like oil from an engine when the oil pan plug is removed. He's sleeping ten hours per night but still feels exhausted. He starts to have headaches and frequent bouts of constipation. His blood pressure rises.

When he goes to the clinic, his doctor asks, "Look Carl, your wife left you just six months ago. Are you sure you aren't depressed?" Carl answers, "Are you kidding? Depression is something women get. I couldn't possibly be depressed." Nonetheless, after an exhaustive work-up, his doctor concludes that depression is causing his physical problems. Nothing else adds up.

Are you experiencing odd changes in your body that you have no explanation for? Table 2-4 shows you some of the various ways that depression can show up in your body.

Like the other three quizzes in this chapter, it really doesn't matter exactly how many of these items apply to you. The more items you checked, the greater the possibility of depression.

If you have trouble getting in touch with your feelings, we have some suggestions for you in Chapter 6. You can learn how to identify your feelings with a little practice.

If your depression shows up primarily in physical terms, medications or some other physical remedy may seem like the best choice for you. See Part 5 for more information on physical solutions.

TABLE 2-4

Depression in the Body Quiz

Check If Yes	Depressed Behaviors
	I have no appetite lately.
	My blood pressure has risen for no apparent reason.
	I feel a bit sick to my stomach frequently.
	My diet is the same, but I'm having a lot of constipation (or diarrhea).
	I can't fall asleep at night even when I'm tired.
	I wake up frequently throughout the night.
	I feel sluggish and tired all day even when I get enough sleep.
	I'm sleeping way more than usual.
	I have a lot of aches and pains.
	I eat constantly to ease my discomfort.
	I've gained or lost 5 pounds and I can't figure out why.
	I feel so tired that I don't even want to get out of bed.

REMEMBER

The items in Table 2-4 may be caused by other health-related problems, not just depression. Therefore, if you're experiencing any disturbing physical problems, you need to see your doctor, especially if they last more than a week or two.

The Faces of Depression

In the "Recognizing the Ravages of Depression" section earlier in this chapter, we outline the four broad ways in which all types of depression can affect an individual. In this section, we turn our attention to the major types of depression to look out for:

>> Major depressive disorder

>> Persistent depressive disorder

>> Premenstrual depressive disorder

>> Depressive disorders and drugs

>> Depressive disorders and diseases

>> Adjustment disorder with depressed mood

>> Other depressive disorders

The American Psychiatric Association publishes a book called the *Diagnostic and Statistical Manual of Mental Disorders* (DSM). Each new edition updates and changes some of the criteria needed to qualify for each diagnosis. The DSM-5 describes and categorizes current conceptualizations of mental disorders such as depression. In the following sections, we describe major types of depression and their symptoms largely based on information contained in DSM-5. However, we present this information in a condensed format without technical jargon. And of course, subsequent editions of the DSM will continue to modify these categories to conform with the latest professional thinking and research.

Understanding what the forms of depression look like can help you figure out whether you're likely suffering from some type of depression. But don't go so far as to give yourself a formal diagnosis; that's a job for professionals.

If you feel that you have significant signs of any of these types of depression, get help. We recommend a visit to your primary care provider to rule out physical problems that could mimic depression. You can sometimes manage to improve minor symptoms of depression by becoming informed and working on your own. However, most forms of depression call for some help from a professional. And if you have feelings of hopelessness or thoughts of harming yourself, get help immediately.

Can't even get out of bed: Major depressive disorder

As with all types of depression, the symptoms of a major depressive disorder fall into the four areas: thought, behavior, relationships, and the body. So what's unique about a major depressive disorder?

Major depressive disorders involve either a seriously low mood or a notable drop in pleasures and interests that unrelentingly continues for two weeks or more. Sometimes depressed people either consciously or unconsciously deny these down feelings and declines in interests. In cases of denial, careful observation by people who know them well usually detects the impairment.

In addition to the low mood and lack of pleasure, in order to qualify as experiencing a major depressive disorder, you generally have to have a wide variety of other symptoms, such as

>> Inability to concentrate or make decisions

>> Repetitive thoughts of suicide or death

>> Major changes in sleep patterns

>> Extreme fatigue

>> Lack of interests in things that were once pleasurable

>> Clear signs of either revved up agitation or slowed functioning

>> Very low sense of personal worth

>> Striking changes in appetite or weight (either increased or decreased)

>> Intense feelings of guilt and self-condemnation

With major depressive disorders, these symptoms occur almost every day over a period of at least two weeks or more. Major depressive disorders vary greatly in terms of severity. However, even mild cases need to be treated. Some forms of major depression are seasonal in nature. For more info, see the sidebar "Seasonal affective disorder: Dark depression."

REMEMBER

The degree of despondency experienced by those with severe cases of major depressive disorder is difficult to imagine for someone who has never experienced it. A severe, major episode of depression grabs hold of a person's life and insidiously squeezes out all pleasure. But it does far more than obliterate joy; severe depression shoves its victims into a dark hole of utter, unrelenting despair that obscures the capacity to love. People caught in such a web of depression lose the ability to care for life, others, and themselves.

TIP

If you suffer from such a severe case of depression, there's reason to hope. Many effective treatments work even with severe depression.

Although all depression is unique to the individual, Edwin's story typifies some of the feelings of major depression.

> The daily pain of living begins the moment the alarm wakes **Edwin** up. He spends most of the night tossing and turning. He only falls asleep for a few moments before waking up to another day of despair. He forces himself to get ready for work, but the thought of speaking to others feels overwhelming. He can't face the prospect. He knows that he should at least call in sick, but can't lift his hand to pick up the phone. He realizes that he could lose his job, but it doesn't seem to matter. He thinks that he's likely to be dead soon.

> He changes out of his work clothes and into sweats; then he goes back to bed. But he doesn't sleep. His mind fills with thoughts of self-loathing: "I'm a failure. I'm no good. There's nothing to live for." He ponders whether he should just end it now. Edwin suffers from a major depressive disorder.

SEASONAL AFFECTIVE DISORDER: DARK DEPRESSION

Some major depressions come and go with the seasons, just like clockwork. People who regularly experience depression during the fall or winter may have *seasonal affective disorder* (SAD). People who have SAD may also experience a few unusual symptoms, such as

- Increased appetite
- Carbohydrate cravings
- Increased sleep
- Irritability
- A sense of heaviness in the arms and legs

Many mental health professionals believe that the reduced amount of sunlight in the winter triggers this form of depression in vulnerable individuals. Support for this hypothesis comes from the fact that this pattern of depression occurs more frequently among people who live in higher latitudes where light fluctuations from winter to summer are most extreme and darkness prevails for a greater portion of the day during the winter. (We discuss evidence concerning treatment of this disorder using bright lights in Chapter 18.)

What do bears do to get ready for winter? Bears frantically forage for food and get as fat as they can. Then they hibernate in a cozy cave. Perhaps it's not a coincidence that people with SAD typically gain weight, crave carbohydrates, have reduced energy, and feel like staying swaddled in bed for the winter.

WARNING

Major depressive disorders generally cause a sharply reduced ability to function at work or deal with other people. In other words, such disorders deplete you of the resources you need for recovery. That's why getting help is so important. If you allow the major depressive disorder to continue, it may result in death from suicide. If you or someone you know *even suspects* the presence of a major depressive disorder, you need to seek help promptly. See Chapter 5 for ideas on how to find professional help for depression.

Chronic, low-level depression: Persistent depressive disorder

Persistent depressive disorder, once known as dysthymic disorder, or dysthymia, looks rather similar to major depressive disorder. However, it's generally considered somewhat less severe and tends to be more chronic. With persistent depressive disorder, the symptoms occur for at least two years (oftentimes far longer), with the depressed mood appearing on most days for the majority of each day. However, you only need to display two of the following chronic symptoms, in addition to a depressed mood, in order for your condition to qualify as a dysthymic disorder:

>> Poor concentration

>> Low sense of personal worth

>> Guilty feelings

>> Problems with appetite and sleep

>> Thoughts of hopelessness

>> Problems making decisions

Compared to major depressive disorder, persistent depressive disorder less frequently involves prominent physical symptoms such as major difficulties with appetite, weight, sleep, and agitation.

Dysthymic disorder frequently begins in childhood, adolescence, or young adulthood and can easily continue for many years if left untreated. Furthermore, individuals with persistent depressive disorder carry an increased risk of developing a major depressive disorder at some point in their lives.

TIP

Although individuals with persistent depressive disorder don't appear as devastatingly despondent as those with a major depressive disorder, they nonetheless languish, lacking in vigor and joie de vivre. These are the people who you may not identify as being depressed, but they sure seem pessimistic and perhaps cynical and grouchy a good deal of the time.

Charlene doesn't remember ever feeling joy. She's not even sure what the words mean. Her parents worked long hours and seemed cold and distant. Charlene studied hard in school. She hoped to gain approval and attention for her academic accomplishments. Her parents didn't seem to notice.

Today, Charlene leads a life that's envied by her colleagues. She earns a great salary and toils tirelessly in her profession as a mechanical engineer. Yet she senses that she's missing something, feels unsuccessful, and suffers a chronic, uneasy discontent. Charlene has a persistent depressive disorder, although *she* wouldn't actually say that she's depressed. She fails to seek help for her problem because she actually has no idea that life can be different.

TIP

People with persistent depressive disorder often see their problems as merely "just the way they are," and they fail to seek treatment. If you suspect that you or someone you care about has persistent depressive disorder, get help. You have the right to feel better than you do, and the long-lasting nature of the problem means that it isn't likely to go away on its own. Besides, you certainly don't want to risk developing a major depressive disorder, which is even more debilitating.

Premenstrual dysphoric disorder: Horrible hormones?

Occasional, minor premenstrual changes in mood occur in a majority of women. A smaller percentage of women experience significant and disturbing symptoms known as *premenstrual dysphoric disorder* (PDD). PDD is a more extreme form of the more widely known premenstrual syndrome (PMS).

Although hormones likely play a significant role in PDD, research hasn't yet clarified the causes. Typically, women who suffer from full-blown PDD encounter some of the following symptoms almost every month, during the week prior to menstruation.

>> Anger

>> Anxiety

>> Bloating

>> Fatigue

>> Food cravings

>> Sensitivity to rejection

>> Feeling overwhelmed

>> Guilt and self-blame

>> Irritability

>> Problems concentrating

>> Sadness

>> Tearfulness

>> Withdrawal from people and activities

The following example illustrates some of the symptoms of PDD. Women with PDD often feel surprised and severely guilty by their emotional reactions to everyday stress. Even though their symptoms are caused by hormonal fluctuations, they find a way to blame themselves.

Denise drives to the grocery store after work. Impatiently, she pushes her cart through the aisle, only to find another patron blocking her way. She feels a rush of annoyance and clears her throat loudly. The other woman looks up and apologizes. Denise hurriedly works her way around the offending cart, giving it a quick shove as she passes.

Waiting in line, her irascible mood worsens. The man in front of her fumbles around for his checkbook and discovers he has no checks. Then he pulls out a handful of cash and realizes he's a bit short. Next, he starts to search his overstuffed wallet for a credit card. Denise finds herself unable to suppress her raging emotions and snaps, "People don't have all day to stand in line waiting for clods like you! What's wrong with you, anyway?"

The man's face turns bright red and he mutters, "Gosh, I'm sorry lady." The clerk intervenes and says, "Wow ma'am. You don't have to be so mean. It can happen to anybody." Suddenly ashamed, Denise breaks into tears and sobs. She feels like she's going crazy. And this isn't the first time Denise has felt this way. In fact, it happens to her almost on a monthly basis.

Premenstrual dysphoric disorder can impact the sufferer's family members as well as well as friends and colleagues. Symptoms usually dissipate a few days after the start of menstruation. Treatment often involves medication.

Major depression after a bundle of joy

Postpartum depression is another type of major depressive disorder that's widely thought to be related to hormonal fluctuations, although no one knows for sure how and why the hormones profoundly affect the moods of some women and not others. Other risk factors include sleep deprivation (common to new mothers), new and overwhelming responsibilities of parenthood, and changes in life roles. This depression occurs within days or weeks after giving birth. The symptoms are the same as in major depressive disorder. (For a complete discussion of these symptoms, see the section "Can't even get out of bed: Major depressive disorder" earlier in this chapter.)

Carmen had tried unsuccessfully to conceive for the past eight years. She and her husband Shawn feel overwhelmed with joy when at last the home pregnancy test registers positive. Their cheerful, cozy nursery looks like a picture in a baby magazine.

Carmen and Shawn weep with happiness at the sight of their newborn. Carmen feels exhausted, but Shawn assumes that's normal. He takes charge the first day home so that she can rest. Carmen feels the same way the next day, so Shawn continues to take over the responsibilities of caring for the baby. Shawn becomes alarmed when Carmen shows no interest in holding the baby. In fact, she seems irritated by the baby's crying and mentions that maybe she shouldn't have become a mother. At the end of the second week, she tells him that he can't go back to work because she doesn't think that she can take care of the baby. Carmen is suffering from postpartum depression.

WARNING

Most women feel a little bit of postpartum depression, or the "baby blues," shortly after delivery. It's not severe and it usually dissipates in a couple of weeks. However, if you begin to feel like Carmen in the earlier story, you need to get professional help immediately.

WARNING

A very small percentage of women with postpartum depression develop psychotic symptoms such as hallucinations or delusions. This condition is quite serious and requires immediate treatment. After a woman has this condition once, she is at heightened risk for developing it after future births.

MAJOR, MAJOR DEPRESSION

Psychosis is a serious symptom of a major depressive disorder in which a person is out of touch with reality. People with depression sometime become so ill that they become psychotic. They may hear voices or see things that aren't really there. In most instances, depression with psychosis requires hospitalization.

People with severe depression also may exhibit paranoid or delusional thinking. Paranoid thinking involves feeling extremely suspicious and distrustful — such as believing that other people are out to get you or that someone is trying to poison you. Delusions range from the slightly odd to bizarre. Most delusions are consistent with depressive thinking and involve feelings of shame, guilt, inadequacy, and punishment. Others involve obviously false beliefs such as thinking the television is transmitting signals to your brain. The problems of psychosis, paranoia, and delusional thinking require professional attention and lie outside of the scope of this book. However, we do detail medications commonly prescribed for these symptoms in Chapter 17.

Depressive disorders and drugs

Dealing with an illness is hard enough without having medications make you feel even worse, but some medications actually appear to cause depression. Of course, distinguishing whether it's merely being sick or the drug that's causing the depression is difficult. Nonetheless, in a number of cases, medications do appear to contribute directly to depression.

TIP

If you notice inexplicable feelings of sadness shortly after starting a new medication, tell your doctor. The medication could be causing your feelings, and an alternative treatment that won't make you depressed may be available. Table 2-5 lists the most common offending medications.

TABLE 2-5

Potentially Depressing Drugs

Medication	Condition Typically Prescribed For
Antabuse	Alcohol addiction
Anticonvulsants	Seizures
Barbiturates	Seizures and (rarely) anxiety
Benzodiazepines	Anxiety and insomnia
Beta blockers	High blood pressure and heart problems
Calcium channel blockers	High blood pressure and heart problems
Corticosteroids	Inflammation and chronic lung diseases
Hormones	Birth control and menopausal symptoms
Interferon	Hepatitis and certain cancers
Levodopa, amantadine	Parkinson's disease
Statins	High cholesterol
Zovirax	Herpes or shingles

You should know that the list in Table 2-5 reflects some of the most common drugs that can trigger depressive symptoms. Many additional medications can do the same. Consult your primary care provider if you have suspicions or concerns.

Abuse of alcohol or prescribed drugs or use of illegal, nonprescription drugs also can lead to depression. Depression may occur during drug use or upon withdrawal. The following is a partial list of these problematic substances:

>> Alcohol

>> Cocaine

>> Amphetamines

>> Opioids

>> Hallucinogenics

>> Inhalants

>> Sedatives

TECHNICAL
STUFF

The official name for this type of depression is *substance/medication–induced depressive disorder* and is most usually diagnosed by a physician or medical provider. Knowing whether major depression leads to substance abuse or substance abuse leads to depression can pose a challenge to sort out. And both can interact with each other. Either way, depression should receive treatment along with any substance abuse issues.

Depressive disorders and diseases

The interaction of depression with illness and disease can be a vicious cycle. Illness and disease (and related medications) can hasten the onset or intensify the effects of depression. And depression can further complicate various diseases. Depression can suppress the immune system, release stress hormones, and impact your body and mind's capacity to cope. Depression may increase whatever pain you have and further rob you of crucial resources.

Chronic illnesses interfere with life. Some chronic illnesses require lifestyle adjustments, extensive time at the doctor's office, missed work, disrupted relationships, and pain. Feeling upset by such disturbances is normal. But these problems may trigger depression, especially in vulnerable people.

In addition, certain specific diseases seem to disrupt the nervous system in ways that create depression. If you suffer from one of these diseases, talk to your doctor if your mood begins to deteriorate. Diseases that are thought to frequently contribute to depression include the following:

>> AIDS

>> Asthma

>> Cancer

>> Chronic fatigue syndrome

>> Chronic pain

>> Coronary artery disease and heart attacks

>> Diabetes

>> Fibromyalgia

>> Hepatitis

>> HIV

>> Infections

>> Lupus

>> Multiple sclerosis

>> Parkinson's disease

>> Shingles

>> Stroke

>> Thyroid disease

>> Ulcerative colitis

REMEMBER

Covid 19 and potentially other pandemic infections pack a double punch for inducing depression. First, its presence in the world causes people to isolate from others, which is a known cause of depression by itself. In addition, the stress of economic losses, loss of family members, and loss of freedom take their emotional toll on people. Finally, some viruses also cause brain inflammation and other damage, which can lead directly to depression. Stay safe!

Adjustment disorder with depressed mood: Dealing with adversity

Life isn't a bowl of cherries. Bad things do happen to everyone from time to time. Sometimes people handle their problems without excess emotional upset. Sometimes they don't.

TANTRUMS: DISRUPTIVE MOOD DYSREGULATION DISORDER (DMDD)

Disruptive mood dysregulation disorder (DMDD) is a new diagnosis found in the depression family of the *Diagnostic and Statistical Manual of Mental Disorders*, Fifth Edition (DSM-5). This diagnosis was basically developed by a few of the contributors to DSM-5 in order to capture a group of children who had previously been misdiagnosed as having a bipolar disorder (manic depressive). The diagnostic criteria include the following:

- Severe, frequent temper tantrums way out of proportion to the situation.

- Irritable or angry mood most days.

- These symptoms occur in at least two settings (such as home and school).

- Symptoms originally appeared before age 10.

- Tantrums are inappropriate for the age of the child.

- Symptoms must be present for at least 12 months.

This diagnosis has received considerable criticism. Many professionals complain that the diagnosis is too similar to another childhood malady called *oppositional defiant disorder* to be useful. Furthermore, the conceptual relationship of this diagnosis to adult depressive disorders is less than clear. Since DMDD is a new diagnosis, research has not yet concluded that it always leads to depression in adults. However, DMDD is now considered a type of childhood depression.

Adjustment disorders are reactions to one or more difficult issues, such as marital problems, financial setbacks, conflict with co-workers, or natural disasters. When a stressful event occurs and your reaction includes a decreased ability to work or participate effectively with others, in combination with symptoms such as a low mood, crying spells, and feelings of worthlessness or hopelessness, you may be experiencing an adjustment disorder with a depressed mood. Adjustment disorder is a much milder problem than a major depressive disorder, but it can still disrupt your life.

James is shocked when his boss tells him that due to downsizing, he's losing his job. He begins a job search but openings in his field are scarce. For the first couple of weeks, he enjoys catching up on sleep, but soon, he starts feeling unusually down. He struggles to open up job application sites on the internet. He begins to feel worthless and loses hope of finding a job. His appetite and sleep are still okay, but his confidence plummets. He's surprised when tears stream down his face after receiving another rejection letter.

James isn't suffering from a major depressive disorder. James is struggling with what is known as an adjustment disorder with depressed mood.

TIP

Although no longer considered as a formal type of depression, adjustment disorder with depressed mood should be treated when it interferes with day-to-day life and lasts for more than a week or two.

And all the rest

At the beginning of the chapter, we noted that depression comes in a variety of forms. Not all depressions fit neatly into clear-cut categories. Let's say you have apathy and depressed mood and are finding it hard to get out of bed. Whether or not your symptoms meet the specific criteria found in a book full of diagnoses doesn't really matter. What matters to you is that you don't feel good and hope to find a way to get better. In many instances, you will want a therapist to help you out, and you are likely to find some techniques in this book quite helpful.

MOTHERS WHO KILL THEIR BABIES

Occasionally, women with severe cases of postpartum depression develop psychoses. *Psychosis* involves serious departures from reality, including *hallucinations* (seeing or hearing things that aren't really there) and *delusional beliefs* (thoughts such as believing that aliens are controlling your mind). *Postpartum psychosis* is psychosis that occurs shortly after giving birth. Psychotic beliefs often focus on the baby and can include thinking that the baby is possessed or would be better off in heaven than living here on earth. The risk of postpartum psychosis increases greatly for any births following an initial diagnosis. Although a very few mothers with postpartum depression with psychosis hurt their babies, they are much more likely to hurt themselves.

In 2013, Kimberlynn Bolanos stabbed her five-month-old baby multiple times. She also attempted suicide by stabbing herself multiple times. The baby died and she lived. She thought that the state was going to take away her baby. She was found guilty but mentally ill and sentenced to 38 years in prison.

In June of 2001, Texas mother Andrea Yates drowned her five children in the bathtub. Yates suffered from a diagnosed postpartum psychosis after the birth of her fourth child, Luke. After the birth of Luke, and before the birth of her fifth child, she tried to commit suicide twice and was treated with medication. However, against advice of her doctors, she stopped taking her medication.

Yates was found guilty of murder. Had she followed through with adequate treatment at the time of her first diagnosis, it's quite likely that this tragedy could have been prevented. She was tried a second time and found not guilty by reason of insanity. Today, Yates is living out her life in a Texas state hospital.

Good Grief! Is Depression Ever Normal?

When you lose someone you love, you're likely to feel pain and sadness. You may lose sleep and withdraw from people. The idea of going out and having a good time will probably sound repugnant. Feelings like these can go on for weeks or a few months. Are these the signs of depression? Yes and no.

TIP

Although grieving involves many of the same reactions that are associated with depression, the two aren't the same. Depression almost always includes a diminished sense of personal worth or feelings of excessive guilt. Grief, when not accompanied by depression, doesn't typically involve lowered self-esteem and unreasonable self-blame. In the early stages of grief, the intensity may come in waves. Memories or thoughts of the deceased cause severe pain. However, the intensity of grief usually diminishes slowly (sometimes excruciatingly slowly) but surely over time. Much later, memories and thoughts of the deceased can bring joy. Depression, on the other hand, sometimes holds on unrelentingly.

A controversy exists among some mental health professionals concerning how to best deal with grief. Some professionals advocate immediate treatment of any disturbing reactions involving grief; these professionals often advise taking antidepressant medications. (See Chapter 17 for more information about antidepressants.) Others contend that grief involves a natural healing process that is best dealt with by allowing its natural course to unfold.

WHEN A CHILD DIES

The loss of a child may be the most profound loss that anyone ever experiences. The grief following a child's death is thought to be more intense, more complicated, and longer lasting than other profound losses. The anguish and loneliness may seem utterly intolerable. Parents may question the value of living. Common experiences of grief of this sort includes extreme problems with concentration, energy, and motivation. Grief can last decades. Innocent questions by strangers such as "How old are your children?" can lead to a rush of grief that can't be avoided.

Others who haven't had such a loss may be sympathetic, but they sometimes fail to understand and appreciate the intensity and duration of this type of grief. We suggest that parents who have lost a child consider contacting a support group such as The Compassionate Friends (www.compassionatefriends.org). This group's mission is to help bereaved parents deal with their loss in a supportive atmosphere.

We tend to agree with this latter group, but if and only if the grief isn't complicated by an accompanying depression. (See Chapter 15 for our discussion about getting through loss and grief.) Still, the decision is an individual choice. In either case, a grieving person needs to be aware that depression can superimpose itself on top of grief. If you're dealing with grief, seek treatment if it goes on too long or includes other serious symptoms of depression.

Digging Out the Causes of Depression

There are lots of theories on the cause of depression. Some experts purport that depression is caused by imbalances in brain chemistry. Advocates of this position sometimes believe that those imbalances in chemistry are due to genetics. Other experts emphatically declare that the cause of depression lies in one's childhood. Still other investigators make the claim that depression comes from negative thinking. You can also find professionals who suggest that depression is caused by impoverished environments and/or cultural experiences. Other researchers have implicated learned patterns of behavior as a cause of depression. Finally, some experts have identified problems with relationships as the major culprit.

In one sense, you can probably come to the same conclusion as the dodo bird in *Alice in Wonderland* and declare that "All have won and all must have prizes." In another sense, nobody deserves a prize. Even though you can find evidence to support each of these positions, nobody truly knows how these factors work, which is the most important, and which ones influence other factors in what ways.

TIP

In spite of the indisputable fact that scientists don't yet know exactly how the multitude of depression-related factors function and interact, you may run into doctors, psychologists, and psychiatrists who have strong opinions about what they believe is "the" definitive cause of depression. If you encounter a professional who claims to know the single, definitive cause of depression, question that professional's credibility. Most sophisticated experts in the field of depression research know that a single, definitive cause of depression remains elusive and likely will never be discovered.

Yet the field of mental health isn't clueless when it comes to understanding how depression develops. Strong suggestive evidence supports the fact that learning, thinking, biology, genetics, childhood, and the environment play important roles in the development, maintenance, and potential treatment of depression. All these factors interact in amazing, but not yet fully understood, ways.

For example, a growing body of studies has shown that medication alters the physical symptoms of depression such as loss of appetite and energy. And antidepressant medication also improves the negative, pessimistic thinking that accompanies most forms of depression. Perhaps that's not too surprising. However, some notable researchers are increasingly arguing that improvements found from antidepressant medication are almost entirely due to *placebo* effects. Placebos are essentially inert pills that nonetheless convey an expectation of hope and promise.

Similarly, studies have demonstrated that psychotherapy alone decreases negative, pessimistic thinking, much like medications do. Some scientists have been surprised by the fact that other studies now demonstrate that certain psychotherapies, even if delivered without antidepressant medication, also alter brain chemistry.

Recent evidence has shown the rate of depression climbing quickly among the population during the Covid-19 pandemic. These people may or may not have had pre-existing risk factors for depression such as difficult childhoods, genetic predispositions, or previous histories of depression. The pandemic presented unique challenges that could lead to depression independently of these other risk factors. (See Chapter 3 for information about the pandemic and depression.)

Taken as a whole, recent studies on the roots of depression fail to support a theory that assigns one specific cause of depression. Rather, they support the idea that physical and psychological factors interact with each other.

BIPOLAR DISORDER: UPS AND DOWNS

Bipolar disorder is considered a mood disorder but no longer a form of depression. However, bipolar disorder is quite different from classic depressions because people with a bipolar disorder always experience one or more episodes of unusually euphoric feelings, which are referred to as *mania*.

In bipolar disorder, moods tend to fluctuate between extreme highs and lows. This fact makes the treatment of bipolar disorder different than most depressions. We want you to be familiar with the symptoms so that you can seek professional help if you experience manic episodes with your depression.

Although individuals with mania may seem quite cheerful and happy, the people who know them can tell that their good mood is a little too good to be true. During manic episodes, people need less sleep, may show signs of unusual creativity, and have more energy and enthusiasm. Sounds like a pretty nice mood to have, doesn't it? Who wouldn't want to feel wonderful and totally on top of the world? Well, hold the phone.

(continued)

(continued)

The problem with manic episodes related to bipolar disorder is that the high feelings spin out of control. During these episodes, good judgment goes out the window. People who have this disorder often

- Spend too much money
- Gamble excessively
- Make foolish business decisions
- Engage in risky sexual escapades
- Talk fast and furiously
- Think that they have super-special talents or abilities

Manic episodes can involve mildly foolish decisions and excesses, or they can reach extreme levels. People in manic states can cause ruin for themselves or their families. Their behavior can get so out of control that they end up in the hospital for a period of time.

Most people with bipolar disorder also cycle into episodes of mild to severe depression. They go from feeling great to gruesome, occasionally within the same day. The depressions that follow a manic episode feel especially unexpected and devastating. The contrast from the high to the low is particularly painful. People with untreated bipolar disorder typically feel out of control, hopeless, and helpless. Not surprisingly, the risk of suicide is higher for bipolar disorder than for any of the other types of depression.

Although it's generally chronic, bipolar disorder can be successfully managed. Both medications and psychotherapy, usually in combination, can alleviate many of the most debilitating symptoms. Scientists are continually developing new treatments and medications.

Warning: Bipolar disorder is a complicated, serious syndrome. The condition has many subtle variations. If you suspect that you or someone you know has any signs of bipolar disorder, seek professional assistance immediately.

Monitoring Mood

Perhaps you have a strong suspicion that you are experiencing some type of depression. Now what? Keeping track of how your mood changes from day to day is one important step in recovery. Why?

>> You may discover patterns (perhaps you get very depressed every Monday).

>> You may discover specific triggers for your depressed moods.

>> You can see how your efforts progress over time.

>> You can quickly determine if you're not progressing, which may indicate that you need to seek help.

TIP

We suggest that you keep a Mood Diary like the one shown in Table 2-6. You can profit from tracking your moods and taking notes on relevant incidents, happenings, and thoughts. Try it for a few weeks.

Use a rating scale from 1 to 100 to rate your mood each day (or at multiple times throughout the day). A rating of 100 means that you feel ecstatic. You feel on top of the world, maybe like you just won $80 million or received the Nobel Peace Prize — whatever turns you on. A rating of 50 means just a regular day. Your mood is acceptable — nothing special, nothing bad. A rating of 1 is just about the worst day imaginable. Interestingly, we find that most people without depression rate their average mood at around 70, even though we define 50 as middle range.

TIP

To keep things simple, use your calendar as a mood diary. Just jot down the number representing your mood. In addition to your mood rating, write down or dictate a few notes about your day. Include anything that may relate to your mood such as

>> Clashes with friends, co-workers, or lovers

>> Difficult times of the day

>> Falling in love

>> Financial difficulties

>> Loneliness

>> Negative thoughts or daydreams floating through your mind

>> An unexpected promotion

>> Wonderful weather

>> Work hassles

Willie has been feeling sad and listless for the past month. He suspects that he may have a problem, so he tracks his mood and finds a few interesting patterns. For an example of one week in Willie's mood diary, check out Table 2-6.

TABLE 2-6   ## Weekly Mood Diary

Day	Mood Rating	Notes (Events or Thoughts, for Example)
Sunday	20	Not a good day. I hung out and worried about getting my quarterly tax payment together by Thursday. And I felt horribly guilty about letting the lawn go without mowing it.
Monday	30 (a.m.) 45 (p.m.)	The day started miserably. I got stuck in traffic and was late to work. In the afternoon, things seemed to go more smoothly, although I can't say I felt on top of the world.
Tuesday	40	Nothing good, nothing bad today. Just the blahs.
Wednesday	30 (a.m.) 40 (p.m.)	I woke up feeling panicked about the new project deadline. I don't know how I'll ever get it done. By the afternoon I'd made a little progress, but I still worry about it.
Thursday	35 (a.m.) 45 (p.m.)	I was thinking about the fact that the days just seem to drag on. I don't look forward to much. In the evening, I enjoyed a phone conversation with a friend.
Friday	50	Miraculously, I got the project done four hours early. My boss said it was the greatest thing he'd ever seen me do. Of course, he probably doesn't think much about my other work.
Saturday	40	I finally got the grass cut. That felt good, but then I had too much time on my hands and started to worry again.

Willie studies several weeks of mood diaries. He notices that he usually feels morose on Sunday afternoons. He realizes that on Sunday, he typically spends time alone and mulls over imagined difficulties of the upcoming week. He also discovers that mornings aren't exactly the best time of the day because he worries about the rest of the day. Interestingly, he also discovers that his worries often involve catastrophic predictions (like not meeting deadlines) that rarely come true. Finally, his mood improves when he tackles projects he's been putting off, like mowing the lawn.

REMEMBER

You can track your progress whether you're working on your own or with a professional. If your progress bogs down, please seek help or discuss the problem with your therapist.

Chapter **3**

When Bad Things Happen

L ife is full of unfairness, tragedy, illness, and setbacks. It's a wonder that so many people face adversity with courage and determination. But what causes those who bravely work through hard times to slide into a state of depression? It may be early learning experiences, genetics, past trauma, or unknown factors. What we do know is that facing fear on your own, alone without support, challenges the best of us. We also know that when stress is chronic and unrelenting, depression may emerge.

Another cause of depression is the *belief* that you have no control over the outcome. There is nothing to be done. You can't problem-solve and find a solution or work harder to make things better. You believe that you have no control over the situation that's getting you down and find yourself feeling hopeless.

In this chapter, we describe some of the situations that lead many to feel depressed. Nonetheless, there is reason to hope. We offer you ideas on how to make the best of your situation and live your life the best way you can. We also cover depression that stems from the chronic stress of major world events. That's because not all depression originates from individual factors such as biology or early childhood experiences. This kind of depression is a normal reaction to highly abnormal times. We give you an overview of how these events lead to depression and some initial ideas for dealing with it. Much more advice appears throughout this book.

Loss and Depression During a Pandemic

According to United States government statistics, previous rates of depression have typically hovered below 10 percent in any given year. During 2020, the first year of the Covid-19 pandemic, these figures skyrocketed. Different studies indicated that about 40 percent of adults experienced symptoms of depression. Clearly, the pandemic managed to overwhelm the coping capacities of many.

Anyone with access to information about the pandemic understandably became anxious. That pretty much means everyone. People worried about finding hand sanitizer, toilet paper, and masks. They stocked up on canned beans, dry pasta, tomato sauce, and cleaning supplies. Although the pandemic created significant anxiety, there was also a sense of electrified attention to the task at hand. Ever so briefly, there was hope that people would rally together, top scientists would discover unique treatments, and the pandemic would soon be defeated.

Unfortunately, that scenario failed to occur. People gravitated toward chronic anxiety or blatant denial. Slowly, over time, depression set in for many as major losses mounted. Social distancing caused loneliness and isolation. People lost the ability to engage in much of life's everyday pleasurable activities, like going out for dinner, seeing a movie, or even going to work. Insecurities about health, finances, the future, and death mushroomed. The following sections describe some of the core issues that may contribute to depression brought on by the pandemic.

Losing connections

Developed countries around the world imposed serious restrictions on gatherings of people. In fact, most were told to stay home, hunker down, and not to leave the house. Occasional outings for necessities such as groceries and medications were allowed, but these outings were rife with anxiety. Wear a mask, don't touch anything, stay away from people, get out quickly, and use hand sanitizer. Errands, once enjoyable, became a possible breach in the cocoon of safety.

People were, more than ever, isolated. At the same time, the field of mental health has known for decades that social connections are critical for sustained emotional well-being. The expected effect of long-term social isolation for most human beings is depression.

DEMENTIA, LONELINESS, AND LOSS DURING THE PANDEMIC

Senior care facilities were ravaged by the Covid-19 pandemic. Less than 1 percent of the United States population resides in a nursing home or assisted living environment. However, these facilities account for about 40 percent of the Covid-related deaths. In order to stem the high rates of infection, measures were taken to protect the residents. These measures include forbidding outside visitation, stopping all face-to-face social activities in facilities, and basically requiring residents to stay isolated in their rooms. Even meals, once a time of critical, valued socialization, are eaten in solitude.

Tragically, these restrictions have also proven deadly. That's because people with dementia need stimulation and connection with others. Loneliness and isolation have increased death rates in otherwise stable patients. There have been increased cases of failure to thrive, a condition in which patients lose interest in eating and drinking. Those people become frailer and are at greater risk of falling. When they do pass away, close friends and relatives are left to grieve on their own, unable to be at their loved one's side.

Losing core freedoms

In February of 2020, we watched a news story about the coronavirus in China. The news report showed large buildings filled to capacity with beds of people who had been exposed to the virus. The government had mandated quarantines to decrease the spread of infection. We mused that such draconian measures would never find acceptance in the United States because of its devotion to freedom and independence. In normal times, such restrictions would be seen as an attack on constitutionally assured liberties. But how quickly things changed. In a matter of weeks, consider a few of the freedoms that were taken away or diminished:

» **Travel:** Borders were closed. People were afraid to fly or travel on crowded buses, trains, or subways. Cruises and tours were cancelled worldwide. National and state parks were closed; when opened, restrictions were applied.

» **Work:** "Nonessential" businesses were closed for months at a time. Restaurants shuttered their doors as did bars, nightclubs, concert halls, barbershops, beauty salons, massage parlors, and movie theaters. Upon reopening, these establishments had to abide by regulations governing the density of patrons allowed in.

>> **School:** Schools were closed throughout the world. When opened, some converted to virtual instruction; others had hybrid programs that mixed virtual with in-person instruction. Many others opened only to be closed because of infections.

>> **Gatherings:** Individual states and communities made different decisions, but large public gatherings were not allowed in most areas. In many cities, any gatherings were restricted to five or ten people.

In the U.S., 50 different states designed 50 different plans. Much of the population accepted greatly increased regulations that restricted their freedom in the interest of saving lives. Others contended that their rights were being trampled on. The later group focused on what they saw as unfair decision-making that resulted in seemingly unfair advantages of some businesses over others (for example, open liquor stores versus closed gyms). At the end of the day, instead of a united country fighting a common foe, the U.S. was further fractured and divided.

All of these losses — the loss of freedom and the loss of unity — can lead to feelings of hopelessness and disconnection, the antithesis of what's needed for good mental health. It's no wonder that many across the world report a chronic sense of despair.

Feeling insecure

A particularly basic human motivation, probably instinctual, is the drive to stay alive. Health pandemics threaten that instinct and not surprisingly, fuel emotional insecurity and anxiety. Compounding the problem is the fact that all too many people desperately seek certainty in their attempts to cope. Yet certainty is never fully obtainable. There are no definitive answers to the following questions:

>> Will I get the virus?

>> If I get it, will I live or die?

>> How can I make myself totally safe from the virus?

>> Will anyone in my family get it?

>> Will the virus come back?

>> Will a vaccine keep me completely safe?

>> If I live through it, will I have lasting health effects?

As health risks and uncertainties about those risks persist over time, depression commonly sets in.

Coping during a pandemic

Everyone struggles during the imposition of pandemic related restrictions. However, for those at risk of sliding into depression and for those who already have, there are a set of strategies you can use. These ideas are based on the premise that it's critical to take actions, no matter how small. See Chapters 11, 12, and 13 for more information on taking concrete actions against depression. Read through the following list and choose a few suggestions to get started:

>> **Make a to-do list.** Break all tasks down into small parts. Make at least some of the items on your list easily accomplishable. Don't overpromise yourself. You can gradually increase your chosen task difficulty over time as your depression slowly abates.

>> **Stay connected with others.** If there are other members of your household, take time to talk to each other and be kind. Nerves can be a bit raw. Forgive. Reach out to friends and family. Connect through meeting software, texting, or social media. The old-fashioned telephone still works too!

>> **Keep moving.** Get outside if you can: Walk, jog, run, bike, or whatever you enjoy. There are also tons of free, easily accessed short workouts online that can be implemented inside or out.

>> **Watch your diet.** Many people report gaining significant weight during lockdowns. Combined with a lack of exercise, a poorly planned diet can deepen depression. On the other hand, it's important to indulge in occasional treats as long as they don't get out of hand. Many people are learning to cook at home because of the restrictions. Take this time to learn new healthy recipes. You'll feel better.

>> **Monitor media consumption.** There are multiple news sources always available. Stay away from constant news watching or scanning. It's good to set aside a limited time to obtain information, such as a half hour in the morning and an hour in the evening. Going beyond that amount of time won't give you much new information and will likely stir up difficult feelings during these tumultuous times. At the same time, do set aside some time to see a great movie, comedy, drama, or even occasionally binge-watch a riveting television series.

REMEMBER

The important principle is to just do it. Take real action. If one thing doesn't do much for you, try another. Focus on accomplishing small steps each day. Reflect on what's important to you and try to live by your values.

WARNING

As always, we recommend seeking professional help immediately if you feel somewhat hopeless or suicidal. And if your moods are keeping you from enjoying everyday life, it's also time to get help. See Chapter 10 for more information about suicide.

During the pandemic, many mental health providers began offering their services via telehealth in order to maintain safe, social distancing while also being able to deliver needed help to patients. Many people find such services a godsend since they feel highly anxious, depressed, and isolated.

TIP

If you're interested in pursuing telehealth services, talk to your insurance provider or primary care physician (PCP) for a referral. Most telemedicine is covered by insurance though you should verify that coverage. There are similar-sounding services offered on the internet with highly variable costs, quality, and insurance coverage.

Financial Stressors

A large research study conducted by the Boston School of Public Health found high rates of depression in the midst of the pandemic. The researchers looked at such factors as loss of a loved one, job loss, or financial stress that might impact the likelihood of people experiencing depression. One finding stood out: If the subject in the study had less than $5,000 in the bank, they were 50 percent more likely to be depressed than those with more than $5,000 in the bank.

This study, consistent with many others, shows the real impact of economic instability on mental health. When financially insecure people lose their jobs, whether due to shutdowns, downsizing, or other reasons, without a safety net, vulnerability to depression escalates rapidly.

Depression arrives with financial stress because of the meaning money holds for people. People believe that their personal worth is related to how much money they have. When they lose a job or can't meet financial obligations, their self-worth plummets. They feel like they are letting others down and have a tremendous sense of guilt.

Depression takes a firm hold when hopelessness sets in. The depression then leads to lack of motivation, feelings of powerlessness, and helplessness. These factors limit the ability to problem solve or take productive action.

If you're mired in depressive thoughts about finances, you are not alone. Financial inequities have never been more pronounced than today. Millions have lost their jobs, and the financial future is uncertain at best. The problem with being depressed about money and finances is that depression leads to inaction. And what is needed is action along with problem solving, which we cover in Chapter 14. In the meantime, take a look at the following sections. Then pick and choose what actions may be useful for your own situation.

Emotional accounting

Know that it is perfectly normal to have negative emotions about financial and job-related problems. These emotions can include anxiety, sadness, and fear. You may lack confidence in your ability to navigate through a crisis.

TIP

Accept those feelings; allow them some space to be felt. These feelings tell you that something needs to happen. Acceptance is not wallowing. Acceptance means allowing feelings in and listening to what they are trying to tell you. Admit that this is a stressful time and be honest with yourself and those close to you.

This is a time to consider how you've managed to get through other difficult periods in your life. Ask yourself the following questions:

>> What coping strategies have worked for me in the past?

>> What support can I get from friends and family?

>> What additional resources can I turn to in the community (food banks or government assistance)?

>> If my emotions feel overwhelming, what are the professional mental health services available to me?

As much as you can, focus on small actions you can do to take care of your emotional well-being. Forgive yourself for the financial situation you find yourself in. Most likely, you are not to blame for your situation. Factors outside of your control such as the job market, the economy, a pandemic, or lack of opportunities contributed to your plight.

Finally, remain flexible. Goals that were highly prized in the past may need to be reevaluated. For example, you may have a high emotional investment in a particular career path. Or you might be hoping and eagerly anticipating a new car or the latest electronic gadget. These goals may need a major overhaul in light of new circumstances. Having the flexibility to pivot and look for new possibilities may be key.

Dollars and sense accounting

If you find yourself in financial trouble, don't put your head in the sand. Although it's tempting to avoid tackling financial issues head on, doing so only allows financial concerns to grow (as well as late fees and interest). It all starts with figuring out how much money is reliably coming in each month and how much goes out. Sounds simple, but if you don't keep careful track, you'll likely miss important information. Take time and go over your income/expense figures multiple times. Recognize that it's amazingly easy to overlook small expenses that wreck your plans.

Once you figure out your income, subtract expenses. If the total is a negative number, you have a problem! If it's a positive number, you're in better shape, but it's quite likely you can find ways to cut those expenses further. As you know, this book focuses on depression rather than finances. However, here are a few tips for gaining better control of your money:

>> **Develop a monthly budget and stick to it.** If at all possible, set aside a bit of money for savings. If you are successful in sticking to your budget after a few months, give yourself a small gift to celebrate your success.

>> **Pay down debt.** Go after high-interest credit card debt first. Always pay more than the minimum if you can. Try to resist using credit cards unless you can pay them off in full each month.

>> **Boost your income.** See if you can get a side job, turn a hobby into a business, or work an extra shift per month. If you have collections or assets that could bring in extra money, consider selling them.

>> **Cut expenses.** Cut out buying coffee on the way to work, and don't go out for dinner except for special occasions. Cut your cable costs, and buy less stuff. Think about downsizing. Whenever you are making a purchase, ask yourself if it is something you absolutely need or simply want. Don't buy it if it is not a necessity.

These are a few general tips. For more information about money, jobs, investing, savings, and getting by on less see *Managing Money All-in-One For Dummies* (Wiley).

TIP

Some people have the luxury of being able to work from home. That ability came in pretty handy when the pandemic hit. Many of these individuals reported an interesting discovery: Specifically, they observed themselves spending far less money each month on items like dining out, clothes, transportation, entertainment, and more. What had seemed so necessary during pre-pandemic times simply wasn't needed. Knowing the difference between a want and a need is a useful lesson for most people, and working from home makes it much easier to learn.

Discrimination and Depression

Discrimination takes many forms. People suffer from discrimination based on race, gender, sexual identity, class, ethnicity, social status, and more. Like other life stressors, unrelenting chronic experiences of discrimination can lead to poor mental health outcomes. Many people cope with discrimination on a daily basis. Here are just a few examples of discrimination:

>> Stop-and-frisk based on profiling

>> Harassment and name calling

>> Waving a hand in class to answer a question and consistently not being called on

>> Hate crimes targeting sexual orientations other than heterosexual

>> Calls to the authorities over someone's benign behavior

>> Being made fun of because of one's accent

>> Being mocked because of a disability

>> Being ignored or excluded in activities and groups

>> Being overlooked for a promotion or a job

>> Not getting job interviews after the age of 50

>> Not getting equal pay for equal work

Whether the discrimination occurs blatantly, or in more subtle ways, the effects often extend to family, friends, and community members. For example, when a hate crime occurs, those who share similar backgrounds can be profoundly angered, hurt, and/or saddened. Or when parents have to comfort a child who has experienced discrimination, the parents generally feels profound distress. They experience both the child's anguish and their own frustration over not being able to protect their child from an unfair world.

REMEMBER

Living in a culture that engages in frequent discriminatory behavior causes those who are targets to feel anxious. However, over time, the frequent, chronic nature of these encounters easily leads to depression.

Defending against discrimination

Most good people agree that all humans are created as equals. Although differences among us are great, so are similarities. We all deserve equal education, opportunities, and fair treatment. Strikingly, the vast majority of people would agree with these statements about universal equality.

However, discrimination, prejudice, and persecution persist throughout the world. Despite attempts at eradicating it, discrimination thrives at great cost to those who are suffer from it. Part of the explanation is that much discrimination occurs at a subtle, almost unconscious level. For example, some people may claim to have no racist attitudes, but their behavior is not consistent with their stated belief. In order to fight discrimination throughout the world, we suggest the following:

>> Learn more about the subtle forms of discrimination, including racism.

>> Don't go along with racist, sexist, or other "humor" at the expense of others.

>> Calmly speak up when people use offensive language.

>> Expose yourself and your children to other cultures. (Don't limit yourself to ethnic restaurants, great as they may be.)

>> Practice doing good works for others.

>> Invite people of other cultures and ethnicities into social, political, and spiritual groups.

TIP

So why will practicing anti-discrimination help for depression? Depression flourishes in disconnected environments, and it fades away when people connect.

Living with discrimination

Discrimination, whether it is teasing or tormenting, hurts. Those who suffer chronic discrimination are at a high risk of developing mental health problems. And unfortunately, many of those with mental health problems do not seek treatment because of poor access, stigma, or distrust of a discriminatory system.

Depression is often the result of chronic, unrelenting negative messages from others. People who have suffered discrimination and have depression can benefit from many of the treatments we describe throughout the book. However, here are a few tips that may be specifically helpful for those with depression and the experiences of discrimination:

>> Surround yourself with people who care about you. Attend support groups or spiritual gatherings that allow you to express your frustrations and grief openly and safely.

>> Accept the emotions you have about your experiences with discrimination. Explore productive ways to express them.

>> Take pride in your own differences.

>> Realize that discrimination originates in ignorance.

A sense of belonging provides a powerful antidote to depression. Search for opportunities to connect and relate with others even if they are different from you. Open your mind and heart to others who have the potential for treating you with mutual respect.

REMEMBER

One aspect of discrimination that makes it particularly difficult for those who experience it is the feeling of lack of control. The victim of discrimination can't change the beliefs or behaviors of those who discriminate. When people feel they have no control over a situation, helplessness and hopelessness often follow. Helplessness and hopelessness are sure pathways to depression.

TECHNICAL STUFF

Discrimination can pile up. A review of research on the mental health of people who are discriminated against at multiple levels was recently reported. Forty different studies were analyzed. These studies specifically looked at racism and discrimination based on sexual orientation (often referred to as *heterosexualism*). These studies showed that the experience of multiple types of discrimination increase chances of depression. Initial evidence also suggests that suicide rates among LGBTQ adolescents who are also racial minorities is greater because of the impact of multiple types of discrimination.

Domestic Violence and Depression

Domestic violence occurs throughout the world. No particular race, class, gender, ethnicity, sexual orientation, or religious doctrine is exempt. Violence between intimate partners is the most common form of domestic abuse, which can include physical aggression, psychological abuse, stalking, harassment, and sexual coercion, among other actions.

Victims of domestic abuse experience high rates of depression, post-traumatic stress disorder, and suicidal ideation. These psychological problems contribute to more substance abuse and poor physical health. Children exposed to domestic violence also suffer psychological problems, including depression, anxiety, and aggression. They are also likely to struggle in school.

If you or someone close to you is in an abusive relationship or feels threatened, the National Domestic Violence Hotline can be reached at 800-799-7233 or visit the website www.thehotline.org. You can also text LOVEIS to 866-331-9474. Trained staff will answer questions and help you stay safe.

Disasters and Depression

Living life on this planet comes replete with substantial risks. Watch the evening news and you're likely to see stores about a variety of environmental disasters:

» Coastal flooding exacerbated by rising sea levels

» Raging forest fires fueled by drought

» Tropical storms and hurricanes made worse by climate change

» Dangerous mudslides caused in part by forest fires

If the human-caused disasters don't get you, there's always natural disasters such as tornados, earthquakes, volcanos, and tsunamis. Finally, there is political strife, social unrest, and crime.

Surprisingly, most victims of disaster do not suffer from depression. They are more likely to become anxious or have a traumatic stress disorder. Humans have a remarkable capacity to endure hardship. Depression tends to become more of a problem when disasters impact a person over a long period of time and resources are limited. For example, a person who lost their home in a forest fire may be able to cope with help from others. But if a couple of years later, another fire threatens their home, weariness sets in and depression can follow. That's especially the case if help from government or other sources is not readily forthcoming.

TECHNICAL STUFF

The United States Global Change Research Program issued a report on the impact of climate change on mental health. They found that a significant number of people who are exposed to climate related disasters develop chronic mental health problems such as anxiety, depression, and post-traumatic stress disorder. Children, pregnant women, and postpartum women are particularly at risk as are disadvantaged people and those with pre-existing mental health problems. In addition, first responders such as firefighters and medical workers are also at risk for stress-related mental illness.

Chapter **4**

Breaking Barriers to Change

When people have headaches, they simply reach for an over-the-counter pain reliever. When people have runny noses, they use a tissue and perhaps a decongestant. It seems like people would deal with depression similarly: Take an antidepressant or get therapy. But most people with depression don't seek help for weeks, months, and sometimes years. A few with chronic depression never get help at all. That's because true change is very difficult, and depression is much more than a headache or a common cold.

In this chapter, we explain why prospects of change pose such a formidable adversary in people's minds — so much so, that they'll do almost anything to keep clear of the idea. And the mere thought of trying to defeat depression often feels even more frightening, partly because depression, itself, typically goes hand in hand with a sense of hopelessness.

We show you the rational fears that fuel procrastination, hopelessness, avoidance, and other self-limiting strategies. And we discuss how certain beliefs, myths, and misconceptions can paralyze people's desire to get to a better place. And, most importantly, we show you how to find out which of these problems may stand in your way and what you can do to push them aside.

> **Alex** has felt moderately depressed for the past two years. His night shift job at a fulfillment center is stressful, and it bores him. He has a degree in business administration but has never tried to find a job equal to his skill level.
>
> Alex often considers doing something about his depression. He actually tried medication for awhile, but he didn't like the side effects. He thinks that therapy is a tiring, long, drawn-out process. He purchased a book to learn more about depression, but it sits on his desk collecting dust. He feels guilty about not reading it, but then he thinks that no book can possibly pull him out of his mind's hazy state. So he ponders his plight and views his situation as hopelessly inescapable.

Because he's fully aware that effective treatments exist, you may wonder whether Alex actually *wants* to remain depressed. Nothing could be further from the truth. Nobody — and we mean nobody — prefers depression to normal moods.

If nobody prefers being depressed, then why does Alex avoid tackling his depression? Actually, he does so for normal, human reasons. In fact, most people with depression refrain from making a change at least for awhile. And when they do initiate efforts to change their situation, they frequently slip back into inaction for short to prolonged periods of time.

At first blush, it may seem bizarre that you would avoid searching for peace and serenity if you suffer from debilitating depression. After all, you know that depression feels horrible, and the alternative certainly appears more attractive. But we suggest that if you find yourself retreating and delaying when you think about trying to battle your depression, it's for good reasons. We now show you how myths, fear of change, and change-blocking beliefs, lie behind this avoidance of taking actions against depression, and these barriers to change make far more sense than you may think.

Flushing Out the Fear of Change

REMEMBER

Fear stands as the No. 1 driving force behind inaction and avoidance. We can understand why you may find yourself avoiding, procrastinating, and feeling hopeless about working on your depression. Do we think that you should stay on the sidelines feeling hopeless and avoid the scariness of change? No.

However, you need to fully appreciate the magnitude of the issues that may stand in your way. If and when you find yourself procrastinating and avoiding the task of getting your depression under control, you have no cause for self-criticism and abuse. Rather, you need to realize that you're experiencing a normal, human fear of change. In the following sections, we tell you about the two most common types of fear that inhibit change.

Fearing more losses

If you have significant depression, you inevitably have experienced profound losses of various types. Such losses include

>> **Belief in positive possibilities:** You have come to believe that only bad things will happen in the future.

>> **Relationships:** You may have lost one or more important connections. You fear that you will inevitably disappoint even those that remain loyal to you.

>> **Security:** You may feel vulnerable and unsteady.

>> **Self-esteem:** You see yourself as unworthy and undeserving.

Your depressed mind fears additional loss; it inevitably overestimates the difficulty of making changes and underestimates your ability to make them. The fear of hope itself is a big obstacle, because you assume that lost hope feels more horrible than never having had hope at all. Perhaps you're like most folks who are mired in depression and believe that

>> If you seek friendship, you'll experience more rejection.

>> If you take a new job, you'll fail.

>> If you take a risk, you'll be humiliated.

>> If you work on your problems, your efforts will be useless.

>> If you dare to hope, you'll fall into an abyss.

If these beliefs apply to you, it's no wonder that you avoid the challenge of change. The fear of additional losses is no trivial matter. It's so easy to conclude that not trying at all is better than trying and failing. Thus, your depressed mind tells you that making no attempt at least preserves a smidgen of self-esteem, whereas working hard at self-betterment and then failing means that you have sunk even further into an abyss of "in's" — incompetence, ineffectuality, incapability, incapacity, insufficiency, and inferiority.

Fearing inconsistency

The *fear of inconsistency* is another type of fear that frequently holds back attempts at recovery. Sounds a little odd, doesn't it? Psychologists have known for decades that people have strong motivations to remain consistent in their behaviors and beliefs. Consistency helps simplify the world. And consistency makes life feel more predictable.

And when you encounter information about yourself that runs counter to firmly held beliefs, you may find ways to reject the new information. This process tends to occur whether you're depressed or not.

The quest for consistency works to sustain depression. If you're depressed, you'll likely find yourself tossing out every piece of positive evidence about you or your world like yesterday's newspaper. You may fear success, especially if it comes with a less-than-Herculean effort, because such an outcome would contradict your long-held negative self-views of inadequacy.

Although you certainly don't like depression, it probably feels familiar and pre-dictable. By comparison, seeking a life of joy likely sounds frightening, unfamil-iar, and unpredictable. Staying in the depths of depression hurts, sometimes horribly so, but at least you feel as though you have a little more control. That's because you've chosen to take fewer risks and stay in the familiar environment of depression.

REMEMBER

We wouldn't be writing this book if we didn't completely believe that you have effective ways to remove yourself from the morass you find yourself in. In fact, each chapter is packed with suggestions, tools, and exercises for doing just that.

TECHNICAL STUFF

HUNKERED DOWN WITH HOMEOSTASIS

Even at a biological level, our bodies attempt to maintain a consistent, stable state — a process known as *homeostasis*. The body works very hard to sustain stable levels of temperature, hormones, fluids, carbon dioxide, blood sugars, and so on. When any of these conditions rise or fall beyond certain close parameters, the body goes into over-drive to reestablish the proper level. Many experts believe that homeostasis operates at all levels, from the cellular level to the psychological level, and even in social situations.

Finding Change-Blocking Beliefs

Depression is usually accompanied by a variety of deep-seated beliefs that support and sustain the melancholy and add fuel to the fears of change. Even though you may have first become depressed many years after passing through childhood, these beliefs generally have roots back to those early years. When you're not depressed, the beliefs hang around in the background, where they usually don't cause huge problems. But when depression strikes, they take center stage and diabolically disrupt your attempts at recovery.

TIP

Change-blocking beliefs are the thoughts and negative expectations you have about yourself and the world that make change seem impossible. Exploring the childhood roots of your change-blocking beliefs can help you discover not only where they came from but also that these beliefs have more to do with a child's interpretation of events than with current day reality.

Occasionally, change-blocking beliefs have roots in adulthood. Usually, traumatic events or chronic, repeated occurrences cause these beliefs to come about later in life. Nevertheless, change-blocking beliefs grounded in adulthood can be dealt with in much the same way as the more common, change-blocking beliefs that originate in childhood.

In the following sections, we describe what we've found to be the most common change-blocking beliefs. We describe each one and give you some tools on dealing with them on a case-by-case basis. Then, in the "Analyzing your findings" section, we provide an exercise that enables you to challenge any or all these beliefs when they get in your way.

REMEMBER

You may be able to think of other change-blocking beliefs than the ones we list here. We suggest carefully reviewing each of the beliefs we list to see if they may be making you feel like avoiding, procrastinating, or viewing your situation as hopeless.

Dealing with dependency and inadequacy

When you believe in your feelings of dependency or inadequacy, you quickly throw the brakes on taking risks. If you feel *dependent,* you probably believe that your depression must be cured by someone other than yourself. And if you think of yourself as *inadequate,* you likely feel incapable of doing anything for yourself. These change-blocking beliefs make taking risks seem particularly scary.

Yet, all efforts to change involve risk — you risk the possibility of failure. Unfortunately, feelings of dependency and inadequacy are almost universal among people who have depression. We can't even think of a depressed client that we've worked with in the past years who felt competent enough to independently tackle difficult, challenging tasks.

The dependency/inadequacy belief usually sends a series of related thoughts running through the mind, such as

>> Whatever I try, I usually manage to screw up.

>> I can't do this without a lot of help.

>> I need help, but no one can help me enough.

>> I don't want to take this risk; I know I'll fail and feel worse than ever.

>> I'm not strong enough to do this.

The dependency/inadequacy belief, and the related thoughts, paralyzes its victims into inaction. And the belief fuels the fear of change because of the assumption that failure will inevitably result. Devin's story demonstrates how his dependency developed in elementary and middle school.

> After **Devin's** father dies when Devin is only 4 years old, his mother becomes increasingly attached to him. As a result, she can barely stand to see him deal with pain or frustration. If he cries or whimpers, she rushes to provide comfort. If he wants candy or a cookie, she fulfills his wish because she doesn't want him to whine. Later, when he can't figure out the answers to his homework assignments, she provides them for him. She has the absolute best of intentions, but she inadvertently fosters the development of Devin's dependency/inadequacy belief.

> Devin never has the opportunity to learn what his real capabilities are, because his mother inevitably steps in before he has a chance to work through his problems. Although the school tests Devin's I.Q. and finds it to be in the gifted range, his teachers describe him as an underachiever. As a result, Devin believes that he's inept. Devin's I.Q. stands in contradiction to his basic belief of inadequacy. He has more than enough brainpower, but his mind tells him otherwise.

Devin's history depicts one of a number of ways that this destructive belief comes into being. Dependency and/or inadequacy can also emerge in childhood when a child receives excessive, harsh criticism. In addition, when parents aggressively push their children toward independence too soon, they can paradoxically cause their kids to feel overly dependent. For example, if parents never provide assistance that is truly necessary, their children may give up too easily. A similar result may occur if parents neglect their children, frequently leaving them alone to fend for themselves at too early an age.

TIP

If you think that you may have some degree of a dependency or inadequacy belief, reflect on your own childhood. Is it possible that

» One or more important people harshly criticized you over the years?

» One or both of your parents stepped in to help you too quickly when you felt frustrated?

» You rarely got help that you truly needed when you asked for it?

» Your parents pushed you way too hard?

» Your parents neglected you and left you alone too often at an early age?

If you answer "yes" to any of the questions in the previous list, please realize that your dependency or inadequacy belief has a very legitimate basis. In other words, you came to this conclusion for good reasons. You need to remember that those reasons don't mean that you're actually dependent or inadequate! If you don't agree, we provide you with some strategies for dealing with this and other dysfunctional beliefs in the "Analyzing your findings" section later in this chapter.

Uncovering an undeserving outlook

The belief that you're undeserving can also derail your recovery train before it works up a good head of steam. Many people who believe that they're undeserving think that something is inherently wrong with themselves. Thus, they beat themselves up for the slightest flaw or mistake. They literally think that they don't deserve to feel good or have good things happen to them.

When people feel as though they're undeserving, they exert little effort to overcome their depression. They may even feel as though depression is what they deserve and expect out of life, and that depression is an appropriate punishment for their perceived miserable existence on this planet.

If you frequently have any of the following thoughts, you may believe that you're undeserving:

» I feel like other people deserve more out of life than I do.

» I don't expect much out of life.

» I think that having needs indicates weakness.

» I feel guilty when people do things for me.

>> Because bad things only really happen to bad people, I must deserve my depression, not happiness.

>> I don't deserve to get what I want.

If you believe that you're more undeserving than other people, you'll likely find your depression more difficult to tackle: You probably fear that any happiness you bring your way will literally lead to punishment, because the happiness is undeserved. You need to clear this belief out of your way before making serious attempts to drain depression from your life.

TIP

You can start working on getting rid of this undeserving outlook by searching for its roots. People don't feel undeserving for no reason at all. A series of childhood events builds the foundation for the undeserving belief. Did any of the following themes permeate your childhood?

>> Were your parents emotionally unavailable to you?

>> Did you frequently feel slighted (compared to one of your siblings)?

>> Did one of your caretakers use *guilt tripping* (criticism and messages that made you feel ashamed) as a major form of punishment?

>> Were you harshly abused or punished?

>> Were your parents exceptionally unpredictable in the things they punished you for?

If these situations ring a bell with you, your undeserving belief is anchored in childhood. You formed this conclusion about yourself because, as a child, you tried to make sense out of the things that happened to you. It's natural to conclude that you're undeserving if your parents shamed you and/or failed to express love consistently. Desiree's story illustrates one way this undeserving belief can form.

Desiree's mother, Charlotte, is what psychologists call a *narcissist.* Charlotte thinks far more about her own needs than her child's. When Desiree exhibits the slightest crankiness at the age of 3, Charlotte whisks her off to spend the rest of the day in her bedroom. Charlotte's motivation is to eliminate an annoyance from her environment, not help Desiree learn self-control. Charlotte deals with Desiree's desires with similar harshness. If Desiree wants something that will inconvenience her mother, Charlotte informs Desiree that she's selfish, greedy, and ungrateful. Desiree decides early on that she's undeserving of good things.

Clearly Desiree deserved as much happiness and good in life as any other child. She didn't think that she deserved happiness, and she still doesn't today as an adult — only because of her upbringing.

Fighting the unfair fight

When people bog down and avoid working on their depression, they sometimes proclaim, "It's unfair; I shouldn't have to work at this! Why did this happen to me?" The belief that depression is unfair and that you shouldn't have to work on the problem is true to a certain degree.

We agree that coming down with depression isn't fair, and we sure wish that you didn't have to put in much work to do something about it. The truth is, we fully believe that:

>> No one truly wants to be depressed.

>> No one deserves to have depression.

>> No one is to blame for having depression.

Depression has many causes (see Chapters 2 and 3 for more on this topic), including genetics, diseases, childhood, tragedy, abuse, pandemics, discrimination, and trauma. You're not to blame for your own depression.

TIP

However, as unfortunate and unfair as it may be, you must work to overcome your depression. You won't find a fairy godmother to come into your life and wave depression away with a magic wand. Even if you choose to treat your depression with the path that often requires the least effort — medication — you still have to work closely with a trusted physician, psychiatrist, or other prescriber in order to monitor your progress and any possible side effects.

REMEMBER

Like other change-blocking beliefs, excessive concerns with unfairness usually have connections to childhood. More often than not, people who focus on unfairness were dealt with quite unfairly by their parents when they were children. Exploring the early causes helps you realize what change-blocking beliefs are about and lays the groundwork for changing them.

Rejecting the victim role

Unfortunately, bad things sometimes happen to good people for no reason at all. Certain negative events have great potential for disrupting people's entire worlds and the ways they view themselves. This disruption usually occurs when:

>> Something really bad happens, such as serious illness or trauma.

>> The negative event was undeserved or unfair.

>> The person feels upset, angry, and/or anguished about the negative event.

When such undeserved events happen to people, their views about who and what they are change. They naturally begin believing that they're sick patients or victims. And beliefs about sickness and victimhood involve an entire set of related self-views and altered behaviors, which we now describe.

People typically shift both their feelings and behaviors — from independent to dependent, from well to sick, from capable to incapable, from in control to helpless, from serenity to rage. This type of change in beliefs, behaviors, and expectations (that come from perceiving yourself as well versus sick) is normal and natural when traumatic events occur.

In a sense, these new beliefs and behaviors about sickness and victimhood require the individual to take on a new role, like an actor in a play. The individual takes on the leading role of patient or victim, and society, friends, family, mental health providers, and physicians carry out auxiliary roles as helpers. These helpers typically have certain expectations for the patient or victim role as well as for their own roles. For example:

>> Helpers feel motivated to help.

>> Helpers don't view the patient as someone who deserves to be blamed.

>> Helpers view themselves as mainly responsible for creating improvement and the patient as a passive recipient of their assistance.

>> Certain helpers may provide compensation to the victim.

>> Helpers believe that it's natural for the patient to feel upset or angry.

>> Helpers usually provide sympathy, concern, and support.

The sick patient and victim roles are legitimate, reasonable, and deserved. In a sense, society created these roles so that people can receive predictable assistance when bad things undeservedly happen to them. We suspect that virtually everyone has occupied one or both of these roles at one time or another. So what's the problem? Nothing at all if you only take on one of these roles for a short period of time.

Determining if you've assumed the victim role

Unfortunately, over time, these roles may become entrenched in the mind. As the belief in one's sickness or victimhood sets in, most people focus more and more on the unfairness and awfulness of what's happened to them. They feel angry and enraged. The worst part is that they frequently feel helpless to do anything about their predicament.

The best way to determine whether a belief in the sick patient or victim role has taken over your life is to ask yourself the following questions:

>> Do I frequently think about how unfair life has been to me?

>> Do I feel enraged by what has happened to me?

>> Do I frequently complain to others about my circumstances?

>> Do I feel helpless to do anything about my plight?

>> Do I feel that doing something about my problems would somehow discount the importance of what's happened to me?

If any of the thoughts from the previous list apply to you, you may have slipped into a victim or sick patient role for more than a short stay. These roles provide no guidance for how to move on, and that's the problem: They keep you stuck.

Shifting to alternative roles

Here are alternative roles that you may want to consider: the role of coper and the role of rehabilitation client. Copers and rehabilitation clients have also experienced bad (possibly horrible), undeserved, unfair events. The people who assume these roles are no more to blame than are victims and sick patients. But they find a way to dig down deep, let go of their anger and rage, and focus on what they can do to improve their circumstances. Rehabilitation sometimes takes months or years of hard work, but most people find that the results are worth the effort. Even chronic, debilitating diseases are often dealt with better by adopting the coper and rehabilitation roles.

If you find yourself trapped with prolonged, unrelenting sickness or victimhood beliefs, seek therapy for additional assistance.

Please realize that we blame no one for taking on a victim or sick patient role. It's a normal, expected, and virtually universal reaction to terrible circumstances. And the more traumatic the events (such as rape, physical abuse, and serious mental illness), the more one is likely to stay in the role for a longer period of time.

However, even in cases of severe trauma, shifting into a coper mode and working arduously to find a better life is the ultimate but highly challenging goal. To accomplish this shift, you need to understand that you deserve peace. And most importantly, you should know that rediscovering happiness in no way discounts or diminishes the awfulness of what happened to you.

TIP

Sometimes people wrestle with the idea that seeking happiness discounts past trauma. They may think that a renewed pleasure and zest for life would somehow mean that nothing truly horrific ever occurred. If this type of thinking sounds familiar, you may want to get back on the road to happiness with a technique we call Putting It in a Vault. This technique is based on a strategy suggested by our colleague, Dr. Robert Leahy, who has written extensively on the topic of why people resist change.

If you've had one or more horrific traumas in your life, try imagining a large bank vault with thick steel doors in your mind. Put your mind's videotape of the trauma into the vault and lock it away. The tape will remain there, and you can play the video of the trauma to appreciate the meaning it has for your life anytime you feel a need to do so. However, when you finish viewing the tape, lock the trauma away and live your life safe in the knowledge that the trauma doesn't need to harm you any further while it's locked in the vault. In this way, you can learn to take charge of your trauma rather than allow the horror to continue controlling your life.

Tackling perfectionism

People who are overly perfectionistic have an increased risk of depression. Because perfection is impossible to achieve, a perfectionist is predetermined to fail. People with perfectionistic tendencies usually have these traits:

>> Are extremely afraid of making mistakes

>> Have excessively high personal standards

>> Judge themselves with severe harshness

>> Harbor serious doubts about the quality of their endeavors

It's no wonder that perfectionists become depressed. The pressure of impossible standards, the fear of making mistakes, and the unrelenting stream of self-criticism leaves the person feeling helpless and hopeless.

TIP

Some people contend that a little bit of perfection is good. In their view, some perfectionism helps motivate hard work and quality effort. However, looked at another way, "a little bit of perfectionism" isn't really perfectionism at all. That's because "a little bit" of perfectionism allows for acceptance and flexibility.

Perfectionism usually begins during childhood. Children with this trait are not given unconditional love. They do not receive the message that they are good enough. Parents who foster perfectionism in their children typically do the following:

>> Show love contingently; in other words, when their children achieve something.

>> Let their children know that their worth is only as good as their performance.

>> Are overly critical of mistakes.

>> Fail to recognize the valuable lessons that mistakes offer.

Perfectionism is thought to be a reasonably stable personality trait. However, with all of the disadvantages associated with perfectionism, it may be worth targeting for change. Therapy is a particularly good and effective way to do that. It's hard work but well worth the effort.

Analyzing your findings

Ridding yourself of change-blocking beliefs isn't the easiest thing in the world to do because, as we mention throughout this section, they usually originated many years ago in your childhood and adolescence. We suggest that reviewing your personal history to more fully appreciate how and why you acquired these beliefs is a good place to start. This knowledge can help you to stop blaming yourself for having the beliefs in the first place.

REMEMBER

Throughout this book, we show you suggested tasks for helping you work on a variety of issues related to depression. You should not view them as required assignments. You may choose to complete some or not. You may also want to work on these assignments in conjunction with a mental health professional. You don't need commands from us to carry out difficult tasks, just to find yourself overwhelmed or feeling like a failure.

TIP

After you figure out which change-blocking beliefs you have, you may want to conduct an Advantages and Disadvantages Analysis of them. This analysis will provide you with important ammunition for challenging these beliefs when they get in your way. To do an Advantages and Disadvantages Analysis:

1. **Get a notebook out and construct a chart.**

   Draw a line down the middle of your paper. Write down the change-blocking belief that you want to tackle at the top of the page. Then label one column "Advantages" and the other "Disadvantages." See Table 4-1 for a sample analysis.

2. **Write every imaginable reason that your change-blocking belief feels advantageous to you.**

   Perhaps it feels like it helps you avoid risks and losses or that other people will like you more if you adhere to this belief.

3. **Write down all the reasons your change-blocking belief gives you grief.**

Perhaps the belief keeps you from exploring new opportunities or prolongs your state of unhappiness.

4. **Review your two lists carefully.**

Ask yourself whether the advantages or disadvantages seem more compelling. Typically, you're likely to find that the disadvantages greatly outweigh the advantages. If so, commit yourself to challenging your change-blocking belief by reading over the disadvantage column frequently. And see Chapter 8 for more ideas on how to challenge problematic beliefs.

Hayden's story shows how he uses this analysis technique to his benefit.

Hayden puts off working on his depression for nine months. He hopes his bleak mood will simply go away all on its own, but his depression only deepens. His therapist suggests reading a particular self-help book. After three more months of procrastination, Hayden reads a chapter. He discovers that he has an entrenched belief that he is undeserving. This belief prevents him from tackling his depression because he literally feels that he doesn't deserve happiness. He currently believes that he's particularly undeserving of pleasure because his depression has caused him to be unproductive in his work as a freelance writer. Although he's a bit skeptical, Hayden conducts an Advantages and Disadvantages Analysis of his undeserving belief. Table 4-1 shows the results of Hayden's advantages and disadvantages analysis.

TABLE 4-1   **Hayden's Advantages and Disadvantages Analysis**

Belief: Undeserving Outlook	
Advantages	Disadvantages
I don't have to feel guilty if I avoid pleasure.	This belief stops me from trying to get to a better place.
People won't think I'm self-centered.	I actually feel guilty all the time, whether I have a good time or not.
I'll be satisfied with less.	I always feel unhappy.
I won't be disappointed by hoping for good things.	I keep myself stuck when I think I don't deserve better.
If I feel undeserving, maybe it will motivate me to be more productive.	Actually, I hate being unproductive, but I think it's my depression that makes me less productive. And if I don't think I deserve better; I'll never be more productive.
	Whenever I feel good, I end up trashing the feeling because I think I didn't earn the right to feel that way. This thinking makes me less motivated to do anything positive.

Hayden concludes that his advantages and disadvantages analysis looks stronger on the disadvantage side of the equation. This inference motivates him to battle his undeserving belief each time it tells him to shy away from doing anything good for himself.

TIP

If you use the advantages and disadvantages technique on one or more of your change-blocking beliefs and it doesn't seem to help, don't get too discouraged. We provide many more ways to bust these and other problematic beliefs throughout the book.

Saving Yourself from Self-Limitations

The earlier sections of this chapter review the considerable fears that change evokes, as well as the powerful beliefs and myths that support those fears. It probably doesn't surprise you that most people avoid anxious apprehensions whenever possible.

TIP

In the case of deciding to deal with depression, avoidance means turning to self-limitation in order to stay clear of your fear of working toward recovery. *Self-limitation* is anything you do that prevents you from working on your depression and therefore reaching your true potential. You may be engaging in self-limitation if

>> You find reason after reason to avoid working on your depression.

>> You view your situation as hopeless.

>> You insist that there must be a perfect solution before trying to do anything at all.

>> You demand to see a guarantee of improvement before you undertake the task of changing.

>> You quit at the very first sign that things aren't working out.

>> You repeatedly engage in harsh self-criticism when you put forth some effort, thereby robbing yourself of motivation.

>> Whenever evidence indicates that things are a little better than you thought they'd be, you immediately discount and discard the data.

>> You wait for the "perfect time" for making changes, which never seems to show up.

>> You become confused, disoriented, or "out of it" whenever you try to deal with your problems.

>> You repeatedly blame other people for your predicament rather than look at what you can do to solve your problems.

If any of the items in this list apply to you when you consider working on your depression, you're not likely to make any progress until you do something about your self-limitation.

TIP

Please be aware that everyone who has depression avoids dealing with the problem and engages in self-limitation at various times in life. Avoid pummeling yourself with harsh judgments, which only work to prolong the sabotaging process.

Instead, read the following sections to find out how to dig your way out of your depression. We discuss a number of ways to stop self-limitation and get your recovery train moving down the tracks. If one strategy doesn't do much for you, try the others.

Tracking saboteurs

Saboteurs prefer to work in the dark. Their chances of success escalate substantially when you can't detect their movements. Therefore, you need to monitor the sabotaging activity that your depressed mind engages in.

REMEMBER

Light (awareness) is the arch foe of your mind's saboteurs; if you start monitoring how these saboteurs work, they won't be able execute their intentions as effectively. Monitoring your thinking increases your awareness of when your mind's saboteurs are at work and therefore enable you to stop them.

TIP

Find a notebook or open a file and consider starting a Self-Limiting Diary. Write the days of the week in a column to the left. Then title a column on the right "Self-Limiting Strategies." (See Table 4-2 for a sample diary.) Each day, write down anything you find yourself doing that keeps you stuck in depression and avoiding doing something about it. Consulting the list of self-limitation strategies in the previous section may help you get started. When you see what you're doing to limit yourself, you're likely to break out of the self-limiting pattern. Morgan's example shows how this technique works.

> **Morgan's** melancholy manages to endure for more than a year before he decides to do something about his predicament. He seeks the services of a psychologist who practices cognitive therapy (see Part 2 for more information about cognitive therapy). The psychologist quickly sees that Morgan, because of a fear of change,

inadvertently sabotages his own recovery efforts at every opportunity. Morgan shows up late to appointments, his mind wanders when he attempts to read self-help materials, he complains about how others treat him, and he insists that his therapist can't do anything to help him.

Morgan's psychologist helps him understand that his behavior only deepens the hole he finds himself in and prevents him from productively working toward improving his condition. It takes some time, but Morgan eventually gets the point. His psychologist then suggests that he keep a diary of his self-limiting strategies. Table 4-2 shows Morgan's results for the first five days.

TABLE 4-2   **Morgan's Self-Limiting Diary**

Day	Self-Limiting Strategies
Monday	I stayed in bed for hours and got to work late. I lost track of time later in the day and showed up to therapy 30 minutes late, which gave me only 20 minutes to deal with my issues. Then I spent 10 of those minutes telling my psychologist how hopeless I am. *Not very helpful I guess.*
Tuesday	My boss said my report was terrific, and I told him it wasn't really that good and proceeded to point out several flaws in it. *What will that do for me?*
Wednesday	I got a speeding ticket. Then I told myself I was an idiot for letting that happen. My insurance might go up, and I'll probably start screwing up other things too. I dwelled on the stupid ticket all day long and had an unproductive day at work. *I guess that wasn't too useful.*
Thursday	I met Sheila last week, and she seemed to like me. I really want to call her again, but I found myself not doing it. Maybe she was just being polite and doesn't like me at all. I started thinking I can't stand any more rejection and put off calling. *Where will that get me?*
Friday	I must have looked at that book my psychologist recommended ten times. But did I pick it up to read it? No, of course not. Then I beat myself up for being such a pathetic loser that I don't even do a simple thing like that to help myself. *I guess that doesn't help my cause either.*

Morgan reviews his diary and finds out how many ways he avoids productive work when it comes to improving his problems. He fears further loss and rejection, so he stays stuck in his depression, thereby insuring that he will fail to find a new relationship. When he hears something positive about his work, he refuses to believe his boss and actively argues with him. His self-criticism only serves to push his mood lower; it hardly helps motivate him to do something better. And his insistence on his own hopelessness only backs him into a corner.

Morgan's psychologist helps him understand that he self-limits for a good reason — the fear of change we review in the "Flushing Out the Fear of Change" section earlier in this chapter. Tracking his self-limitation does seem to help him tackle his problems. As Morgan sees the myriad of ways he avoids efforts to recover and maintain his current sad state, he starts to recognize his self-limitation before the fact. Then he ever so gradually stops backing away from change and starts taking on his problems.

If you find yourself avoiding and self-limiting, try keeping a self-limiting diary. But don't use your diary as a trigger for self-criticism and abuse. Beating yourself up will only perpetuate self-limitation by making you feel worse about yourself.

Suspending judgment

If you bog down in a web of self-limiting thoughts when reading this book or participating in therapy, suspend judgment for a while. Experiment with the idea that just maybe therapy can work for you. While you're suspending judgment, work as hard as you can at following the techniques that we describe throughout this book or that your therapist suggests.

TIP

The deeper your depression, the more we recommend starting with Part 3. That's because getting yourself moving is important, and Part 3 gives you a variety of ways to jump-start into action. After you start moving, your energy will likely pick up and give you a boost for tackling the rest of the important techniques.

As you work on the various antidepression tools we provide you, you may find yourself practicing self-limiting from time to time. Fight it with all you can muster. Although simply repeating positive, self-affirming statements to yourself won't do much for curing depression, sometimes repeating certain ideas can serve as important reminders. Therefore, consider repeating one or more of the following statements to yourself on a regular basis:

>> What do I truly have to lose by trying? I don't have to tell anyone what I've been doing, so no one will even know if my efforts don't work.

>> The only real failure comes from never trying.

>> Focus on progress, not perfection.

>> When I dump on myself, it doesn't help. I will try to focus on what I do right more than what I do wrong.

>> Don't judge, just do.

Going slow

You can also limit yourself in a rather surprising way — by working too hard and fast on your depression. Believe it or not, tackling your depression head-on at full speed can cause unexpected problems. Be sure to go slow. Going too fast sets you up for unrealistic expectations. Focus on small successes. If you happen to experience a big success, that's great. But savor it a bit and pull back from pushing ahead for just a little while.

REMEMBER

You're more likely to overcome your depression by taking a gradual, steady approach rather than swinging away for home runs.

Pacing yourself has another advantage — it can help keep you from feeling overwhelmed by the tasks at hand. Some people look at a book such as this one and notice that it contains more than 300 pages along with numerous exercises. They then conclude that they could never get through it all. If you think that you may not be able to get through this book, consider the following ideas:

>> You don't need to read every single chapter and do each and every exercise to derive significant benefits. If a particular exercise doesn't look that pertinent to you, don't do it! And certain chapters may not be important for you to read. For example, if you have a very good relationship, you may not want to read Chapter 16.

>> Looking at the whole picture at once can lead to self-limitation because doing so can feel overwhelming. Focus on one small step at a time. For example, if we focused on writing this entire book as though it had to be completed in a single week, we'd stop writing this instant!

WARNING

If you have a serious level of depression that includes thoughts of death and hopelessness, or you work on the strategies in this book without experiencing success, please consult a professional for additional assistance.

Appreciating how progress proceeds

Many people who come to us for help with depression expect to improve, and they're correct to have that expectation. But all too often they also expect to see prompt progress that proceeds in a smooth, steady, upward fashion. The only problem with this second expectation is that we have yet to see it happen! Why?

To be honest, we're not entirely sure why, but we do know that humans almost inevitably progress gradually, with many peaks and valleys along the way. It's important not to expect your change efforts to move ever steadily upward. Change just doesn't progress in that manner. Your progress will likely resemble Figure 4-1.

As you can see in Figure 4-1, progress contains both peaks and valleys. Like the stick figures on the chart, you're going to occupy various positions as you work to overcome your depression:

>> **Standing on a peak:** When you occupy this position, you're more likely to form unrealistically positive expectations about how you will progress in the future. You need to remind yourself that you will experience both ups and downs.

>> **Walking in a valley:** At this point, you may be tempted to conclude that you have never been at such a low spot before. The truth is, you may have made progress, but at these downturns, it may be impossible to see the progress you made — especially after being on the higher peak earlier. Try to resist making judgments on your progress during the inevitable downswings.

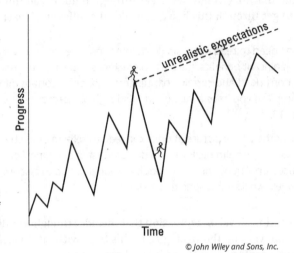

FIGURE 4-1:
The usual path of progress with depression.

REMEMBER

When you're on an upswing, you can probably assess your progress fairly realistically, but you need to resist the temptation to predict a too rosy progression in the future. And when you've taken a dip, try not to judge how you've been doing overall, because it won't be possible at those times.

TIP

Finally, we want you to know that the inherent downswings in the process of change has its advantages. That's because each decline, though unpleasant, can provide you with useful information about the events that trigger your low moods. You can see what to do with such events in Chapters 5 and 6. The key lies in expecting these downturns and not bashing yourself for experiencing the inevitable ups and downs in overcoming depression.

Rewriting your reams of failure stories

If you're depressed, you've probably written hundreds of failure stories of doom and gloom. Oh, you may not have actually put the words on paper, but your mind undoubtedly has pictured rejection, shortfalls, wasted efforts, botched attempts, and humiliation more times than you care to recall. And those images more than likely include a rich detail of your anticipated bungling along with an itemized list of horrors that would have resulted from your failure.

Stories about potential failures can cause people to avoid efforts that are aimed at improving depression. In essence, the stories become another form of self-limitation. So, how about considering something different?

TIP

Get out your notebook and a pen. Or, if you prefer, bring up the note-taking app on your phone or computer. Write a story about how you just may actually succeed at something! Include details about how you're going to approach the challenge, your plans, and the difficulties you anticipate.

Write down how you imagine you're going to overcome those difficulties. Be sure to include any thoughts about your fears, but also include strategies for working your way through the fear. If you have trouble coming up with ideas for getting around the obstacles, ask yourself what someone else might do. Make your story long enough to include the specifics; don't skimp.

LOW SELF-ESTEEM HELPS BUILD BARRIERS TO CHANGE

A group of researchers at the University of Washington and the University of Waterloo in Canada conducted a series of studies on self-esteem and its effects on the motivation to break bad moods. In one of these studies, the researchers put a group of students (some of whom had low self-esteem and others had normal self-esteem) in a bad mood by making them listen to depressing, sad music. Then the researchers offered the students a choice of videos to watch, including a comedy. All the students believed that the comedy would do the best job helping them get into a better mood. But surprisingly, slightly less than half the students with low self-esteem chose to watch the comedy, whereas about three-fourths of the other participants chose the comedy. The students with low self-esteem appeared to believe that it's not particularly appropriate to change a bad mood. Furthermore, the students with low self-esteem also seemed to think that their bad moods were more acceptable than the other students did.

Low self-esteem usually accompanies depression. This fact supports the idea that people who are dealing with depression and low self-esteem typically fall into inaction. Therefore, you need to work on breaking your mind's barriers to change before you attempt other recovery techniques.

Chapter **5**

Finding Help for Depression

A re you feeling blue? Okay, we're going to guess that, because you're reading this book, you or someone you love has been feeling depressed to one degree or another. Perhaps you merely feel a little down in the dumps, or maybe you're desperately despondent. The good news is that you can find help in a number of places, from the bookstore to the therapist's office. The bad news is that the shear number of choices can be confusing. In this chapter, we clear up the confusion by laying out your options for obtaining help and giving you the tools you need to make an informed decision.

We provide you with background information on two primary options for dealing with depression — psychotherapy and medication — so that you can figure out what's right for you. We help you decipher the differences among the various mental health professionals and determine whether you have a good match with the professional you choose. And we also talk about self-help which can augment medications or psychotherapy, and in mild cases, may prove sufficient.

Stumbling onto a Solution

People often neglect to think through their decision to seek help or investigate their options carefully. Sometimes this approach works out just fine — even though the options for dealing with depression are numerous and strikingly different.

> Consider **Veronica**, for example. She takes a job as a head librarian in a new city. She feels excited about her new position. Nevertheless, she misses her friends and family far more than she expected. At the age of 52, she's considerably older than her co-workers, and she finds it difficult to relate to them. After talking to her adult daughter on the phone one evening, she's surprised to find tears welling up in her eyes. Over the next few weeks, her mood deteriorates, and she begins to cry frequently. She feels rising guilt and remorse for having moved away from the ones she loves.
>
> Veronica receives a new shipment of books and notices one about fighting depression. She begins to leaf through it. The book's message resonates with her. After reading a few chapters, she concludes that her mood reflects an adjustment disorder with depressed mood. Over the next six weeks, she picks the book up many times and tries out its many suggestions. Her mood gradually brightens, and she starts to enjoy her new job and the new city.

Veronica stumbled upon the self-help option, and it worked for her. Her depression was quite mild and related to her move. As she became more adjusted to her situation, she was able to cope. Other folks find their way into therapy or medication, and they find that treatment works over time.

TIP

Unfortunately, many people don't find the best option for dealing with their depression on the first try. It's important to consider all your options for help and weigh the information carefully so that you can make an informed choice. But, if your first attempt doesn't work, don't give up. Try something else. Sometimes it takes a few tries to find your best treatment.

Pursuing the Psychotherapy Option

Psychotherapy involves work with a therapist using psychological techniques to alleviate emotional problems. And psychotherapy works well for treating depression. Incredibly, psychotherapy comes in literally hundreds of different forms and types; it's also practiced by a wide array of professionals. Yikes! How are you ever going to figure out how to get the help you need in this maze of options?

Never fear. In this section, we give you the information you need to find your way through the maze. First, we discuss the types of psychotherapy that are known to work for treating depression, and then we tell you how to sort out who's who among mental health professionals.

The effective therapies

Feel free to read the vast literature that encompasses hundreds and hundreds of articles on the effectiveness of psychotherapy for treating depression. We're guessing that you probably don't want to read all that info, so we did the research for you. (Don't feel too bad for us; it's our job.) From this literature, we zero in on four empirically validated therapies for depression.

What does empirically validated therapy mean? Empirical refers to an approach that systematically tests a therapy's effectiveness through careful observation using well controlled research studies. When a therapy is validated, it can be trusted to deliver consistent results. Many studies are required before scientists fully endorse a therapeutic approach as empirically validated.

REMEMBER

The following therapies have been proven to be effective and, for many, produce excellent results within a reasonable time frame:

» **Cognitive therapy:** In brief, cognitive therapy operates on the assumption that the ways in which people think about, perceive, and interpret events plays a pivotal role in how they feel. For the treatment of depression, no psychotherapy has received as much support as cognitive therapy. Flat out, it works. It works at least as well as medication does for treating depression, and it appears to provide a degree of protection against relapse — something that medication can't do. See Part 2 for a wide array of techniques and ideas based on cognitive-therapy principles.

» **Acceptance and Commitment Therapy (ACT):** ACT has many similarities to cognitive and behavior therapies. However, it places greater emphasis on accepting all feelings and emotions rather than trying to rid yourself of them entirely. ACT suggests that attempts to eliminate or avoid all bad feelings almost always backfire and merely make bad feelings more intense. Accepting feelings, paradoxically, helps soften them. It also works on value clarification and commitment to living a life based on your personal values. ACT has been found to be an effective treatment for depression. Chapter 9 is based largely on the premises of ACT.

>> **Behavior therapy:** Studies have found that changing your behavior can also improve the way you feel and alleviate depression. Behavior therapy focuses on helping you to change behaviors (such as increasing your pleasurable activities and teaching you ways to solve problems). Most practitioners of behavior therapy also include at least some cognitive techniques in their work. Many of these professionals call themselves cognitive-behavioral therapists. See Part 3 for a review of various behavior-therapy–based techniques.

>> **Interpersonal therapy:** This type of therapy attempts to help people identify and modify problems in their relationships, both past and present. Considerable evidence supports the value of interpersonal therapy for decreasing depression. Like cognitive therapy, this approach has also been shown to alleviate depression about as well as medication. Sometimes this method of therapy delves into issues involving loss, grief, and major changes in a person's life, such as retirement or divorce. A fair portion of this approach also involves the relationship between the therapist and client (like learning to relate to the therapist in ways that may help you with other relationships), which a book can't provide. Check out Part 4 for strategies such as learning to replace losses that are derived in part from interpersonal therapy.

Most people aren't aware that hundreds of different types of therapy exist. If you cast around, you may run into practitioners of psychoanalysis, hakomi therapy, eye movement desensitization reprocessing (popularly referred to as EMDR), client–centered therapy, transactional analysis, and Gestalt therapy, just to name a few. We believe that many of these therapies likely have value, and some may work for depression. However, the scientific literature is limited on these other types of therapy as applied to depression. We suggest that you start with therapies that have been fully established as effective.

Who's who in psychotherapy

REMEMBER

Most people don't realize that, in the majority of states, just about anyone can call themselves a therapist without getting into trouble with the authorities, because the title "therapist" isn't typically covered by licensing laws. Instead, states regulate specific professional titles and the right to practice psychotherapy or prescribe medications.

In the following list, we review the most common professional titles controlled by state professional licensing boards. We also describe the usual training required to obtain each type of professional license, although requirements vary slightly from state to state. You need to ask about a practitioner's specific training in particular types of psychotherapy, because not all professionals have been trained in the types of psychotherapy that have been found effective for depression (which we outline in the preceding section).

- **» Clinical psychologists:** To become a licensed clinical psychologist, an individual has to earn a doctorate degree in psychology. In addition, she must complete a yearlong internship followed by one or two years of supervised postdoctoral training. Doctoral programs in psychology generally emphasize the science of human behavior and provide training in psychotherapies that have been validated by research. Nevertheless, you need to check on the psychologist's expertise in an empirically validated therapy before you commit to working on your depression with her. In some states, clinical psychologists who have completed additional training are allowed to prescribe medications as well as conduct therapy.

- **» Counselors:** Licensed, independent counselors have a master's degree and two years of postgraduate supervision. In a few cases, counselors may only have bachelor's degrees in education, psychology, or theology. *Pastoral counselors* have theological training in addition to their training in counseling. Most counselors provide a range of psychotherapies. Inquire about their specific experience with the types of psychotherapy that have been found to be successful for depression.

- **» Psychiatrists:** Psychiatrists earn a medical degree and participate in a four-year residency program that trains them in the treatment and diagnosis of emotional disorders, including depression. Their training typically emphasizes biological treatments. Therefore, many psychiatrists strictly deal with medication management and/or alternative biological therapies such as electroconvulsive shock therapy (see Chapters 17 and 18). However, some psychiatrists do receive extensive training in psychotherapy. If you're interested in obtaining psychotherapy, be sure to ask if the psychiatrist you're thinking about working with offers it.

- **» Social workers:** Social workers sometimes go by various titles such as *licensed social worker* and *independent social worker.* The titles *qualified clinical social worker* and *diplomate in clinical social work* are given to folks who reach the most advanced levels of training. To become a qualified clinical social worker, the applicant must have earned at least a master's degree in social work, worked two years under supervision beyond the master's degree, and passed a comprehensive national examination. Social workers provide a range of psychotherapies, although some of them focus on arranging social services and helping people access resources. A social worker's title doesn't necessarily indicate the extent of his psychotherapy training. So just ask to find out whether the social worker you're planning to work with offers psychotherapy and has been trained in therapies found effective for the treatment of depression.

TIP

Various states may also license a number of other types of mental health professionals. For example, many states license marriage and family therapists or psychiatric nurses to provide therapy. Check with your state's professional licensing board or your insurance carrier. If a therapist is not licensed, beware.

Finding the right therapist for you

Some people take less time choosing a therapist than they do picking out the best cantaloupe at the grocery store. That's too bad, because the right therapist can help you recover and reach new levels of adjustment and well-being. And in the worst case, the wrong therapist can take your time and money, actually causing increased emotional distress.

REMEMBER

The following are important issues to consider when you look for a therapist:

>> **Finances:** Ask how much the therapist charges and whether your insurance covers that specific professional. Some insurance companies have lists of so-called preferred provider therapists that they cover. Some policies allow you to see almost any licensed therapist, while others restrict access to a very narrow panel of providers. Though unusual, a few companies only cover psychotherapies known to be effective, such as the ones reviewed in this book. Be sure to check your coverage rather than make an expensive mistake based on your assumptions. Some people choose not to use insurance because they want to see a particular professional or they have special concerns about privacy.

TIP

Investing money in therapy ultimately pays off in numerous, unexpected ways. For example, studies have shown that psychotherapy actually reduces medical doctor visits; it also appears to improve physical health in addition to mental health.

>> **Reputation and recommendations:** Therapists can't provide you with the names of satisfied customers, because they're bound to respect confidentiality. In most states, you can access information from your state government's website to see if there have been any formal complaints or ethical violations against a practitioner. In addition, you can inquire about therapists' reputations from other sources. Ask around. Talk to your friends and your family physician.

WARNING

Beware of advertisements in the newspaper, television, or phone book: They *are not* especially reliable sources of information about therapists' reputations.

>> **Scheduling:** Some therapists have extremely full practices with very limited options for appointment times. You may need to find someone who sees people in the evenings or on weekends. Be sure to ask what hours the therapist keeps.

>> **Training and licensure:** We discuss the general training requirements for various licensed mental health professionals in the "Who's who in psychotherapy" section earlier in this chapter. Consider this entry on our list as a reminder to ask about training and experience in the therapies that are

known to work for depression, such as cognitive therapy, behavior therapy, and interpersonal therapy. (For a definition of these therapies, check out the "The effective therapies" section earlier in this chapter.)

TIP

The Covid-19 pandemic spawned the rapid growth of what's known as telehealth and/or teletherapy. Teletherapy uses computers or smartphones to allow therapy to be conducted remotely. During the pandemic, teletherapy seemed like the right thing to do for obvious reasons. And preliminary studies indicate likely benefits from teletherapy, but considerably more research is needed to confirm this finding. On the other hand, many people greatly prefer face-to-face therapy. The times are changing, and we'll have to wait and see if remote therapy will ultimately replace much of in-person care.

Deciding whether your therapist is a good match

Most of the time when people choose a therapist, they feel a good connection, and they get better. Therapists generally are bright, kind, and skillful. However, therapists and clients sometimes just don't make a good match.

You may find that your therapist is a poor match for you. Maybe the therapist looks just like your ex-spouse, and every time you go to therapy, you feel a flood of painful memories. Or maybe you don't feel connected to your therapist for some reason that you don't understand. The quality of the therapeutic relationship has been found to consistently predict good or bad therapy outcomes, so it's critical that you feel comfortable.

TIP

Here are some questions you may want to ask yourself to help determine your comfort level after you see your therapist a few times:

>> Do I feel like I can tell my therapist just about anything?

>> Does it seem like my therapist cares about me?

>> Is my therapist reasonably optimistic about my likely progress?

>> Does my therapist understand me?

>> Does my therapist seem interested in my problems?

>> Does my therapist seem to set strict agendas and won't let me bring in something new that's important to me?

>> Does my therapist hear what I'm trying to say?

>> Is my therapist reliable and usually on time?

» Does my therapist keep discussion of personal issues to a minimum?

» Is my therapist open and accepting of criticism?

» Do I trust my therapist?

» Is my therapist nonjudgmental and noncritical with me?

» Do I feel safe discussing my problems with my therapist?

If you answer any of these questions with a strong "no," or you answer several of them without a clear "yes," discuss your concerns with your therapist. If you feel that you can't discuss these issues with your therapist, ask yourself why.

REMEMBER

If you have good reasons for feeling so unsafe that you can't imagine speaking frankly, you probably need to search for another therapist. On the other hand, if your reticence comes from shyness or embarrassment, please realize that therapists are trained to hear your concerns, and you have an absolute right and need to express them.

TIP

How your therapist reacts to your concerns about the quality of your client-therapist relationship will tell you if the relationship can be repaired. Following is an example of how a good therapist might respond to a client's concerns:

Client: I need to talk to you about something.

Therapist: Sure, what is it?

Client: I've been feeling like I can't be honest with you because I'm afraid you'll be critical.

Therapist: I'm glad you brought that up. Can you help me understand when it's felt like I've been critical of you?

Client: Well, last week I told you about my plans to look for another job and you said I shouldn't do it.

Therapist: That must have sounded like criticism, as if I wasn't supporting you.

Client: Yes, it did. It felt like you thought I was stupid.

Therapist: That must have felt awful. Can you think of any other reason I might have made that suggestion?

Client: No. Was there one?

Therapist: Well, yes. I've simply found that when people make major life decisions while they're in the throes of a major depression like you, they often regret their action later. It's just so hard to look at things objectively at times like this. On the other hand, I certainly want to explore your unhappiness at your job. Come to think of it, I probably didn't ask you enough about that. Would you like to tell me more now?

That exchange seems to work out fairly nicely, doesn't it? The therapist listens carefully to the client's concerns, acknowledges having failed to adequately explore the issue, and demonstrates interest in doing so. If your therapist responds to you in this manner, we suggest that you remain in therapy a little longer to see if the relationship can become more productive.

TIP

But sometimes therapists have their own problems, and they don't respond very well to clients' concerns. Here's an example:

Client: I need to talk to you about something.

Therapist: Sure, what is it?

Client: I've been feeling like I can't be honest with you because I'm afraid you'll be critical.

Therapist: Well, I certainly don't think I've ever criticized you. What would make you think such a thing?

Client: Well, last week I told you about my plans to look for another job, and you said I shouldn't do it.

Therapist: That's because you're in no condition to be looking around for work. You're far too depressed to do something like that. You really thought I was criticizing you?

Client: Yes, I did. It felt like you thought I was stupid.

Therapist: That's just not true. You're obviously feeling overly defensive. We need to work on that.

Client: To be honest, I'm just not feeling heard by you.

Therapist: Well, I'm clearly listening to you now.

In this case, the conversation does nothing to repair the strained relationship. The therapist reacts defensively and shows no support, empathy, or connection with the client. If your discussions with your therapist often sound like this one, you probably should consider going to another professional.

TIP

You should know that most therapists won't react like the one in the preceding example. Therapists tend to listen well, express empathy, and react to criticism with openness.

Debunking myths about therapy

Myths and misconceptions about therapy and self-help resources are another major reason why many people avoid seeking help for depression. We sometimes hear people discuss therapy in uncomplimentary terms. Of course, rarely do these same people actually undertake a regimen of therapy. They avoid therapy like the plague because they truly view the process as misguided and useless. If they do begin therapy, they typically avoid full participation and then quit too early because of their misperceptions. These people buy into the many myths and misconceptions about therapy. In this section, we discuss each of these myths and why we believe that they're inaccurate.

Therapy is a long, complicated process

Therapy and self-help involve some work. However, numerous studies have demonstrated that most cases of major depression can be treated successfully with about 20 sessions of the types of therapy we discuss in this book. Other studies have shown that, for a few people, self-help alone can provide sufficient assistance for overcoming mild cases of depression. Studies have also shown that self-help can be a valuable addition to therapy.

But if you're battling chronic, long-term depression, you may indeed discover that you require a relatively lengthy course of therapy. However, you'll likely experience a lift in mood within a few months of starting your therapy, and odds are good that you'll feel that the long-term payoff from continued work is more than worth the effort.

Therapy just provides excuses

People who ascribe to this myth often view themselves as inferior and believe that they deserve to suffer from depression. Other folks who view therapy as an excuse generator believe that certain therapies (especially cognitive therapy; see Part 2) simply push positive thinking. The truth is that these therapies don't ask you to simply see everything as positive. Rather, they guide you to collect and examine evidence (much like scientists do). When you discover evidence that supports a negative aspect about yourself or your world, you work to change what you can and accept what you can't change.

Therapy and self-help merely trivialize depression

Throughout this book, we state that depression is a serious problem — sometimes deadly serious in that suicide poses a significant risk. All good therapists understand the seriousness of this condition.

On the other hand, we do realize that therapy gives you techniques that are fairly straightforward and not particularly complex. These strategies may indeed feel trivial. After all, you may have battled profound depression for years, and the idea that some simple techniques may help you overcome your depression can feel very discounting. But therapists try to take complicated ideas and information and break them into easily understood, digestible units. If you were to ask anyone to comprehend and execute all of this information at once, most folks would naturally feel overwhelmed by it all.

Sometimes you may feel that a therapist is asking you to change too quickly or easily, which can make you feel diminished, as though your depression is simple and easily changed. If you're in therapy, discuss these feelings with your therapist. If you're attempting to treat yourself with self-help and you feel as though you're being asked to change too quickly, you may benefit from adding therapy to your efforts.

Therapy ignores the importance of emotions and feelings

The mental health field appreciates the agony and pain behind depression. That's why this field has devoted decades of professional exploration and research to finding ways to alleviate the pain of depression.

Emotions and feelings are of paramount importance to therapists. Nevertheless, sometimes therapists ask you to focus on your thoughts in addition to the emotions generated by those thoughts. As a result, it may feel like your emotions aren't fully appreciated. If you're in therapy, discuss this feeling with your therapist. If you have this reaction while reading a self-help book such as this one, you may want to supplement your efforts with a therapist who can listen to and appreciate your feelings more completely than an author can from afar.

Neither therapy nor self-help can give me what I need

Well, this thought has some truth to it. No therapist or book can possibly give you everything you need. Most therapists and authors realize that they have limitations. For example, you very well may feel disappointed by one or more parts of this book. And we want to hear from you if that's the case.

But try to approach both therapy and books with the realization that your needs will only find partial fulfillment. Your needs are more likely to be met through multiple sources: books, therapists, friends, relatives, and so on. And, unfortunately, we don't know of anyone who can truthfully report feeling 100 percent fulfilled all of the time.

Therapy doesn't work

Literally hundreds of studies have demonstrated the effectiveness of the therapies we describe in this book. As we discuss each of these therapies, we also briefly make note of the research behind them. However, not every type of psychotherapy has convincingly demonstrated such effectiveness. If you get therapy, make sure it's one we discuss in this book.

I can't change who I am

I can't change unless I feel totally understood, and no author or therapist can ever understand the complexity and depth of my problems. The idea that no author or therapist can ever completely understand every aspect of your depression is absolutely true. In fact, many mental health professionals haven't experienced a major depressive episode, so they can't truthfully say that they fully grasp the entire entanglement of your torturous emotional experience.

However, most therapists do their best to listen and connect with the devastating impact of depression. Hopefully what they write reflects a reasonable understanding of what they hear. And research shows that therapy works quite well even though most therapists can't claim a 100 percent understanding of the agony you may be experiencing.

People who go to therapy are weak

Although this thought effectively blocks more than a few people from seeking help, we fully believe that it is grounded in falsehood. In truth, seeking help is a courageous act. It requires letting down your guard and pondering your vulnerabilities. Think about it. Who is more courageous? Someone who feels compelled to present a false front and avoid exploring any personal vulnerability, or someone who owns up to problems and decides to face them head-on? We think the latter is more courageous.

People just go to therapy to whine and complain

The vast majority of people who seek help do reveal some "complaints" about their lives, but then they set about trying to do something about their problems. Therapy has about as much to do with whining and complaining as rapidly flapping your arms has to do with flying.

Talking to a Professional about Antidepressant Medication

The actual decision regarding whether or not to use medication for your depression is a complex one to make. In Chapter 17, we review both the upside and the downside of treating your depression with medication in detail. However, if you opt for antidepressant drugs, you still need to know who to get them from. A variety of different professionals prescribe medications for depression.

As you may imagine, physicians prescribe most antidepressant medications. Two types of physicians prescribe these medications far more frequently than other physicians:

>> **Primary care physicians:** These physicians are the ones most people go to for their routine care such as annual physicals and treatment for colds and flu. This group includes specialists, such as family practice physicians, internists, geriatric physicians, and sometimes even gynecologists. Talking to your family physician about symptoms of depressions can be a reasonable way to start your treatment.

In fact, you may be surprised to know that primary care physicians write more than 60 percent of the prescriptions given for emotional disorders. Nevertheless, if your depression is quite severe or complicated by the presence of other problems, such as anxiety or substance abuse, you need to consult a psychiatrist or a prescribing psychologist.

TIP

Before you ask for antidepressant medication from your primary care physician, be sure to find out whether your doctor is comfortable with these medications. Some general practitioners have considerable training in using medications to treat emotional disorders, while others know relatively little about this specific area.

>> **Psychiatrists:** Keep in mind that psychiatrists receive more extensive training in the biological treatments of depression than any other prescribing group of professionals. In addition, they regularly see patients with depression and other emotional disorders. Thus, they have considerable experience with the tricky side effects and drug interaction issues involved with antidepressant medication.

A few other professionals, in addition to physicians, are allowed to prescribe antidepressant medication:

>> **Nurse practitioners and physician assistants:** A majority of states allow these professionals to prescribe antidepressant medication in addition to other medications. Most of these practitioners have quite limited training in the treatment of emotional problems such as depression, though some do. Be sure to ask. If your depression isn't severe or complicated by the presence of other emotional problems (such as physical maladies, substance abuse, or suicidal thoughts), you may consider obtaining antidepressant medication from these mid-level providers.

>> **Prescribing psychologists:** Most psychologists do not prescribe medication. However, a growing number have completed additional training that enables them to do so. You need to check with your individual state to see if psychologists have specialty training in psychopharmacology.

>> **Pharmacists:** In several states, pharmacists are lobbying for the right to prescribe certain types of medication. Usually this privilege involves collaboration with a primary care physician. Pharmacists also have quite limited training in the treatment of emotional problems, but you can consider obtaining your medication from a pharmacist if you have a mild, uncomplicated form of depression. (See Chapter 2 for more information about the different types of depression.)

TIP

If you decide to take medication and also receive psychotherapy from another provider, encourage your therapist to communicate with the health care professional who is prescribing your medications. Communication ensures that both professionals are working on the same page.

Exploring the Self-Help Option

Everyone who is dealing with depression can benefit from self-help. *Self-help* refers to efforts you make on your own, without professional assistance, to deal with your depression. Scores of studies have demonstrated the value of self-help for a variety of emotional, behavioral, and medical difficulties. For a few individuals, self-help appears to be all they need. However, frequently, self-help may not be enough. But even if your own efforts fall short, self-help can provide a potent addition to therapy, medication, or a combination of both.

Deciding whether self-help is a solution

Should you consider self-help as an exclusive means of overcoming depression? In most cases, probably not. But before making the decision to try self-help alone as your strategy, ask yourself the following questions:

>> **Am I having any suicidal thoughts?** If the answer is yes, you need to obtain an evaluation from a mental health professional. That person will likely recommend psychotherapy, medication, or a combination of the two in addition to self-help.

>> **Is my depression seriously interfering with my life in areas such as work, relationships, sleep, appetite, or recreation?** Once again, if the answer is yes, you may be suffering from a major depressive disorder, which means that you probably need more than just self-help.

If you answer "no" to both of these questions, self-help *may* be the right place to start. However, you need to consider another question before you begin: "Do I have the desire and motivation to work on the advice I receive from self-help sources?" We're not talking about hours of study every day. But self-help does require more than a quick read of an article or book. And you, like plenty of folks, may do better when you have a coach or leader inspiring you. Only you can answer this question. If you can't confidently answer "yes" to this question, talk to a mental health professional about your options.

If you make the decision to stick with self-help, that's great. This book is a terrific place to start. Then if you want to obtain extra self-help resources, you can choose additional books, videos, self-help groups, or whatever combination of resources you think will help. Work for a while at applying what you learn, and monitor your progress carefully. You can use the mood monitoring form (the Mood Diary) that we outline in Chapter 2 to help keep track of your improvement.

WARNING

If you don't see progress through self-help after a month or two of effort, look into additional assistance. And if at any point you feel discouraged, start having suicidal thoughts, or your depression worsens, get additional help.

Reviewing the resources

Choosing the right self-help approach depends in part on your personal preferences and style. The fact that you're already reading this book suggests that the written word may appeal to you. The following list covers the most common self-help options. (We provide additional specific suggestions in the appendix.)

>> **Books:** This is the only book in the entire literary world that has value in helping people with depression. Just kidding, folks! Reading several different self-help books is a pretty good idea. Even though you may hear some suggestions more than once, repetition helps you remember, and all authors have slightly different ways of explaining concepts. The best books for dealing with depression give you information about treatments that are known to work (such as cognitive therapy, acceptance and commitment therapy, behavior therapy, interpersonal therapy, and medication).

Books are an inexpensive way of getting help and general information, which is an obvious advantage. But more importantly, books can also provide you with a whole lot of information that would take a therapist many sessions to cover. And you can refer to the information as often as you need to. Finally, if you combine reading with therapy, it may just take you less time to get better.

REMEMBER

Make sure that the authors of any self-help book that you purchase have credentials and experience helping others deal with depression.

>> **Videos:** For folks who learn best by hearing or seeing, videos have merit. Look for the same author credentials and information on effective approaches that we note for books.

>> **Self-help groups:** Self-help groups offer support and understanding. People with common problems gather in these groups to share information and experiences. The members help themselves and each other by expressing feelings and solving problems together. Unfortunately, we don't know of any major, organized groups like Alcoholics Anonymous or Take Off Pounds Sensibly with a nationwide network of self-help groups for people with depression. However, the National Alliance for the Mentally Ill (www.nami.org) is a self-help support and advocacy group for people with emotional problems and their families. They offer information concerning the availability of local support groups. In addition, your local chapter of United Way likely has a directory of community resources.

>> **Websites:** You can find a wide range of resources related to depression on the internet. You can join a chat room or download articles. But take particular care if you venture away from the websites we list in the appendix. First, the internet has more than its share of unqualified, though well-meaning, individuals serving up advice. Second, outright frauds also market their products and ideas on the internet.

WARNING

Numerous unscrupulous entrepreneurs hawk various types of books, herbs, videos, and other types of merchandise that promise prompt relief from depression with little or no effort. Buyers beware! No miracle cures exist for overcoming depression.

2

Understanding and Accepting Thoughts and Feelings

IN THIS PART . . .

Figure out the relationship between thoughts and feelings.

Recognize how thinking gets distorted.

Uncover new ways to think.

Accept difficult emotions.

Get help if you have suicidal thoughts.

Chapter **6**

Understanding the Thought/Feeling Connection

P eople with depression feel horrible. They are overwhelmed with sadness. They feel lethargic, despondent, and unmotivated. With these feelings, it's almost impossible to believe that anything will ever change. It's totally understandable that when people with depression ask for help, first and foremost, they want relief from those terrible feelings. In fact, relief from painful feelings represents the main goal of most depression treatment seekers.

Surprisingly, it's also the wrong target. Why? Emotions or feelings are important ways the body communicates with your mind. They inform and guide your behavior.

REMEMBER

Believing that you absolutely need to rid yourself of distressing feelings *prevents* you from learning how to tolerate discomfort and learn from your emotions. Paradoxically, acquiring the ability to tolerate and accept distressing feelings can lead to greater comfort.

In this chapter, we explain the relationship between emotions, thoughts, and behavior. Emotions are responses or labels that follow physical sensations and interpretations of those sensations. For example, you feel sluggish and fatigued. You may interpret those sensations as sadness and depression. On the other hand, you might interpret those same sensations as a result of a poor night's sleep. Throughout the following pages, we lay out the interactions of these sensations, feelings, and interpretations. We give you tools for examining and understanding your own emotional life.

Understanding Emotions

Emotions are signals to our minds about our responses, bodily sensations, interpretations, reactions, and current conditions. For example, you may respond to a critical comment with shame and feel sad or worthless. Or you may react with outrage and feel anger. You might see a spider and feel intense terror. Or perhaps you find spiders interesting and feel a sense of curiosity.

Alternatively, imagine you're sitting outside on a breezy summer day with a cold iced tea feeling peaceful and contented. Or maybe you are sitting outside on a breezy summer day with a cold iced tea feeling restless and bored. Same situation; two different sets of emotions.

REMEMBER

Emotions give you information about how you're responding to various events and situations. Pay attention to your emotions, as they have much to tell you.

TECHNICAL STUFF

For our purposes, we use the terms emotions and feelings pretty much interchangeably. Some argue that emotions arise primarily out of body sensations; others believe that thoughts or interpretations occur first. We suggest that you let psychologists and philosophers debate about those distinctions. Ultimately, the goal is to observe thoughts, emotions, and bodily sensations and listen to what they're trying to say.

Feelings emerge from your body

Believe it or not, experiencing a full-blown major depression but remaining unaware of sad feelings is possible. People with that lack of awareness tend to have multiple physical symptoms of depression such as low energy, problems with sleep, changes in appetite, and tension. In addition, they are likely to lack motivation and feel overly pessimistic.

Other people with depression try to suppress, deny, and/or avoid unpleasant feelings. They try to feel better by not feeling at all. And this strategy could even make a certain degree of sense — except that denying feelings doesn't work and only makes things worse.

TIP

Stuffing your feelings down inside is like filling a grocery bag with too many cans. Eventually your bag is going to rip apart, spilling its contents all over the place. The bottom line from research: Denial and repression are linked to poor emotional health, whereas expressing and allowing awareness of feelings improves both body and mind.

When people find *denial* and *repression* (either conscious or unconscious attempts to avoid thinking about uncomfortable emotions and thoughts) failing to blot out their unpleasant feelings, they sometimes turn to other strategies, such as immersing themselves in their work or abusing drugs and/or alcohol to drown out their sorrows. Unfortunately, avoidance of bad feelings by distracting yourself through excessive work or by ingesting substances only provides fleeting, temporary relief. In the end, they both actually cause you to dig yourself into a deeper hole and, ultimately, increase the intensity of depression.

A lot of people (with and without depression) have trouble finding their feelings. If you often don't know what you're feeling or people say that you're out of touch with your feelings, you can change things with a little work.

TIP

If you start tuning into your bodily sensations, we think you're likely to find feeling words to capture what's going on. It may take you some time, but tapping into what your body is telling you will facilitate your efforts in getting to a better place. You can start tuning into your bodily sensations by paying attention to the following:

>> Muscle tension

>> Your breathing (Is it fast, slow, deep, or shallow?)

>> A sense of heaviness in your chest

>> Dizziness

>> Posture (Are you relaxed, rigid, or stiff?)

>> Queasiness

>> Fatigue

>> Insomnia or excessive sleepiness

>> Changes in appetite

>> A constricted sense in your throat

>> Discomforts of any type

Spend 5 minutes a day actively tuning into such bodily sensations. Everyone experiences sensations like these, so just start tuning into your body and recognizing when you have them. Try to think of feeling words that capture your complete physical and mental state. Here's a partial list to start you out:

Afraid	Irritable
Apprehensive	Low
Despondent	Morose
Disturbed	Melancholy
Embarrassed	Nervous
Empty	Obsessed
Frustrated	Sad
Guilty	Shaky
Heavy	Somber
Hopeless	Tense
Inadequate	Worried
Insecure	Worthless

Feelings sprout from your thoughts

In addition to coming from your body, feelings also emerge from your thoughts. That works out just fine when your thoughts are correct interpretations of reality. However, when you are depressed, thoughts are often at variance with actual events and happenings. Here are examples of two people responding to the same event to illustrate this connection:

Leticia and **Raul** work on the same team for a marketing platform company. During the pandemic, they both work at home. In an online meeting, their supervisor suggests that his team needs to improve their data tracking systems. Here are Leticia and Raul's reactions to that comment.

Leticia thinks, "Well, he's probably right about the data tracking system. We need to make some minor adjustments and improvements. In the long run, this feedback will help us in our work."

She feels energized and enthusiastic about the task. Her emotions are positive. She feels happy and ready to focus on finding a solution.

Raul, by contrast, thinks, "That supervisor is always on our case. We can never be good enough. I think he's singling me out for criticism. He doesn't like me anyway. Who knows how long I'll last on this team. I might be looking at a demotion."

Raul feels defeated, depleted of energy, and has difficulty concentrating. He can hardly think about solving the problem. He feels discouraged and despondent. His motivation plummets. Raul suffers from chronic depression.

TIP

We hope by now that you are beginning to get a sense of how thoughts and feelings interact. Try to recall or notice patterns in your thinking and feeling. We give you more strategies for investigating those patterns throughout the book.

Feelings guide your behavior

Feelings also influence behavior. Many times, feelings push you toward appropriate actions. Emotions act as road signs that lead you in the right direction — well, much of the time.

For example, fear calls out for caution and alertness. When afraid, you must quickly determine whether you need to fight, flee, or freeze. That's an important survival tool. While driving, when you suddenly hear sirens behind you, your attention is alerted and you either quickly pull over to let an emergency vehicle pass, or perhaps if you've just robbed a bank, maybe you punch the gas pedal.

Anger, a response to mistreatment or threat, motivates you to take action. Hopefully the action is a productive, assertive response that helps solve a problems or protect you from a threatening situation. However, anger can also be misdirected and even dangerous.

Anxiety is an emotion that pushes you to pay attention to what lies ahead. Similar to fear, it may lead you to avoid a potentially dangerous situation. Unlike fear, anxiety sometimes motivates you to prepare to cope in advance. For example, you might fear public speaking. Anxiety gives you the incentive to practice before giving a speech. Anxiety also can lead you astray. For example, those with social anxiety may avoid socializing with others. That avoidance may contribute to feelings of loneliness and isolation.

Depression also guides your behavior. When you are depressed, you tend to withdraw, shut down, and retreat. In fact, depression usually stops goal-directed behavior, or, at the least, it certainly makes it harder to get moving. Sometimes, this withdrawal is a good coping mechanism, especially when depression is grief based. You need time when grieving to slow down and mourn. In the short run, depressed behavior may help draw on sources of empathy and support. Unfortunately, in the long run, it may serve to push others away.

And when depression is chronic, it's behavior-stopping tendencies can often lead to more problems. Those behavior-stopping feelings get in the way of productive work or daily responsibilities. Not getting things done then leads to more negative feelings. Thus, depression uninterrupted feeds on itself and deepens over time.

Interpreting Thoughts

Research shows that people with depression are tormented by a variety of negative thoughts. These thoughts intensify feelings of sadness and hopelessness. However, some depressed people declare with total conviction, "I don't have any negative thoughts in my head! I just *feel* horrible."

If you have that reaction, we believe you and know that you may not hear specific words and sentences running through your mind like many people do. However, we're referring to thoughts in a broader sense.

Consider thoughts as your *interpretations* or *perceptions* of the important events in your life. They're the way you see or look at happenings. In other words, thoughts are the *meanings* you consciously or unconsciously assign to what's going on around you.

TIP

You may not be aware of an actual dialog going on in your head when something happens to you, but humans have a way of assigning meaning to the occurrences in their lives. If you feel a sudden rush of feelings, try asking what event immediately preceded the feelings and ponder your perception or interpretation of the event.

For example, if someone says to you, "I like your outfit," you may not be aware of any particular thoughts. However, you will immediately have a feeling. It could be positive or negative or basically neutral. That feeling didn't come out of the clear blue sky.

To determine what thoughts are driving your feelings, ask yourself how you interpreted that event. Did you hear the message as a compliment about your clothes? Or did you hear the comment as sarcastic, meaning that your outfit is hopelessly out of style? Or, perhaps you heard the statement as a mere attempt at politeness. Those interpretations are your thoughts. And they'll all result in different feelings about the comment.

You may find these questions useful for helping you figure out your thoughts about events:

>> What meaning does the event have for you in your life?

>> What concerns do you have about the event?

>> What implications does it have for your future?

>> Does this change the way you see yourself?

>> Does this remind you of anything that happened to you in the past?

>> What do you think the event could mean about you?

>> Does this say anything about how others see you?

>> What passed through your mind as you noticed the event?

TIP

Sift through these questions and use them to figure out what thoughts, perceptions, and interpretations you're having in response to important situations or events. You may be surprised at how busy your brain has been working to make sense of your experiences.

Distinguishing thoughts from feelings

More than a few people have trouble discriminating between thoughts and feelings. When asked about their thoughts about an event, they may reply with a description of their feelings. And other people, when asked about their feelings, respond with a sample of thoughts. Imagine a couple of friends sitting, socially distanced, outside having coffee:

Emily and **Rich** have been close friends for years. Rich is sharing with Emily some struggles he is having with his girlfriend. He describes a fight they recently had about finances during which his girlfriend accused him of being a freeloader.

Emily exclaims, "Wow, that's really cruel. How did you feel?"

"I felt that she was being her usual bratty self and that I actually have good job possibilities coming up, and then I'll make some real money," Rich replies.

Clearly, Rich has confused his thoughts with his feelings. It may be that he doesn't really get in touch with his feelings easily. Many people are like that and struggle to accept and deal with how they feel. If you have trouble with understanding your feelings, refer to the earlier section, "Understanding Emotions."

On the other side of the coin, some people are unaware of the thoughts behind their feelings. Here's what that looks like using another conversation between friends, Aubrey and Wayne.

> **Aubrey** and **Wayne** are hiking in the foothills together. They're chatting about Wayne's recent negative work evaluation. Aubrey asks Wayne what he thinks caused the bad evaluation. Wayne replies, "Well, I felt horrible about it. I was angry at myself and my boss. I felt helpless and inadequate."

Wayne clearly feels bad, but it's hard to know what his actual thoughts are about the evaluation. For example, perhaps he's thinking that he'll lose his job. Or maybe he's being treated unfairly and will never get a promotion at this company. Or he may believe that he deserved the evaluation. In any case, without information about both thoughts and feelings, considerable, useful data is lost.

Emotions and thoughts: A two-way street

REMEMBER

Thoughts strongly influence feelings, and feelings affect thoughts. The interconnectedness of thoughts and feelings both play a role in depression.

But the story doesn't end there. Physical factors that help shape feelings also play a role in depression. Factors such as fatigue, illness, and blood chemistry can produce dismal feelings, which, in turn, sow the seeds for dark, depressing thoughts.

> For example, **Carlo** tosses and turns through a third night. He's not sure what's causing his recent bout of insomnia, but every time he thinks he's about to fall asleep, another part of his body itches, or a position becomes uncomfortable. Carlo's day begins with a long rush-hour drive; his usual calm acceptance dissipates into irritability. His fatigue compounds his growing worry. He starts to think, "What's wrong with me? I'm not going to be able to get through another day. I feel horrible. I can't focus or concentrate on work. I'm going to lose my job. What's wrong with me?"

Carlo's thoughts have spiraled out of control. Why? Too many days in a row of poor sleep shift his thoughts into negative gear. One good night of sleep just might allow Carlo to return to normal. Or not. Sometimes, a physical event can start a cascade of bad thoughts and feelings that may just stay and visit for awhile.

No one knows how to determine which of the three components (feelings, thoughts, or physical factors) kicks off depression for any particular person. But the good news is that you can interrupt the cycle of depression in various ways with treatment no matter what started the downward spiral.

The goal of most psychotherapies for depression is to help you be fully aware of your negative thinking when it occurs and then actively rethink those thoughts in more realistic terms. After you've done so, your depression is quite likely to lift.

Exploring Emotion-Driven Behavior

As we discuss earlier in the section "Feelings guide your behavior," emotions push you to act or not act in a certain way. For example, fear and anxiety are likely to activate a flight or fight response. Joy and happiness often activate a desire to approach an event or situation. Depression, on the other hand, usually leads to withdrawal and avoidance.

These emotionally driven action tendencies involve evolutionarily adaptive survival instincts. However, not all actions that follow emotions are adaptive. When people have chronic depressive disorders, withdrawal is not an adaptive response and actually makes depression worse.

For example, if you feel depressed and that keeps you from exercising, not doing so will have two negative consequences. First, you will have missed an opportunity to feel better after endorphins fill you with positive feelings. Second, you will likely feel guilty for not exercising. And that's not a great way to lift your mood, right?

Depressed people often want to wait until they feel better to do things like going out, exercising, completing tasks, or getting together with family and friends. However, they may end up waiting a very long time. Good feelings rarely spring from inaction. See Part 3 for information about getting moving again.

Feelings are not facts

Most people with depression have countless negative thoughts about events. Then the mind uses emotions as cues or evidence for supporting the truth of those thoughts. The temptation to view feelings as facts is called *emotional reasoning.* The emotional reasoning goes something like this:

>> I've done something wrong. I *feel* guilty, so I must have done something wrong.

>> Something is wrong with me. I *feel* ashamed, so there must be something defective about me.

>> I'm hopeless. Because I *feel* so horribly hopeless, I must truly be hopeless.

>> I can't clean the garage because I don't *feel* like cleaning the garage.

>> I can't work on my depression because I don't *feel* like working on my depression.

The problem is that feelings all too often occur in response to distorted views of events. So the very feeling that you're using as a way of proving your thought probably came about in connection with a negative or distorted thought in the first place.

REMEMBER

Feelings are *not* facts. Just because you *feel* something doesn't make it true!

Frankly, if all those suffering from depression constantly catered to the directives of their feelings, few would ever improve with therapy. If you're depressed, you most likely don't feel like devoting energy toward doing anything about your condition because you have little energy to start with. And if you listen uncritically to feelings of hopelessness, you'll likely similarly conclude that you have no reason to improve your lot.

But don't get the wrong idea. Feelings and emotions *are* important. Positive feelings give you information about what you like and don't like. Negative emotions alert you to danger and assist you in knowing that something isn't right in your life. Feelings make us human. We value and respect feelings. Much of the intent of this book is to help you find ways of feeling better.

However, we suggest that you resist using feelings as though they're facts. A common example of such flawed reasoning is to determine your personal worth based on feelings. Thus, if you *feel* awful, you conclude that you must *be* awful. Not a very useful conclusion.

TIP

Start tracking your use of emotional reasoning. Tune in when your mind tells you to avoid an undertaking merely because you don't *feel* like it. Ask yourself if you've felt that way in the past but successfully plowed through the feeling anyway. Did you end up feeling better when you pushed on, or when you gave in to the feeling?

REMEMBER

Don't conclude that we're saying negative feelings are wrong and positive feelings are correct. If that idea were so, people should consume fattening foods, certain drugs, and alcohol in copious quantities simply because they feel good! We simply mean that feelings can distort your perception of reality and yourself if you let them.

Feelings drive avoidance

Most people with depression desperately want to reduce their suffering, which manifests itself in the form of sadness, loneliness, despair, despondency, guilt, and so on. Unfortunately, depressed feelings push people to avoid doing what they need to in order to start feeling better. It takes courage and hard work to get yourself to tackle depression head on and fight it. You will need to eventually do the following:

>> Notice, identify, and label your feelings.

>> Accept your feelings.

>> Become aware of your thoughts.

>> Challenge your thoughts.

>> Become aware of your actions.

>> Engage in anti-depressant actions.

Throughout this chapter, we have focused on understanding your thoughts and feelings and how they affect each other. In upcoming chapters, we show you how thoughts can be distorted and ways to rethink them.

PINK ELEPHANTS AND NEGATIVE THOUGHTS

When you hear that negative thinking increases negative emotions, you might think of a quick solution — just stop thinking negatively. In other words, just shove any dark thoughts out of your mind the moment you detect them. You're cured! Well, not so fast.

Drs. Richard Wenzlaff and Daniel Wegner reviewed research on the topic of this technique, which is known as *thought suppression.* Years of research has demonstrated that suppressing unwanted thoughts doesn't work. Even worse, attempting to do so virtually assures that you'll end up experiencing the very thoughts you were trying to avoid in the first place, and to a greater extent than if you hadn't tried to suppress the thoughts at all. It's a bit like the old saying, "Don't think about pink elephants." Suddenly, you find yourself seeing pink elephants in your mind, whereas if no one had told you not to think about them, you probably wouldn't have done so!

You may think that psychotherapy advocates thought suppression because one of its goals is to help you think in less distorted, negative ways. But we urge you not to attempt ridding your mind of negative thinking merely by suppressing sad thoughts. Instead, figure out how to use the skills we provide you with for developing new thinking habits. It's worth the effort.

Chapter **7**

Defeating Distorted Thinking

T he mind is an extraordinary thinking machine. It conjures up fabulous stories, creative solutions, and exquisite poetry. The mind recalls the past, deciphers the present, and predicts the future. When functioning well, the mind gives you the gift of intelligent and untroubled functioning. But when the mind is clouded by depression, it takes the past and makes it full of regrets and guilt. The mind makes the present a living hell, and it predicts the future as full of gloom and unhappiness.

In this chapter, we show you how the depressed mind distorts reality — past, present, and future. We present the most common types of thought distortions. Understanding and tracking your own distortions helps you challenge them. Then we show you how people with depression tend to make their lives more difficult by being overly critical of themselves and engage in excessive self-blame. We give you a couple of tools you may want to try in order to smooth out your self-blaming, critical tendencies.

REMEMBER

Throughout this book, when we describe various tools for coping with depression, realize that the decision to actually try them out is up to you. Just reading about them may help you carry out similar tasks with a therapist at some point. The last thing you need to do is engage in self-loathing because you didn't carry out an exercise that we recommend.

Cognitive therapy, or *thought therapy,* is the most widely researched approach to the treatment of depression. Numerous studies have repeatedly confirmed that thought therapy alleviates depression and reduces recurrences of depression. The content of this chapter is largely based on the principles of cognitive therapy.

Cognitive therapy is a type of psychotherapy. All psychotherapies involve work with a therapist using psychological techniques to alleviate emotional and behavioral problems. Cognitive therapy primarily uses techniques designed to change thoughts in order to improve the way you feel. A common misperception about cognitive therapy is that feelings don't matter, but in reality, the main point of changing your thinking is to improve the way you feel.

A major idea underlying cognitive therapy is the interconnected nature of feelings (which we also refer to as emotions) and thoughts. Thoughts strongly influence feelings, and feelings alter thoughts. So thoughts and feelings both play a role in depression.

Recognizing Thought Distortions

A primary premise of cognitive therapy rests on the well established idea that certain thoughts you have in response to events, situations, or perceptions lead to depressed feelings. In this section, we show you how those depression-causing thoughts are almost always distorted. By *distorted,* we mean that these thoughts don't accurately reflect, predict, or describe events or situations. In this section, we help you analyze your thoughts for these distortions. In doing so, you can start on the road toward seeing your world in more realistic, accurate terms.

By asking you to examine your thoughts for various types of distortions, we are *not* trying to get you to *rationalize* everything bad that happens to you. The goal of cognitive therapy is to teach you how to ponder, reflect, and weigh your distorted thoughts in order to later rework them in such a way that they match reality. (See Chapter 8 for information on developing accurate, replacement thoughts.) When reality sucks, we don't want you to deny that fact. Rather, we want to help you to cope when events turn negative.

You may find it helpful to know that people with depression don't own exclusive rights to distorted thinking. Every single human on this planet has significantly distorted thoughts at times. Depression merely makes these distortions more frequent and intense. Even those people who aren't especially depressed could likely benefit from taking a look at our strategies for ironing out such distortions. And if you are depressed, discovering new ways of thinking may lead to a far more joyous existence.

REMEMBER

If you find yourself objecting to the material in this chapter because the information sounds overly simplistic or that it seemingly discounts the importance of your feelings, please read (or reread) Chapter 4, which discusses common barriers to change. In Chapter 5, we describe various myths about therapy. The depressed mind very well may resist hearing some of the information that follows. If you're depressed, take your best shot at reading this material, and take your time before you form conclusions.

In the following sections, we discuss each of these types of distortions and show you how they can shape your perceptions of reality as easily as you can mold cookie dough into shapes of people, trees, or monsters.

Meeting the reality scramblers

Reality-scrambling distortions involve twisting reality in ways that make events appear as bleak as you feel. The human mind has a rich variety of ways for distorting incoming information. And the depressed mind escalates these distortions to the point that reality morphs into a tangled mess of mangled misinformation.

In the sections that follow, we discuss each of the most common types of reality-scrambling distortions. We then show you examples of how these distortions gang up on you and work together to deepen depression. Understanding how these distortions operate can start the process of more accurate thinking.

TIP

Everyone scrambles reality from time to time. Depressed minds just use reality scramblers more often, and they more fully buy into them. In the following sections, we review common reality scramblers — the tactics that the mind has for scrambling signals from your world. Read carefully to see if your mind ever resorts to using these reality scramblers.

Although we present the reality scramblers separately, you should know that they tend to overlap. And any given event may be interpreted through the lens of multiple distortions.

Catastrophizing

Your mind uses this scrambler to magnify or *catastrophize* the importance or awfulness of unpleasant events. The small problems in your life become huge catastrophes. Here are some examples:

>> Imagine that your computer crashes and you need to reboot. You instantly have a strong fear that all of your files are lost. When you talk to the IT guy, he asks for your recovery key. You have no idea what he's talking about. You can't believe this will ever work out. You are doomed.

>> You have a slight headache and you assume that you probably have an inoperable brain tumor. You imagine a slow, lingering death.

>> Your partner is 30 minutes late from work and you assume that he is having an affair or possibly dead in the middle of some street.

People who catastrophize make mountains out of mole hills. You can see that catastrophizing can lead to upticks in both anxious and depressive thoughts.

TIP

If you engage in catastrophizing, take a few deep breaths and consider another perspective.

Filtering

The depressed mind typically searches for dismal, dark data while screening out more positive information. The not-too-surprising result? The world (or yourself) looks dreary and bleak. Here are a couple examples of mental filtering that typically accompany depression:

>> You are having a great conversation with good friends about favorite movies. Warm feelings and laughter abound. During the conversation, one of your friends says something about your lack of taste. On the way home, you focus entirely on that one comment and disregard the mostly great time you had.

>> You are a college student with a good grade point average. You get one test back with a B-minus grade. You are convinced that you are stupid and shouldn't be in college. Your job prospects now seem bleak. You have forgotten about all of your previous good grades.

TIP

As you can see, mental filtering can create a dark, negative perception when the overall reality is relatively positive. Most distortions fail to capture nuances that incorporate a mixed array of positive and negative evaluations.

Seeing in black-and-white, all-or-none terms

This reality scrambler views events and your character in absolute terms, with no shades of gray. Everything becomes all or nothing, black or white, good or bad. The following are examples of all-or-none reality scramblers:

>> I had a couple of potato chips and I'm not supposed to eat empty carbs. I'll never get my weight to where I want. I may as well give up.

>> The coach said I'm in danger of losing my starting pitcher role. I'll never get that college scholarship, and I can't afford college without it.

>> Anyone in that political party must be horrible.

>> People come in two versions, either good or bad.

The problem with such polarized thinking is that it sets you and others up for inevitable failure, disappointment, and abuse. All-or-none thinking imposes standards that no real human could reach.

TIP

Most people, events, and situations are not at the extreme but somewhere in the middle. Take some time to search for a middle ground in all of your interpretations.

Dismissing evidence

This scrambler looks at evidence that just might contradict the mind's negative thoughts and dismisses that evidence as inadmissible and/or completely irrelevant. Even when that evidence is strong and supportive, your depressed mind rejects it. Take a look at these examples:

>> Suppose you have the thought that you're a failure. Then your boss gives you a promotion for your performance. You assume that your boss just gave you the promotion because she needed to fill the empty job slot quickly, and you happened to be available. Your mind concludes that the promotion was meaningless and that your inadequacy runs deep. You dismiss any positive feedback that comes your way.

>> Let's say you win the audition for your city's symphony orchestra. You conclude that the organization is a low-paying, ill-supported group that anyone with minimal musical talent could join. You take what should be a proud moment and trash it.

The way this reality scrambler works is sort of like being accused of a crime, and the judge throws out every single piece of evidence that proves your innocence as irrelevant. We suppose you can guess the verdict. In this case, your own mind is throwing out evidence and determining the verdict.

TIP

Before you throw out evidence, consider spending some time evaluating its veracity.

Overgeneralizing

This ploy involves looking at a single, unpleasant occurrence and deciding that this event represents a general, unrelenting trend. Thus, when something bad or unfortunate happens, you assume that it will continue to happen and probably get worse. Here are a few examples:

>> You drop your fork on the floor and conclude that you are a clumsy klutz who's always dropping things.

>> You break up with your first lover and conclude that you will never find another good match.

>> You get a bad grade on a math test and conclude that you are lousy at math.

>> You get rejected by a friend and conclude that nobody likes you.

>> One person cuts you off in traffic and you declare that every driver in town is reckless.

>> Your kids leave the fridge open and you yell at them that they never close the door.

Words like *always* and *never* are tip-offs to this reality scrambler.

Mind reading

Mind reading occurs whenever you assume that you know what others are thinking without checking it out. Couples are notorious for attempting to mind read their partner's intentions. Here are some examples:

>> A wife assumes her husband doesn't love her because he seems distant.

>> Someone assumes that an unanswered email or text means the recipient is rejecting him.

>> Someone may not ask out a new acquaintance because "I just know she wouldn't go out with someone like me."

>> A grocery store clerk assumes that angry customers are mad at her rather than merely annoyed at having to wear a mask.

It's helpful to step back when you engage in mind reading. Check with the person you're trying to mind read. You just may discover you had the story all wrong.

Looking at reality scramblers in action

We've given you some tips in the preceding sections on how to decrease the impact of reality scramblers. However, the most important task in decreasing distortions in thinking is to learn how to identify these scramblers in action. You can do that by examining your thoughts for scramblers. We suggest that you jot down a list of reality scramblers in your phone, tablet, or computer. (You might put it in a reminder app.) Then, when something is upsetting to you, pull out the list and think about whether or not a reality scramble is in play. You also might want to do this work in a more formal way. If so, follow these steps:

1. Open a file or a notebook.

2. Divide it into three columns.

3. Write down the upsetting event in the left column.

4. In the middle column, record your thoughts about the event.

5. In the right column, list the reality scramblers you feel may be influencing your thoughts.

6. Reflect on whether there's a more balanced perspective that conforms better with reality.

7. Notice if that reflection helps shift your view and possibly lessens your upset.

We'll show you several examples of how this process works. Brandon's story illustrates how reality scramblers distort his thoughts and intensify his negative feelings. Then we show how Brandon and his psychologist use this information to begin the slow process of reshaping his thoughts.

> **Brandon** works as a general contractor for a large developer. He arrives home from work one day to find a note from his wife saying that she's decided to file for divorce and has taken the kids with her. The note says that she's had enough of his long work hours, and she plans to find happiness some other way than with him. Brandon is shocked and hurt. His grief fails to dissipate, and he slowly sinks into a deep depression over the following year. What began as a normal reaction to loss, morphed into a chronic sense of sadness, worthlessness, and despair. At this point, his boss strongly urges him to see a psychologist for help, out of concern for his obvious distress.
>
> Brandon's psychologist diagnoses a major depressive disorder and decides that cognitive therapy will likely help. First, as part of this therapy, the psychologist discusses the types of reality scramblers that the depressed mind usually employs. Brandon isn't sure that he distorts anything in his life, but he agrees to look into the possibility.
>
> Next, the psychologist works with Brandon to help him see that his thinking is indeed distorted by reality scramblers. Check out Table 7-1, which shows their work.

TABLE 7-1   Brandon's Reality Scrambler Tracker

Events	Thoughts (or Interpretations)	Reality Scramblers
My wife left me.	I've been a totally horrible husband. I'll never find another person to care about me and I can't survive on my own. She never really cared about me.	Catastrophizing Overgeneralizing Mind reading
A bookkeeper at the office that I like said I looked worn out.	I've had a thing for her, and now she says I look like hell. I've made a complete fool of myself. She probably thinks I'm the last man on earth she'd go out with. No one's ever going to see me as attractive.	Catastrophizing Black and white Mind reading Overgeneralizing
I bounced a check.	I'm messing everything up lately. My credit rating is going to plummet if I do things like this! I'll never get that car loan I need.	Overgeneralizing Catastrophizing Black and white
I got a very positive job evaluation.	The department head is just trying to butter me up. He wants me to work more hours, and I just can't do it. Next time, I'll probably get a terrible evaluation if I don't do everything he wants.	Dismissing evidence Mind reading

Do you see in Table 7-1 how consistently Brandon's depressed mind scrambles his thoughts or interpretations of the things that happen to him? Time and again, his mind catastrophizes about the meaning of negative events and puts them into all or none terms. Even positive events are either filtered out or dismissed. Is it any wonder that he ends up feeling fear, despair, sadness, and apprehension? The following list spells out each of Brandon's events and the reality scramblers that apply to the way he interprets those upsetting happenings.

>> **First event: Brandon's wife leaves him.** His reaction contains three types of reality scramblers. He is *catastrophizing* when he says that he can't survive on his own. After all, he'd been a content single bachelor for five years before he met his wife. He *overgeneralizes* when he claims that he was a totally horrible husband. For the first two or three years, the couple was fairly happy with each other. He was *mind reading* when he thought that she never cared for him.

>> **Second event: A bookkeeper that Brandon likes told him he looks worn out.** Again, Brandon *catastrophizes* by thinking that she was actually saying he looked like "hell." He engages in *black and white* thinking when he says that he made a complete fool of himself. He *mind reads* when he assumes that he's the last man she'd ever go out with. Finally, he *overgeneralizes* by predicting that no one will ever see him as attractive.

>> **Third event: Brandon bounces a check.** He *overgeneralizes* by claiming that he messed up everything. He *catastrophizes* when he thought that his credit rating would plummet. Finally, he thinks in *black and white* when he states that he'll never get a car loan.

>> **Fourth event: Brandon gets a positive job evaluation.** Brandon *dismisses evidence* when he thinks that the boss is just trying to entice him into working more hours. He's also *mind reading* his boss's motives.

You can probably see why Brandon feels depressed. His mind systematically makes bad things worse and good things not so good. But perhaps you're wondering, if, just possibly, Brandon's thoughts are *not* actually distorted by reality scramblers. Possible? Yes, of course. However, you can tell that reality scramblers are at work by the fact that Brandon doesn't use qualifiers, such as "possibly," "maybe," or "perhaps." And he fails to factor in other considerations, such as the likelihood of his assumptions in relation to other possible outcomes.

This is just the beginning of therapeutic change for Brandon. He needs help to see how these reality scramblers are partially responsible for his sadness. Then he can begin to reinterpret his world with more balanced thoughts.

TIP

Although these strategies are straightforward, most people with depression will benefit greatly by working with a professional therapist who can guide them through the process. If you decide to seek therapy, you can easily use these tools together.

Start tracking your feelings and see whether you can connect them to the events in your life and the interpretations you make of those events. Then subject those thoughts to scrutiny. Find out whether your mind scrambles the meanings of the various occurrences that pop up each day.

TIP

If you find it easy to spot these reality scramblers, you're one step ahead of the game. You'll probably soon start seeing doubt creep into the unquestioned truth of your depressed mind's reflexive interpretations of events. In other words, it's not a big leap to go from seeing that those interpretations might contain distortions to realizing that a less twisted view of happenings might be more valid, as well as make you feel better to boot. That's the purpose of looking for distortions in thoughts — doing so starts to shake the hold that your depressed mind has on your thinking. (We show you many other ways to actively untwist distortions in your thoughts in Chapter 8.)

Table 7-2 contains three more sample events and sample thoughts (or interpretations) and feelings about these events. It also has a space for you to think about possible reality scramblers embedded within those thoughts. See if you can figure out which scramblers apply. After you've filled in the reality scrambler column, check out the correct answers that follow.

TABLE 7-2   **Practice Finding Reality Scramblers**

Events	Thoughts (or Interpretations)	Reality Scramblers
You arrive home an hour late from work and your husband says, "Gosh honey, I was worried about you. What happened?"	He's actually being paranoid that I was out having an affair. He's always jumping on me about things. I think maybe he wants me to have an affair so that he can get out of this marriage. After all, with my depression, I haven't been such a great wife lately.	
You're a coauthor of *Depression For Dummies,* and your project editor emails you that he really likes the first submission and reminds you the next portion is due in two weeks. But you're running behind.	I'll never get this in on time. And when I don't get my part finished, my coauthor (and wife) will be really angry. And the editor is bound to lower the boom. We might even lose the contract. It won't matter that the editor liked the first part if the second portion comes in a few days late.	
You ask someone out for a date. She tells you, "Sorry, I'm busy that night. Perhaps some other time?"	Obviously, she thinks I'm a zero; she's just being polite when she says "perhaps some other time." I'm never going to find someone to go out with. What's wrong with me?	

Here are the answers to this quiz:

>> **First event, arriving late:** Enlarging, overgeneralizing, mind reading, filtering

>> **Second event, running behind on work due:** Enlarging, filtering, dismissing evidence, overgeneralizing, mind reading

>> **Third event, turned down for a date:** Enlarging, mind reading, filtering, overgeneralizing, black and white

Making Misjudgments

The depressed mind, more often than not, acquires a nasty habit of making harsh, critical judgments about almost anything you do, thus deepening depression with each fault-finding episode. We can't remember the last time we worked with a seriously depressed client who didn't resort to harsh self-judgments. Thus, the fact that guilt is an important symptom of major depression is no coincidence. Even people who have little or no depression often judge themselves more negatively than they need to, but those with depression sometimes walk around as though they have a scarlet "G" for *guilty* tattooed on their foreheads.

The "making misjudgments" type of thought distortion comes in three forms:

» Shoulds

» Unfair comparisons

» Self-labels

TIP

Like the reality scramblers earlier in this chapter, all three of these distortions occur instantly, reflexively, and without careful consideration of reality. Keep reading for detailed info on each form and how they lead to bad feelings. When you see how often you resort to using "shoulds," "unfair comparisons," and "self-labels," you're likely to use them less often and feel better as a result.

Shoulding on yourself

Psychologist Dr. Albert Ellis (1913–2007) deserves the credit for the phrase "shoulding on yourself." We're amazed at the extent to which people use the word to pummel themselves for the slightest misdeed. You've probably heard people say the following:

» I *should* have known better.

» I *should* be more careful.

» I *shouldn't* even have thoughts like that!

» I *shouldn't* have eaten that cake!

If you think that people don't use this word a great deal, start listening to what people say. Tune in and notice whenever you hear the word *should*. Some folks use it so often you'd think someone had offered them a dollar for every time they used the word. The depressed mind not only uses the word *should* frequently, but it also takes it quite seriously.

REMEMBER

But what's so bad about *should?* Nothing much, if you only mean it in the sense of conveying an expectation of what's to come, such as, "The package should arrive today." But when used to judge yourself or your behavior, the word can add a mound of unnecessary judgment and harshness to your self-evaluations.

Ah, but some folks think that using "shoulds" as a way to motivate themselves to do better is a good idea. The only problem with that approach is that motivation based on guilt doesn't work very well. For example, imagine two types of teachers — R.F. (for rewarding, yet firm) and G.I. (for guilt inducing). R.F. treats his kids kindly and with warmth, but responds with firm guidance when they steer off course. G.I. judges her students harshly, tells them they shouldn't be so lazy when they aren't working hard enough, and humiliates them with dunce caps when they perform poorly.

Which teacher would you prefer? Which one would make you feel more motivated to do good work? Psychologists know, in general, that kind reinforcement, offset with firm limits as needed, works better than guilt induced by *should* statements. But which approach do you take for yourself? All too many people judge themselves with contemptuous, critical evaluations for even the slightest misdeed.

TIP

Start tracking your "shoulds" today. See if you can substitute terms such as "I'd rather," "I want to," "it would be better if," and "I'd like to." See the following examples for ideas:

> **Should statement:** I *should* have done a better job on that project.
>
> **Alternative statement:** I *would like to have done a* better job on that project.
>
> **Should statement:** I *shouldn't* have eaten that doughnut.
>
> **Alternative statement:** I *wish* I hadn't eaten that doughnut; I'll try to make up for it in other ways later.
>
> **Should statement:** I *should* never lose my temper.
>
> **Alternative statement:** I *would like to have better control of my temper;* I'll try to work on that by learning some methods of self-control.
>
> **Should statement:** I *should* exercise every day.
>
> **Alternative statement:** I *would* like to exercise every day, but with my busy schedule, it is not possible. I do the best I can.

TIP

Another approach to "shoulds" is to ask yourself where you've seen it written that you *should* do this or that. Is the rule you've made for yourself with your personal should statements chiseled in granite somewhere? If not, you may want to rewrite the rule. Finally, ask yourself if "shoulding on yourself" helps you or just makes you feel bad. Keep in mind, as we note earlier in this section, that guilt and shame do little to motivate positive behavior, especially when used to excess.

By the way, if you're an astute reader, you're bound to catch us using the word *should* from time to time in this book. Although we usually try to avoid "shoulds," the word is so engrained in everyone's psyche that we, too, slip once in a while. Of course we know we *shouldn't,* but we suppose we're human just like everyone else.

Critically comparing

If you really want to make yourself depressed, or deepen your depression, comparing yourself in unfair ways to others will do the trick about as easily as anything we can think of. Many people make these comparisons with frightening frequency and without forethought. And their feelings of personal worth slowly disintegrate with each putdown of the self that occurs every time they contrast themselves negatively with someone else. Do any of the following comparisons sound familiar to you?

>> You have a friend who has far more successes than you do. Therefore, you conclude that you've failed.

>> You're a student, and you receive an A- grade on an exam, but you denigrate your performance because a few others did even better.

>> You don't get as many dates as a few of your friends, so you conclude that you're undesirable.

>> You're a teenager who isn't as popular as some kids, so you assume that you're a total reject.

>> You're a pretty successful writer of self-help books, but a friend of yours writes a *New York Times* best-selling book, so you conclude that your writing sucks.

>> You're overweight, and you have a friend who is as skinny as a rail, so you conclude that you're a fat pig with no self-control.

>> Your neighbor buys a new luxury, electric car, which you can't afford, so you think of yourself as inadequate as well as deprived.

This list contains some really great ways to pound yourself into the ground! But you may wonder how such comparisons distort reality. After all, in each case, one or more people stand higher on the totem pole than you do for a given success or self-quality. But the distortion doesn't lie in seeing others who do better than you do. That fact is true and alright as far as it goes. The problem comes about in the self-destructive conclusion that if you don't equal or surpass others, you amount to nothing. The issue is similar to all-or-none, black-and-white thinking we discuss earlier in this chapter in the "Meeting the reality scramblers" section.

Further distortion occurs in the fact that these comparisons focus on a single factor that the other person has, which you don't have. The comparison zeroes in on one isolated issue and ignores the bigger picture. For example:

>> The highly successful friend also happens to overwork himself to the point that he feels miserable.

>> Your skinny friend happens to spend money like water and is saving nothing for retirement.

>> The neighbor with the new, expensive car happens to have $45,000 in credit card debt.

If you focus on a single end result, you can always find someone you know who either is or could be better you. For example, we have no doubt that neither of us has a sole quality, trait, success, or achievement that someone else couldn't best us on. Whether we concern ourselves with our intelligence, personality, writing, appearance, income, or accomplishments, certainly we'd have no trouble finding others in the world who rate higher. If we compared ourselves on each isolated quality, we could quickly dig ourselves into a black hole by summing up these comparisons as personal failures.

TIP

When you find yourself making comparisons to others, try thinking in the following ways:

>> Realize that focusing on single issues where others do better is a waste of time and only saps your feelings of worthwhileness. Instead, learn to appreciate both your strengths and weaknesses as a totality.

>> Don't just compare yourself to the top. Look at the whole picture. How do you stack up against the middle, or even the bottom?

>> Allow yourself to accept average, normal, and even less-than-average qualities into your self-perceptions. All humans have a few or more qualities that lie in that range, and we assume that you're human.

Labeling libelously

The final distorted method for making misjudgments involves finding a particularly obnoxious label to apply to yourself, such as *disgusting, pathetic, idiot, pig, bungler, clod, misfit, freak, oaf, nerd,* and so on. And don't make the mistake of thinking these labels have no consequence. The old adage your mother may have told you, "Sticks and stones may break my bones, but words can never hurt me," sounds great. But it isn't true. People use words to hurt themselves (as well as others) all the time.

What do you say to yourself when you stumble, trip, or drop something? Do you call yourself a total klutz or a clumsy oaf? Labels like *klutz* and *clumsy oaf* erode your sense of self-worth. And low self-worth is a symptom of depression. In the following example, Aaron uses lots of negative self-labels and feels rather rotten as a result.

> **Aaron** works as a DJ at a popular radio station. People know him all over town because, as the station's marquee DJ, billboards exhibit his face everywhere. But Aaron doesn't feel particularly notable, special, or accomplished. He's a lifelong perfectionist who berates himself for every mistake. After a single mispronunciation, he calls himself a jerk. If he inadvertently says something that a few listeners take offense to, he thinks he's an idiot.
>
> Labels like *freak, monster, a nobody,* and *fool* regularly ramble through his mind. His self-worth erodes to the point that he believes his audience is only temporarily fooled; someday soon, they'll all turn away from him. Thus, he turns down a high-paying job in a larger city because he knows that the more sophisticated listeners in that city will see right through him and understand what an imposter he really is.

TIP

If you're a bit like Aaron, start tracking your self-labels. See how often you apply them to yourself in response to mistakes, failures, and quirks. We call this tool the Label Replacement Strategy.

1. Grab a notebook or open up a note on your phone or computer.

2. Divide the document into three columns.

3. Write down the event in the left column.

4. In the middle column, state the label you attach to yourself.

5. Then in the right column, try reworking your labels with alternative, less extreme phrases.

TIP

Whether you do this on paper, in your device, or in your imagination, this strategy can help change a troublesome habit. By doing this activity, you can start to view yourself more realistically and stop the pain brought on by negative self-labels. See Table 7-3 for examples of replacing your labels.

TIP

Self-labels may run through your mind so often that you can't possibly catch them all. If so, don't worry. Just write down the ones that particularly grab your attention and see if you can replace them with other kinds of thoughts. If you find this exercise difficult, you may want to read Chapter 8 and return to it afterward.

TABLE 7-3   **Label Replacement Strategy**

Event	Label	Label Replacement Thought
You gained a few pounds.	I'm a *pig!*	Okay, I gained a few pounds. I'll try to work on that.
You wrecked the car.	I'm a *pathetic loser.*	Well, I didn't like wrecking the car, and it was my fault. Guess I'll have to try to be more careful. Statistics say this happens to most people at one time or another in their lives.
You didn't get the hoped for promotion.	I'm a complete *failure.*	Although I didn't get the promotion, I've had plenty of successes. I have to learn to take the bad with the good.
You get turned down for a date.	I'm a *nerdy freak.*	One person turned me down. How does this make me a freak? If I'm going to succeed at dating, turndowns will happen.

Assigning blame to the wrong source

Another type of thought distortion involves blaming the wrong source(s) for your problems. This distortion can take one of two forms:

>> Most often, people with depression *personalize* problems and blame themselves entirely for their current plight.

>> Alternatively, some people place blame for all their problems on others, thereby disowning any responsibility for making changes in their lives.

TIP

Neither of the these strategies is productive. As an alternative, try combing through all the possible causes of your particular problem at hand and allocating responsibility in a reasonable, fair manner. Generally speaking, you can only work on the portion of your problem that you own — the part that you actually are responsible for.

Rachael complained to her psychologist that her son was having major problems with his behavior at school. Rachael's conclusion? She was a *bad mother,* period. In addition to using a global self-label, Rachael was personalizing the entire problem as totally resulting from her poor parenting.

So her psychologist asked Rachael to list all the possible causes for her son's misbehavior. With some thought, she realized that Logan's father had a lot to do with how he's behaving, that he spent hours and hours playing games, and that he was hanging around with a rough bunch of kids at school.

Then her psychologist asked her to consider what overall proportion of the problem she may have caused and due to what specific things she'd done in raising Logan. Finally, he asked her to think about what she could do with her part of the issue.

We call this the Responsibility Reallocation and Action Strategy. This strategy helps you work through unwarranted guilt and blame. When you have an issue that you feel overwhelming guilt about and other factors are involved, ask yourself the following questions:

>> What is the situation that I feel guilty about?

>> How much am I responsible for this outcome?

>> Are there any other possible reasons for this outcome?

>> What was my role in this?

>> What are other possible factors?

>> What can I do to improve the situation now?

>> What can I do in the future?

TIP

With the Responsibility Reallocation and Action Strategy, you avoid immersing yourself in guilt and self-blame. Rather, the approach allows you to take responsibility for an appropriate portion of the problem and do what you can with it. If it involves something that's over and done with, no action is possible. But you can try to let go of the guilt because feeling guilty will lead nowhere and holds no advantages for you.

The following example shows you the answers that Rachel came up with. When she finished the exercise, she realized that there were many other factors that influenced her son. She was able to let go of some of the guilt and move on to more productive actions.

>> **What is the situation that I feel guilty about?** I feel horrible about my son Logan being in so much trouble at school. He's aggressive and talking back to his teachers.

>> **How much am I responsible for this outcome?** I'm his mother, so I feel responsible. I know I spoiled him. He got away with all sorts of misbehavior.

>> **Are there any other possible reasons for this outcome?** Well, his father was never around. When he did show up, he was pretty critical. Actually, he was always yelling at Logan. Logan was afraid of him.

>> **What was my role in this?** I couldn't get his father to back off. So I was constantly babying Logan after he got in trouble with his father. Otherwise, I was basically a good mother. Logan knows he is loved.

>> **What are other possible factors?** I guess there's a chance that Logan takes after my father. He was always in trouble at school too. There is a possibility that genetics plays a role. Also, Logan is pretty addicted to violent video games. I don't know if that is good or bad. He's hanging out with a bunch of rough kids too. Oh, and Logan has to assume some responsibility for his actions.

>> **What can I do to improve the situation now?** Obviously, I need to set clear, firm expectations for Logan. I'll work with the school psychologist and see what help she can give me. I don't want Logan to become like his father. I can also find Logan a therapist so that he can work out some issues. He's a bright boy and has so much potential.

>> **What can I do in the future?** I think I tend to blame myself for everything. When I do that, it makes me depressed and I withdraw. So instead of solving the problem, self-blame makes it worse.

When Rachel takes a look at the answers to the questions, she realizes that she is not the total reason her son is having problems. She feels ready to take action rather than wallow in self-blame.

REMEMBER

Guilt and blame are common emotions found in people who suffer from depression. They are often unwarranted. Furthermore, they tend to lead to unproductive solutions and keep people stuck. Forgiveness of the self leads to healing.

Chapter **8**

Rethinking Thoughts Lurking Behind Depression

I t is quite common for depression to emerge in response to health crises. In fact, depression is particularly likely to occur following heart attacks or strokes. Even though the depression may seem and probably is in part purely physiological, working on changing the way you interpret events is an effective way to deal with depression. The following story of George is an accurate portrayal of how depression follows a heart attack.

After six months of delightful retirement, **George's** golf handicap has decreased by three strokes. He swings his nine iron and grins as the ball flies down the fairway. He resists renting a cart; walking the course is part of his exercise routine. Today, though, he notices an uncomfortable tightness in his chest. He ignores the sensation but then begins to feel nauseous and starts to sweat. He's suddenly dizzy, and pain radiates from his chest down his right arm. He collapses on the grass.

Five weeks later, after successful bypass surgery, George sits at home depressed and hopeless. He believes that life will never be the same. He can't imagine ever being able to play golf again. His retirement will surely be one of illness, misery, and dreary boredom.

His doctor prescribes rehabilitation at the hospital's gym and predicts that George will be out playing golf in a few months. George cancels his rehabilitation appointments. He can't muster the energy to get dressed in the morning, let alone go to a gym. His dreams destroyed, George contemplates suicide.

George experienced a triggering event (his heart attack) that set off a slew of gloomy thoughts about his future health and retirement. Those thoughts led him directly into a depression. However, the good news is that his thoughts can be changed in ways that will make him feel better. He merely has to practice a series of skills we discuss later in this chapter in the section "Rethinking from start to finish."

In this chapter, we tell you how to develop a *Thought Tracker*, which helps you see relationships between your interpretations of events and your emotions. Once you have collected a series of events, feelings, and thoughts, we explain how to subject your thoughts and perceptions to scrutiny using objective evidence. You can then use this evidence to construct new "evidence-based" thoughts. Furthermore, we give you a large toolkit for repairing distorted thoughts, which will lead the way to feeling better.

Building a Thought, Feeling, and Event Tracker

The goal of cognitive therapy is to help people develop realistic thoughts. In order to do that, you must learn to pay attention to the situations, thoughts, and feelings that occur when you are feeling depressed. People with depression, as we describe in Chapter 7, often have distorted thoughts that increase negative feelings. We have a tool for you to use in order to begin the process of rethinking thoughts. It is called a Thought Tracker.

REMEMBER

Feelings are the words you use to describe your physical sensations and thoughts related to an event, situation, memory, or prediction.

TIP

Use the Thought Tracker when you experience troubling feelings. It can help you track and understand the connections between your thoughts, feelings, and the events that trigger them. In addition, the Thought Tracker can help you become more aware of the types of events that trouble you and prepare you to do battle with your problematic thoughts. Turn to a page in the notebook or open a file on your device. Divide it into three columns. Fill each column out with the following information (and check out Table 8-1 for a sample):

>> **Feelings:** Use the left column to write down bad *feelings* (not thoughts) and rate them on a 1 (very mild) to 100 (extremely severe) scale. People often notice their feelings before anything else, even though thoughts usually precede the feelings, so focus first on what you're feeling. (Besides, bad feelings are what depression is all about.) Sometimes you'll notice yourself experiencing more than one feeling. Record all the bad feelings you notice. If you are having trouble with identifying words to capture your feelings, check out Chapter 6.

>> **Events:** Use the middle column to write down the *event* that preceded or triggered the feeling. Such events are usually things that happen to a person, but sometimes, they involve a daydream or image that floats into the mind. If you notice the event before the feeling, feel free to fill out the event first. In either case, events do occur before the feelings, so if you first notice an unpleasant feeling, ask yourself what happened in the preceding moments to minutes. Only occasionally will the feeling emerge more than a half hour following the event; most times, the feeling comes on almost instantly.

TIP

When writing down the event, try to be as specific as possible: Include where you were, who was there, and what happened.

>> **Thoughts:** Use the right column to record the thoughts or interpretations you have about the event — in other words, how you see the thing that happened. These thoughts generally occur automatically without careful, conscious reflection. Be sure to take time and reflect on all possible reactions or interpretations you have.

Sometimes you'll have slightly different thoughts that relate to different feelings that all stem from the same event. Look at the thoughts you have that relate to each feeling you list under the feelings column.

For example, if you recently got promoted and your new boss asks you to rush a report to her desk, you may have feelings of both fear and despair. Fear-related thoughts may center on concerns of being reprimanded if you don't finish on time, and despair-related thoughts may focus on the belief that you're overwhelmingly inadequate for handling this new promotion.

On the other hand, perhaps you got promoted and your new boss asks you to rush a report to her desk, you may have feelings of joy and excitement about the opportunity to show your boss how capable you are. Same event, different feelings.

Here's an example of how the Thought Tracker works. **Sharif** works at a software engineering firm. He tends to be quite a perfectionist, which adds further stress to his already highly demanding job. When one of the computer programs he's working on repeatedly crashes, Sharif crashes. He can't sleep; he can't eat; and thoughts of suicide enter his mind. Sharif confides his despair to a close friend. His friend strongly urges him to see a therapist. Sharif objects at first, but his friend insists.

His therapist suggests that Sharif fill out a Thought Tracker whenever he finds himself feeling down. Take a look at Table 8-1 to see what Sharif came up with.

TABLE 8-1   **Sharif's Thought Tracker**

Feelings (0 to 100)	Events	Thoughts (or Interpretations)
Despair (80) Helplessness (95)	The computer program I'm working on crashed again.	My boss is going to figure out that I don't know what I'm doing and fire me. I'll never be able to figure this out.

You can see how Sharif's thoughts probably contribute to his bad feelings and overall depression. We suggest you fill out a Thought Tracker for a week or so. Try to capture at least one or two problematic events each day. After you've accomplished this task, you'll be ready to tackle the thoughts that lead to your depression.

Finding Adaptive Replacement Thoughts

The investigation of depressive thinking begins with tracking down thoughts, emotions, and events that relate to depression with a Thought Tracker. This tool helps you see various examples of how feelings naturally flow from your thoughts. Thoughts also stand accused of seriously distorting reality.

Now, we take the basic Thought Tracker a significant step further and demonstrate how to take your depressive thoughts to what we call *Thought Court*. The goal of Thought Court is to put your thoughts on trial and, if you find them guilty, to develop accurate, believable replacement thoughts (not overly positive spins on the events). Although Thought Court is a mildly playful term we use to describe the rethinking process, keep in mind that the strategy is both serious and powerful.

TIP

Thought Court forms the core work of cognitive therapy. Therefore, we suggest that you keep using these strategies frequently, regularly, and persistently. The good news is that you don't have to spend huge amounts of time. Generally speaking, devoting 10 to 20 minutes, 4 or 5 times per week, will provide a noticeable boost to your moods within 8 to 12 weeks. And after your moods start to lift, we suggest that you continue the work for at least another 8 weeks or so to be sure that your new ways of thinking have plenty of practice.

WARNING

As with other suggested exercises in this book, feel free to try it out. However, if you bog down or start to struggle, consider seeking help from a professional mental health therapist. Furthermore, if you have feelings of hopelessness, intense despair, or suicidal thoughts, get help immediately.

Here's a brief summary of the Thought Court process for you to review. We give you the complete rundown in the sections that follow.

1. **Use the Thought Tracker:** This part of Thought Court consists of recording all your thoughts, interpretations, or perceptions of the event that triggered your ultimate cascade of difficult feelings. You also rate the severity of the resulting feelings.

2. **Weigh the evidence:** This step involves gathering evidence that both prosecutes and defends the truthfulness of your thought. We ask you to carefully examine your thoughts and weigh the evidence to determine whether you should hold onto your thoughts or judge them guilty of distorting reality and making you unnecessarily depressed, which means they should be tossed in jail.

3. **Find replacements thoughts:** This step occurs if you find your thought guilty. You develop a reflective replacement thought that seems believable, not unrealistically positive. These thoughts often include a small portion of the original negative thought, but they incorporate credible positive information as well.

TIP

You need to develop replacement thoughts because having no perspective on or interpretation of the events in your life is impossible. In other words, the human brain is always attempting to explain what events mean.

4. **Rate the results:** Take your reflective replacement thoughts for a test drive. It's important to know if your replacement thoughts feel better than your old, depressive thoughts. Therefore, this step asks you to rate how you feel with the new thought versus the old one.

Persistence is key to successfully prosecuting negative, depressive thoughts. Practice regularly and keep at it until your feelings of depression have quelled for quite a while. Realize that improvements take time. But if things get worse instead of better, consider seeking professional help.

TIP

Try to avoid using these techniques simply "in your head." Work in the head makes a great supplement to the work you do in written form, but it's even better to also write it down on paper or a device. Writing all the elements down in a notebook or putting them into a file helps you utilize the objective part of your mind, which you need for this task. Furthermore, writing facilitates memory.

Review doesn't hurt either, and we recommend going over your thought records from time to time for additional help. In one sense, any good principle of education is a good principle for cognitive therapy, including summaries and a little repetition.

With the Thought Court process, we're not suggesting that negative thoughts and feelings have no validity whatsoever and that you should banish such thoughts and feelings from your life. Before we go any further in our discussion, we want to clear up these possible misconceptions. Consider the following points:

>> **Negative thoughts often (though not always) have a grain of truth.** We want you to appreciate any such truth. Denial isn't a useful undertaking. When things are truly bad and difficult, you're better off finding ways to cope than rationalizing and fooling yourself.

>> **Sadness isn't the same as depression.** Losses and adversities of various types will make you unhappy, and we wouldn't dream of suggesting that you shouldn't feel sad when such occurrences come to pass. The death of a loved one, loss of a job, severe illness, financial reversals, and physical disabilities all present serious challenges, emotional upheaval, and profound sadness or despair.

TIP

Typically, reactions to losses don't cause a deterioration in your basic sense of self-worth, and they do ease over time. Sometimes, it takes a very long time, but the feelings do get better eventually. See Chapter 2 for more information about the difference between grief and depression. And see Chapter 15 for ideas about working through loss or grief.

Tracking feelings and thoughts

You must find the accused party before going to trial. Recall a time when you felt strong negative feelings such as sadness, despair, guilt, or shame. What's to blame for those feelings? A Thought Tracker can tell you by uncovering the links between events, thoughts, and feelings. A Thought Tracker will show you that most of the time, your unpleasant emotions come from the thoughts or interpretations you make in response to events that have happened to you.

To understand the relationship between thoughts, feelings, and events, you need to record your thoughts along with the events that came before them and the feelings that followed. Rating the intensity of those feelings in order to know just how much trouble your thoughts are stirring up is also a good idea.

Ramon's story illustrates how to track down the thought suspects and prepare a case. We follow Ramon throughout this chapter to show you how the entire process works.

Ramon reluctantly reaches out for help after feeling seriously depressed for a month. He isn't sure how his depression started but feels its impact on his sleep, energy, interests, and concentration. He's starting to show up late for his college classes and decides to drop two of them in order to keep his head above water. At the strong urging of one of his friends, Ramon calls the student mental health center.

The counselor at the center recommends cognitive therapy because it has the longest and best established track record for treating depression. Furthermore, the approach helps prevent relapse. The counselor asks Ramon to start noticing the times when he feels especially sad, depressed, and/or upset. Then he tells him to record these feelings on a Thought Tracker that he gives to Ramon. After Ramon fills the form out completely, the therapist suggests that Ramon underline the most troubling, inflammatory thought — the one that stirs up the most difficult emotions. Table 8-2 shows one of Ramon's records.

TABLE 8-2   **Ramon's Thought Tracker**

Feelings (0 to 100)	Events	Thoughts (or Interpretations)
Shame (90) Guilt (80) Despair (85)	I failed the English midterm last week. I scored in the 38th percentile for the class as a whole. Two classmates next to me saw my grade when the instructor plopped it down on my desk in full view of the entire world.	I should never have taken this class in the first place. This F means that I'm stupid and that I'll never graduate from college. I really studied for that exam, and the best I can do is an F. Now I look like a fool to everyone in the class.

Ramon diligently records the specifics of his unpleasant event and carefully rates his feelings. He contemplates what thoughts instantly passed through his mind after receiving his exam. At first, all he comes up with for thoughts are that he shouldn't have taken the class to begin with. However, when he considers the implications for his future and what he thinks the grade means about him, he finds more information to write down under his thoughts column. Finally, he reviews his various thoughts and concludes that one of them troubles him the most by inflaming his feelings of shame, guilt, and despair. That inflaming thought is that an F on an exam means that he's stupid and will never graduate.

Checking the evidence

After you identify a particularly troubling thought, take that thought to court. In this court you play the role of defense attorney for the thought as well as the prosecutor. Your job is to prepare a case for both sides. The depressed mind usually has no difficulty coming up with evidence for the defense of the negative thought (that is, evidence in support of the thought). You're likely to have more trouble coming up with evidence for the prosecution (evidence that refutes the negative thought).

We have a list of evidence-gathering questions to help you prepare the case for prosecuting the troubling thought:

>> Do I have any experiences or evidence from my life that would contradict my thoughts in any way?

>> Have I had thoughts like these in the past that didn't pan out as true?

>> Is this event as awful as I'm letting myself believe that it is?

>> Is this negative thought illogical or distorted in any way? (See Chapter 7 for a list of common thought distortions.)

>> Am I ignoring any evidence that would dispute this thought?

>> Is my thought based on facts or reflexive, critical judgments?

TIP

Using a Thoughts on Trial form (see Table 8-3 for a sample), record the evidence both for and against your problematic thought on a page in your notebook. Divide the page into two columns: "Defense" (evidence in support of your thought) and "Prosecution" (evidence against your thought).

Now we return to Ramon to demonstrate how this process plays out. Ramon's counselor suggests that he take his inflammatory thought (that an F on a test means he's stupid) to court. To do so, he asks Ramon to play two roles — first, as the defense attorney and then as the prosecutor.

Next, the counselor gives Ramon a Thoughts on Trial form to fill out as carefully as he can. Table 8-3 shows what Ramon turns into his counselor after pondering both sides of the case.

TABLE 8-3   Ramon's Thoughts on Trial Form

Accused Thought: *This F means that I'm stupid and that I'll never graduate from college.*

Defense: Evidence in Support of Thought	Prosecution: Evidence Refuting Thought
An F is clearly considered a failing grade in college.	Well, I suppose one F doesn't have to mean that I'll fail.
If I accumulate too many F's, I will no doubt fail.	I'm sure that a few smart people have failed an exam or two.
Generally speaking, only stupid people fail.	
This class was only freshman English. If I fail early classes, I'm sure to fail later ones.	
My mother said that I obviously either didn't try or wasn't cut out for college, so that means I'm stupid.	

As you can see, the defense attorney side of Ramon's thought has the upper hand with his initial efforts. He's obviously struggling to develop a plausible case for the prosecution in order to overthrow the negative thought. Here's a dialogue between Ramon and his counselor that shows how a few of the right questions can help.

> **Therapist:** So Ramon, you failed this English midterm and concluded that you're stupid and will never graduate; is that right?
>
> **Ramon:** Well, yes. What other, how do you say it, ah, conclusion could there be?
>
> **Therapist:** Think hard on this question. Can you think of any evidence that would suggest you're actually pretty smart? Anything at all.
>
> **Ramon:** I suppose so. I did get practically all A's in my high school. But it must have been a really bad school.
>
> **Therapist:** Okay, I'll get back to the quality of your high school in a moment. But do you have any other evidence that says you might be smart?
>
> **Ramon:** I guess I did get an A in calculus, an A- in Latin American history, and an A in biology. But I know those subjects really well. They do not count for much.
>
> **Therapist:** So explain that to me. If you know a subject really well, it doesn't count? Is it possible that you're using the thought distortion known as *discarding positives*? How do you know a subject really well unless you've studied and mastered it? And can you really do that if you're stupid?

Ramon: Okay, you have a point there. Maybe I am discounting important information. But I still failed English.

Therapist: Oh yes, you did. And that reminds me, where did you go to high school?

Ramon: In Buenos Aires, why?

Therapist: How long have you spoken English?

Ramon: I took my first class two years ago, why?

Therapist: Is it possible that English would be a little more difficult for you than for most students, since you've only started learning the language in the past two years?

Ramon: I suppose, but I've always excelled at everything I do.

Therapist: And when you excel, does that mean you're doing so because you're just lucky or because you're smart?

Ramon: I suppose, sometimes, I'm smart.

Therapist: By the way, didn't you tell me that more than 40 percent of the class failed the exam? And didn't most of the students speak English as their primary language? If that's the case, is it possible that you're being a little harsh with yourself, to say the least?

Ramon: Okay, I get your point. Maybe I am, as you say it, ignoring positive information and focusing on negatives. Perhaps a little more work in English, possibly even a tutor, would help.

Armed with this nudge from his therapist, Ramon develops a list of additional evidence for the prosecution side of the case against his negative thought that an F means he's stupid and will never graduate from college. His list of evidence for prosecuting his negative thought now includes the following:

>> I did get very good grades in three other classes that most of the students found difficult.

>> I have usually succeeded in most of what I do.

>> Because I usually succeed, I probably fall apart when I don't.

>> How can I expect to excel in English when I just started learning it two years ago? I just need some extra work and help with the subject.

>> My mother criticizes me all the time; just because she thinks I'm not cut out for college doesn't mean anything. Besides, I think she may just be trying to get me to return home. I will eventually, but not now.

>> I suspect very smart people fail sometimes when they take classes that they know very little about and find challenging. I need to look at the big picture.

TIP

At first, most people find it difficult to come up with good evidence for refuting their thoughts. If that happens to you, try these tactics:

>> **Take your time.** You can go back to the form over a period of several days if you need to. The goal isn't to feel better immediately, but to discover the skill of subjecting your thoughts to careful, objective analysis. Figuring out skills takes time.

>> **Carefully review the evidence-gathering questions we list earlier in this section before the Thoughts on Trial form.** Ponder each question and push yourself to find evidence that can contradict your negative thought.

>> **Consider seeking help from a professional to get you started.** Professional assistance can help you discover that the vast majority of your negative moods are fueled by thoughts that rest on a foundation of sand.

After Ramon completely fills in his Thoughts on Trial form, with his new evidence, he's ready to make a verdict. He declares his thought, "This F means that I'm stupid and that I'll never graduate from college," guilty of fraud and deception. He now sees that the thought causes him enormous shame and pain, but with little basis for doing so.

Finding replacement thoughts

TIP

After you judge the thoughts leading to your depressed feelings guilty as charged, you need to develop an alternative perception, a *reflective replacement thought*. These thoughts are *reflective* because they require effortful consideration. And the reflective replacement won't help if it, too, is based on falsehood.

Pollyanna perspectives, overly positive spins, and simplistic dismissals of negative thoughts look very different from reasonable, reflective replacement thoughts. A *Pollyanna perspective* is a view that's overly optimistic without basis. An *overly positive spin* is a clumsy attempt to make a bad event or situation seem like a good thing (politicians are pretty good at positive spins). And *simplistic dismissals* are ineffective attempts to minimize the meaning of unpleasant events.

Returning to Ramon, and his discarded negative thoughts about his F grade, check out these examples of three *ineffective* types of replacement thoughts, followed by the later *reflective* approach:

>> **Pollyanna perspective:** So I got an F on this test; I'm sure I'll get an A next time.

>> **Overly positive spin:** One F on my transcript will show job recruiters that I'm human; it's really a good thing.

>> **Simplistic dismissal:** So what? An F is meaningless. I know I'm smart.

>> **Reflective replacement thought:** An F doesn't mean that I'm stupid; I have too much evidence to suggest otherwise. It does mean that I should take a serious look at this class and see if I need remedial work, a tutor, or whatever, in order to master this subject. I'm intelligent enough to get through this if I get the needed help.

REMEMBER

After you've taken your thoughts to court and gone through the painstaking work of finding them guilty, don't replace them with equally bogus alternatives. Rather, craft a new perspective based on reason, logic, and solid evidence. In other words, develop a perspective that's a reflective interpretation of what's occurred in your life.

Such reflective interpretations include any partial truth contained in your negative thoughts. For example, Ramon realized that an F did mean something important, just not stupidity. And these interpretations are best if they include realistic positive information. In Ramon's case, that means recognition of his intelligence.

Rating your replacement thoughts

If you find your thoughts guilty of fraudulent negativity and replace them with new evidence based on reflective replacement thoughts, you've made a great start. But the exercise is only useful if it does you some good!

TIP

We suggest that after you take your thoughts to court and replace them with alternative thoughts, you rate the outcome. How? It' simple. List the feelings you originally rated as stemming from your negative thoughts. Then re-rate those feelings to see if they change.

Ramon wrote down each of his feelings and found these results:

>> **Shame** went from **90** to **55**.

>> **Guilt** went from **80** to **40**.

>> **Despair** went from **85** to **65**.

These ratings indicate that Ramon's work on replacing his thought shifted his feelings significantly. However, the difficult feelings didn't go away entirely. And the fact is you can expect that some residual unpleasant feelings typically will remain. You'll have to practice this exercise a lot before you find them diminishing to the point that they feel almost inconsequential.

But what if the feelings remain the same or, even worse, increase? This outcome occurs occasionally, so try not to panic. Consider the following possibilities instead:

» **You've identified the wrong event.** To check out this possibility, ask yourself what else had been going on around the time you experienced the troubling feeling. Possibly, the event was actually a daydream, image, or thought that had just floated through your mind, and you failed to notice it. If you're able to capture another triggering event that seems more likely to have started the downhill slide, start over and run through the Thought Court process again.

» **You've arrested the wrong thoughts.** It could be that you've put a thought on trial that isn't as upsetting to you as some other thought about the event. For example, if you feel ashamed and inadequate after dropping a pass while playing touch football with your friends, perhaps you thought it was because you were a bit clumsy. So you take that thought about clumsiness to Thought Court and don't feel better after disputing it and developing a replacement thought.

But maybe the event involves additional, more troubling thoughts. In addition to thinking that you were clumsy, perhaps you were bothered by seeing how upset your teammates were and thinking that you horribly disappointed them by letting them down. If so, you need to take the more troubling thought through the Thought Court process. If you don't benefit from Thought Court, be sure to ask yourself if you may have additional, more troubling thoughts to arrest and put on trial.

» **You may have additional thoughts that you need to deal with.** We told you to take your very most disturbing thought to Thought Court. However, you may want to take remaining thoughts through the same process. Do so with any such thoughts if they seem to arouse a lot of unpleasant emotion.

» **You came up with an unbelievable reflective replacement thought.** Ask yourself if your replacement thought is too much like the *Pollyanna perspective*, the *overly positive spin*, or the *simplistic dismissal* we discuss in the "Finding replacement thoughts" section earlier in this chapter. Develop a reflective replacement thought that seems truly believable.

» **You have a sense that you don't actually want to change your feeling about the situation.** If this concern seems correct to you, you may want to read Chapter 4, which deals with breaking barriers to change. You may very well find certain beliefs blocking your way toward feeling better. If so, you'll most likely find it helpful to work on those beliefs first.

WARNING

If you work on the entire Thought Court process, as well as the potential change-blocking beliefs in Chapter 4, and you still struggle with feeling better after a number of weeks, please seek professional help. You should seek help sooner if you feel hopeless and helpless and don't pull out of those feelings fairly quickly. This book can still provide a useful accompaniment to therapy, but you shouldn't try to use it alone in such cases.

Rethinking from start to finish

We introduce this chapter with a story about **George** and his bypass surgery, and we didn't want to end his story on such a down note. Plus, recalling George's progress provides another example for you on how to complete the Thought Court process.

George's cardiologist recently attended a continuing education conference that featured discussions about how often depression follows heart attacks and even increases the likelihood of additional heart problems. After additional research on cognitive therapy, the cardiologist suggested to George that he see a clinical psychologist. George agrees, and after a few sessions with his psychologist, George decides to take his thoughts to court. Here's how George makes the most out of his Thought Court process.

First, George fills out a Thought Tracker form, as shown in Table 8-4.

TABLE 8-4   **George's Thought Tracker**

Feelings (0 to 100)	Events	Thoughts (or Interpretations)
Despair (85) Hopelessness (85)	Heart attack, bypass surgery, hospitalization, and the prospect of lengthy rehabilitation.	I'm old. I'll never recover from this heart attack. Rehabilitation sounds grueling. I can barely get out of bed. And I could never be happy without being able to play golf again.

George's thoughts that arouse the most despair and hopelessness include the idea that he'll never recover and that he could never be happy without playing golf again. He analyzes these thoughts with a Thoughts on Trial form, as shown in Table 8-5. To do so, he ponders the evidence-gathering questions. (See the section "Checking the evidence" earlier in this chapter for the list of questions.)

Based on George's Thoughts on Trial form, he formulates a reflective replacement thought: "The odds are pretty good that, with work, I can recover from this bypass surgery. It won't be easy, but it's better than the alternative. And if I don't recover to the extent that I hope, I can still find some interesting things to do."

TABLE 8-5   **George's Thoughts on Trial Form**

Accused Thought: *I'm old. I'll never recover from this heart attack. And I could never be happy without being able to play golf again.*

Defense: Evidence in Support of Thought	Prosecution: Evidence Refuting Thought
I've seen good friends whither and die after a heart attack.	I guess I've also seen people get a lot better after bypass surgery and live a number of good, active years.
Rehabilitation does take months, and that assumes it would work.	I have thought things looked bleak in the past, and things got better. I thought I'd never recover from the loss of my wife. It was very hard and I still miss her, but I managed to feel happy again.
I don't have the energy for rehabilitation; maybe I'll go when I feel better.	I suppose maybe I'm ignoring my doctor's prognosis; he said I should recover.
If I don't get better, I'll never play golf again.	I think maybe I'm trying to make conclusions because of how I *feel* rather than the facts.
	They say that energy only comes after you start moving and that the body deteriorates when you lay around. Maybe that's true.
	Although it's true that I'll never play golf again if I don't get better, I'll never get better if I don't get moving.
	Even if I don't play golf again, I do know some friends who seem pretty content, even though they have physical limitations.

Finally, George rates the results from his new reflective replacement thoughts by re-rating his feelings:

>> Despair was at **85;** now it's at **30.**

>> Hopelessness was at **85;** now it's at **10.**

George continues working with the Thought Court process for several months. He ultimately recovers from his surgery and plays golf again. His handicap never gets as low as it once was, but he feels good about the outcome.

Opening a Thought-Repair Toolkit

Going to court and weighing the evidence that supports and refutes your problematic thinking isn't the only method for dealing with problematic thoughts. We've designed a toolkit for detecting and ironing out any distortions and twists in these thoughts. You may want to review each one of these tools and try them out on your own thoughts.

Refer to Table 8-1, the Thought Tracker shown earlier in this chapter, and fill it out for yourself in your notebook. Underline the thought that arouses the most difficult emotions. Then run the thought through one or more of our thought repair tools in the following sections. As with Thought Court earlier in this chapter, the goal is to develop accurate, believable replacement thoughts rather than overly positive spins on events.

Giving your problem to a friend

TIP

What? Are we suggesting that you find a way to dump your problems over onto a friend? Not exactly. This thought-repair tool involves imagining that a good friend of yours ran into the identical event that you did and experienced the same exact thoughts and feelings. Giving your problem to a friend allows you to view the thoughts from a different, more objective perspective.

Thus, you literally imagine that friend sitting in a chair next to you, telling you about those negative thoughts. What would you say? Keep in mind that we're not asking you to simply make your friend feel better by lying or distorting the facts. Rather, we think that you should tell your imagined friend what you actually think makes sense. Paige's story illustrates how you can put this tool to good use.

> **Paige's** childhood consisted of a barrage of criticism from her father; that is, when he noticed her at all. Now, as an adult, she serves as an assistant director of a large social service agency. Unfortunately, she has little confidence and finds fault with anything she does. In addition, she magnifies her mistakes and sees them as larger than life. However, her boss, impressed with her report on project development, insists that she make a presentation to the executive board of the agency.
>
> Filled with fear, Paige complies with the request. She does a credible job, and several board members make positive comments. However, she forgets to pass out handouts until her talk is over, and one of the members suggests that her presentation would have made more sense with the handouts in advance. Paige feels horrible, so she fills out a Thought Tracker (see Table 8-1) and realizes that her feelings of shame and self-loathing relate to her unquestioned thoughts, which have concluded that her performance was an utter failure, and her job might be in jeopardy.
>
> Although skeptical, Paige agrees to try the tool of giving her problem to a friend. She imagines her friend Kayla sitting in an empty chair next to her. Kayla relays the information about the speech and declares that she failed abysmally and might even lose her job. After all, the person with the critical remark was her agency's chairperson of the board of directors!

Oddly, when Paige hears those thoughts from the imagined Kayla sitting in the chair, she finds different, more reflective thoughts flowing through her mind. She tells Kayla, "What? Didn't you hear the boss say that he was so impressed with your report that he wanted you to make the presentation in the first place? And why are you discounting the positive comments made by several of the influential board members? Of course, it's true that remembering the handouts in advance would've been nice. Most likely, your anxiety got in the way. But other than that, you did a great job!"

You're probably thinking that this strategy is too easy to believe. How can something this simple possibly work? The tool helps because it allows you to back away from your problem a bit and ponder the issue from another perspective. After you've done that, you may find it easier to be a little more objective. In any event, many people benefit from this strategy.

Putting time on your side

It's amazing how much anguish people can generate over the things that happen in day-to-day living. When disagreeable events slap you in your face, gaining perspective can be a challenge.

TIP

Putting time on your side is a strategy that asks you to view your problem at a distant, future point in time. You consider how important your problem and your thoughts about your problem will seem weeks, months, or even years in the future. It's amazing how many of the things people find upsetting look insignificant in the future. Jacob's story shows how he makes use of this tool.

> **Jacob** has a rather serious problem with anger. He's abrasive, curt, and hostile — more so than he even realizes. He has few friends, and his blood pressure has soared in the past year. He's depressed, and his psychologist tells him that anger contributes to his lack of friends and depression. His psychologist suggests that Jacob start using a strategy she calls putting time on your side.
>
> She says, "It's pretty simple, actually. Jacob, what I'd like you to do is notice what's going on whenever you feel angry. Then take a moment to step back and ask yourself a question. How upsetting will this situation feel and how important will it be a year from now? Rate that importance on a scale from 0 to 100, where 0 represents no consequence at all and 100 is equivalent to terrorists capturing you and telling you that they plan to slowly torture you to death over the next two weeks, and the torture has just begun."

It takes Jacob awhile to start catching his angry moments and stepping back enough to answer the question. However, as he does so, he discovers that very few of the anger-arousing moments in his life manage to rise above a level of 10 on that 100 point scale a year later. Slowly but surely, he finds his anger going down.

TIP

Putting time on your side works especially well with anger-arousing events. However, it can also put a better perspective on other happenings that arouse different feelings, such as sadness or upset. See how it works for you.

Putting thoughts to the test

Many of the thoughts that disturb you can be put to the test. In other words, you can run various experiments to see if they really hold water. We have three such experiments for you to perform.

Playing out negative predictions

The depressed mind makes lots of predictions about the future. And these predictions typically look ominous and foreboding. In part, those predictions look bleak due to various distortions discussed in Chapter 7, such as filtering out positive information and magnifying negatives. Thus, positive possibilities are excluded, and negative outcomes aren't only assumed but are also enlarged.

If you're depressed and listen to your mind's forecasts, you'll probably avoid activities and events that hold the remotest chance of unpleasant outcomes. Try to push yourself to experiment with these predictions, though. In other words:

>> Go to that party and see if you actually have a bad time like you're assuming.

>> Make yourself volunteer to give that speech and see if you survive.

>> Call your friend and see if she actually wants to have lunch with you even though you think she won't.

REMEMBER

If you plan to use this strategy, your best bet is to test out at least ten of your negative thoughts and predictions. Some of them may very well prove true. But most of the time, nearly all of them prove false. Even when they do turn out to be true, the actual experience usually doesn't feel as awful as the prediction says it will. See Chapter 13 for more information about challenging negative predictions.

Performing a survey

You can also test out thinking by actively collecting data and information. In other words, you can carry out a survey of family, friends, or colleagues. For example, perhaps you believe that most people see money and status as the measure of a person's worth, and you just had to take a job at lower pay. You could ask a group of friends (or strangers for that matter) what they think makes someone important and worthwhile in their eyes. Is it earning power, prestige, or other qualities, such as honesty, friendliness, and so on? You may be surprised at what they tell you.

Or if you have a concern specific to a particular individual, you can approach that person and check it out. Tyler uses this tool to overcome a pervasive worry that his wife is losing interest in him.

> **Tyler** notices that his wife has shown less interest in sex lately. He assumes that she no longer finds him desirable. So he withdraws from her out of fear of rejection. The more he withdraws, the more she seems to lose interest. He becomes irritable, and the relationship deteriorates further. His psychologist suggests that he ask her what's going on. He doesn't want to, but with prodding, he realizes that he has little to lose.
>
> So he asks his wife what's going on. Tyler approaches his wife and says, "Honey, I've missed you lately. It seems we both work too much. How can we find more time for us?" He's surprised to find that she misses him and has been holding the same negative assumption (that he has lost interest in her). She explains that work was really intense for a few months, and her sex drive had waned for a while. When her interest returned, he seemed to have gone away. This discussion led to an improved relationship.

REMEMBER

If you use this tool, be sure that you don't set your experiment up to fail. In other words, had Tyler approached his wife in an accusatory manner, the outcome likely wouldn't have been so positive. How do you think she would have responded if he'd said, "How come you don't ever want to have sex anymore? Don't you care about me or our marriage?" When you check something out, be sure to consider how your wording will sound.

And if you unfortunately encounter negative data when you check things out, at least you know what you're dealing with. Even if Tyler's wife said she was having an affair, he would now know what's going on and could decide what to do. We find again and again that avoidance rarely spares pain in the long run.

Honing your acting skills

A final method for putting your thoughts to the test involves acting "as if" you don't believe them. In other words, if you think that you'll be rejected every time you approach someone, play a new persona for a week or two. Imagine that you're someone who won't get rejected. Act as if you're that person and see what happens when you approach people. Don't take our word for it; try it out. Doing this exercise will increase your chances of social success because you will be putting yourself in a *position* to succeed. If things don't go well, you won't be crushed. Instead, you'll just try again with the next person. Go ahead. See for yourself.

Revisiting your all-or-none thinking

As we mention in Chapter 7, the depressed mind thinks in all-or-none, black-and-white terms all too frequently. Perhaps you've fallen prey to this kind of thinking from time to time. If so, you may think that you must achieve perfection, or else you're abysmally and totally inadequate. Similarly, you may think that you must

>> Achieve everything possible, or else you're a complete failure.

>> Live a totally moral existence, or else you're an egregious, guilty sinner, deserving of hell and damnation.

>> Always think of others, or else you're completely selfish.

We aren't suggesting that you can't have high standards for yourself. It's just that the all-or-none thinking that usually accompanies perfectionism sets you up for misery. No one is perfect.

TIP

You're likely to derive benefits from redefining and recalculating your all-or-none thinking. When you find yourself immersed in all-or-none, black-and-white thinking (and almost everyone does now and then) try the following:

1. **Carefully define what you're talking about.**

   Clearly define and elaborate on what you mean by any labels you apply to yourself, such as "failure," "loser," and so on. Without having a clear idea of what these labels mean to you, you can't perform the second step.

2. **Recalculate your new definition on a percentage or continuum basis.**

   Here's how you do the recalculation: Whenever you hear absolute terms in your mind, such as "always," "never," "failure," "loser," "horrible," and so on, try thinking in terms of a continuum, or a rating scale. In other words, recalculate and estimate a *percentage* of the time your negative thought is true.

   Thus, if you think that you're a failure, estimate what percentage of the time you've succeeded and what percentage you've failed and what failure really means to you, rather than a global label. If you think that you're a horrible person, recalculate and ask yourself what percentage of your actions are truly "horrible," as you defined the term in the first step, what percentage are "good," and what percentage are "neutral."

REMEMBER

Few things in life exist in all-or-none terms. Redefining and recalculating can help you see the shades of gray that your depressed mind may have blocked from your sight. When you define your terms and put your self-evaluations on a continuum, you're likely to find that your recalculated assessment feels a lot better — and, more importantly, better reflects reality.

> **Erin** complains to her counselor that she's an inept mother because her kids are acting up in school. The therapist asks her to explain what an inept mother is; what does such a mother do that other mothers don't? Erin replies that an inept mother is one who doesn't know anything about parenting, is mean to her kids, and neglects them. The therapist asks Erin if that definition fits her, and Erin says, "Well, not really. I guess I mean that I just don't always know how to handle them."
>
> "Okay, then instead of asking how often you're an inept mother, because that doesn't fit, let me ask you how often you don't have any idea of how to handle your kids versus how often you do know what to do?" her therapist inquires.
>
> After considerable thought, Erin concludes that she probably knows what to do with her kids about half the time. This more realistic redefinition and recalculation of her problem leads to a fruitful discussion of how Erin might discover more about parenting and increase the percentage of time she feels competent in knowing how to handle her kids. She figures that, with work, she can increase the percentage to 60 percent of the time, and further work can keep the percentage going up.

Facing the worst

Facing the worst is one thought-repair tool that's especially important. Cognitive therapy doesn't work as well when you stick your head in the sand like an ostrich. Rather, you have to think about the worst possible implications and potential outcomes of your thoughts.

Putting your worst face forward

It's surprising how often people manage to see that they could cope with their worst imagined fears, if they had to. Of course, no one would want to, but you're likely to discover that it's more possible than you think.

TIP

You can identify your worst imagined fears by asking yourself what you're most afraid of. Then, if what you fear actually happened, what would it be like for you? After you identify these scenarios, answer some fear-coping questions. These questions can help you deal with your feared worst-case scenarios. These questions include the following:

> » How likely is it that your worst feared fantasy will come true? (Consider assigning a probability from 0 to 100 percent likely.)

>> If the worst fear actually happens, what possible ways could you cope with it?

>> If the worst occurs, can you think of options or alternative plans of action?

TIP

If you get stuck when reflecting on these fear-coping questions, you may find it helpful to review other thought-repair tools, as well as the Thought Court process discussed earlier in this chapter. And if anxiety and fear complicate your depression, consider reading another book we wrote, *Anxiety For Dummies* (Wiley).

Putting the worst to work

Sometimes, what seems like "the worst" actually happens. When that occurs, it can be useful to predict the various negative outcomes and the coping possibilities. Jack's story illustrates how this process of facing the worst goes.

Jack celebrates his 45th birthday with a sense of gloom and doom. He's worked at a high-tech chip manufacturing company for the past 15 years. During those years, he's invested 90 percent of his retirement fund into his company's stock. For a while, that decision looked pretty darn good to Jack as his fund soared to heights he'd never imagined, well over $2 million.

Then the tech bubble popped, and the value of Jack's company's shares plunged so fast that he couldn't do anything to save his retirement fund from devastation. Jack naturally lamented the loss, and he fears that retirement may lie far into his future. His therapist suggests that Jack track his thoughts on a Thought Tracker, which he does (see Table 8-1). The event is the demise of his retirement fund; his feelings are despair rated as 80 and self-loathing rated as 85. Jack records his thoughts in response to the event as:

- I may not be able to retire before I'm 80 years old.

- I was stupid to invest so much money in my company.

Of course, Jack and his therapist could've worked on these initial thoughts to see if they contain distortions and to gather evidence for refuting them. And in fact, they did so by using many of the techniques illustrated in this chapter. However, Jack experienced only a minor lifting in his troubling emotions of despair and self-loathing. Therefore, his therapist asked Jack the following:

Therapist: Even though we see evidence to the contrary, let's assume that you were stupid to invest so heavily in the company and that you won't be able to retire until you're at least 80 years old. What's the worst possible meaning that these thoughts hold for you if they did happen to be true?

Jack: It would mean I'd be ridiculed.

Therapist: Okay, and let's say you receive ridicule. What about ridicule feels so awful? What would happen next if that were so?

Jack: Everyone would see me as an idiot and a fool.

Therapist: So if you truly were an idiot and a fool, what makes that feel so horrible to you? What's the worst imaginable thing that would happen if that were so?

Jack: Everyone I care about would leave me and no longer love me; I couldn't stand that.

At this point, his therapist has reached some of Jack's truly core fears — abandonment and loneliness. So Jack's thoughts hold even greater meaning for him. They mean that not only is he stupid and can't retire for a long time, but that everyone he cares about will leave him and that he couldn't stand living on his own without them. Jack's therapist poses the following questions to him in order to help him gain a better perspective. Jack's answers follow the questions.

- **How likely is my worst feared fantasy to actually come true?** Actually, as I review the evidence, it seems quite unlikely that my family would conclude that I'm an idiot and leave me. Even if they thought I did something stupid, I have lots of evidence of their absolute loyalty. So I give this scenario about a five-percent chance of happening.

- **If the worst fear actually happens, what possible ways could you cope with it?** Ugh, this would be very difficult. But I guess I would find a way to deal with the loss. People do. Perhaps I'd join a support group. I could stay in therapy longer. And I could immerse myself in some useful distractions, such as reading and exercise.

- **If the worst occurs, can you think of options or alternative plans of action?** I'd try to stay in touch with my kids, even if they despised me. I could always find a group of supportive friends. Even if my current friends think that I'm a fool, it doesn't mean other people will think similarly because they won't know about what I did with my retirement money. And I could master new job skills or find work in another tech company. Some of them are still hiring, and I'm not that old. I have time to rebuild my finances. Finally, over time, I could possibly find another wife. I'm not that bad looking after all.

REMEMBER

Cognitive therapy works best when you don't deny, rationalize, or avoid the worst thoughts in your mind. Rather, this therapy delivers maximum results when you deal with the most dreadful possibilities directly.

Chapter 9

Accepting Thoughts and Feelings

Being aware of the present moment is the goal of *mindfulness*. In a mindful state, you're aware, engaged, connected, and nonjudgmental. Mindfulness is a central aspect of Buddhist teachings, but you don't need to practice Buddhism to benefit from mindfulness.

You may be wondering what mindfulness is doing in a book about depression. Fortunately we have an answer to your question: A couple of decades of research on mindfulness and depression have shown that the practice decreases depressive symptoms, which appears to be related to mindfulness reducing ruminative thoughts. *Rumination* involves thinking the same thing over and over in an endless loop. People with depression often suffer from negative, repetitive thinking. In addition, mindfulness lessens worry, helps people change their way of handling depressive thoughts, and decreases avoidance. Furthermore, literature indicates that mindfulness helps prevent relapse of depression.

In this chapter, we try to help you become more mindful. To start you on the path toward mindfulness, we begin with a discussion about avoidance. Then we explain and describe the difference between *you* and *your mind.* Next, we show you the clutter that clogs up your mind and how to clean it out. Finally, you can discover how to apply mindfulness to your day-to-day life. Doing so can both decrease depression and help prevent depression from making an unwelcome return.

Avoiding Avoidance

When you are in emotional distress, it is only natural to want to be rid of it. The term *avoidance coping* refers to attempts to deny or minimize dealing with negative emotions or current stressful challenges. Everyone wants to avoid pain or stress. From an evolutionary standpoint, that instinct probably has some value. Avoidance coping encourages you to move away from dangerous or unknown risks. Sometimes, that makes sense, and in the short run, avoidance can be adaptive. For example, if you get a spot on your face, instead of rushing to the dermatologist, you might wait a couple of weeks and see if it goes away (unless it's very painful or it looks particularly ominous). If it does go away, the avoidance saved you a lot of time, hassle, and money. If it doesn't go away, you most likely didn't make it worse.

Sometimes, you may receive horrible news or suffer a great loss. In those cases, short-term avoidance helps you cope until you can gather your resources. For example, many people following the death of a loved one feel numb. That reaction protects them from overwhelming grief, which usually shows up shortly after the loss. The time of denial allows them to begin to process their grief.

However, there is a cost to chronic avoidance. People who use avoidance coping as a strategy over years are at greater risk for eventually developing depression. When you deny or avoid feelings about a situation, you . . .

>> Pretend that everything is okay.

>> Turn away from unpleasant painful aspects of what's going on.

>> Try to distract with drugs or alcohol.

>> Minimize the significance of the problem.

>> Attempt to not think about the problem at all.

>> Try to project the problem on someone or something else.

These attempts to avoid only delay problem solving and coping. They can interfere with taking action or getting help when needed. Problems grow under the glare of avoidance. The following sections will show you how to accept rather than avoid. Acceptance opens the gate to positive change.

Drawing the Line Between You and Your Mind

As we said before, the human mind is a *thinking machine.* Your mind continuously uses language to form judgments, evaluations, and analyses of yourself and the world. Language (like the written word) is uniquely human. If you don't think so, try sending an email to a three-toed sloth and see what kind of response you get.

REMEMBER

But human minds tend to make too many judgments and evaluations. These judgments become your sense of reality. And when the mind is depressed, these judgments can be overwhelmingly negative. Believing that you *are* the same thing as those negative evaluations and thoughts becomes too easy. So, as important as your mind is, in this section, we want you to realize that *you* are something more than your mind.

Okay, maybe we're getting a little deep here, but bear with us. Take a few moments to reminisce about yourself as a child. Choose any age you can recall. What was your life like? What did you feel? What did you do? What did you like and dislike? Where did you live?

Do you have an image of yourself as a child; are you able to see yourself? If so, you probably can't remember a lot about your thoughts back then. When people try to remember themselves as a child, they usually recall their lives. The *you* in your memory consists more of your experiences — what you did and how you felt — than the thoughts running through your mind.

Another way to see the difference between you and your mind is the following experiment: Sit still for a few moments and listen for a thought to come into your mind. Perhaps it will come instantly or it may take a little while. When your mind generates that thought, listen. *You* are the one listening. *You* aren't the same thing as your mind and your thoughts.

The *you* that isn't your mind is the part of you that observes, experiences, breathes, and lives without judgment and analysis. It's funny that the term mindfulness was coined to describe this state of awareness *without* thoughts and judgment. We think that the term *mindlessness* is far more descriptive. But alas, we succumb to convention in this chapter and stick with the term mindfulness.

Losing Your Mind

Those with depression find that their minds are filled with a pessimistic, self-defeating stew of thoughts. Those thoughts often consist of bleak assessments of the self and the world. Here are just a few examples:

>> It's payday and I don't have enough to cover the bills. I guess I'm a failure. Here I am, 35 years old, and I still don't make enough money. What's wrong with me? My life sucks.

>> Look at that gray hair. God, I look old. I'm an out-of-shape mess. People must look at me and think I'm a loser.

>> I've been stuck at home for seven months because of the pandemic. Life will never be the same. I can't stand the isolation.

>> I was a terrible wife. I regret cheating on my husband, and I'm not sure I can forgive myself. I don't deserve another chance.

>> I've been depressed for so long that I see no way out. No one can help me. And I can't help myself.

Have you ever heard thoughts like these run through your mind? The mind never stops. It produces this steady stream of evaluations and judgments throughout your waking day. And this chatter sometimes even creeps into your dreams. If you're like most folks, you've probably had at least a few dreams where you feel unprepared, embarrassed, or humiliated.

Mindfulness is about seeing the difference between you and your mind. In this section, we show you how to stop viewing thoughts as facts and start viewing them merely as mind chatter. We give you some tools to shake up your conviction that negative, self-evaluative thoughts are true. And we also show you how the mind keeps you out of the present by feeling guilty about the past or worrying about the future.

WARNING

If your thinking is particularly dark and hopeless, be sure to get professional help immediately. Mindfulness may form a part of your treatment, but you need more than self-help efforts.

Thinking about negative thoughts as facts

When we sat down to write this morning, we felt pretty good because we had what we thought was a great way to introduce a particular concept. But we soon realized that we both completely forgot what the idea was about. "That's okay," we said, "we'll just look through our notes and find it." No such luck. We then had a slew of negative thoughts:

>> How could we forget something like this?

>> We're way too disorganized.

>> How could we be so stupid as to not make a note and file the idea?

>> We're completely stuck and can't come up with another idea.

>> This is going to ruin our day.

You may guess that our moods sank like a stone dropped into a lake. But that didn't happen. Instead, we took our dogs for a walk and noticed what a wonderful day it was. We observed the unbridled joy of our dogs as they sniffed every bush, barked at the birds, and watered a few choice spots.

How did we remain in a good mood and enjoy the walk? Although it's taken us a while, we view our thoughts less seriously than we used to.

REMEMBER

Thoughts are just thoughts, not facts. By letting go and not dwelling on our negative thinking, we simply came up with another idea for presenting the issue.

All too often, the human mind responds to thoughts as though they truly reflect reality. Imagine cutting into a fresh lemon with a sharp knife. Now, pretend you are bringing the lemon to your lips and squeezing out a little juice. Are you salivating? If so, your mind is responding to these words and associated images almost as though they were actually a real lemon. Nothing wrong with that.

However, if you believe that all your negative thoughts are somehow as real and solid as this book you're holding, you're probably setting yourself up for some mental anguish. In Chapters 7 and 8, we discuss in detail how frequently thoughts contain distortions. In this chapter, we ask you to take these ideas further and to view thoughts merely as thoughts. Psychologist Steven Hayes goes so far as to call your mind's incessant stream of thoughts *mind chatter*. In the sections that follow, we have some ideas for dealing with this mind chatter in ways that can help you start taking these thoughts less seriously.

Thanking your mind!

TIP

When you hear negative, self-downing thoughts rambling through your mind, thank your mind for developing such an interesting idea! In case you're wondering, we recommend you carry out this strategy with a significant dose of sarcasm directed at your mind — remember, you aren't your mind. You can also tell your mind how creative it's being. Take a look at some responses you can make when you hear your mind chattering away:

Your mind's thought: I am such a jerk!

You: Thank you, mind, for that lovely thought!

Your mind's thought: I'll never find someone to love.

You: Excellent job, mind! Thanks!

Your mind's thought: I'm hopeless.

You: Very good. How in the world do you come up with these ideas, mind?

Your mind's thought: I can't stand this feeling!

You: Thank you, mind, for making my day that much more interesting!

Getting the idea? Try this technique each and every time you hear your negative mind chatter. You do have a choice. You can decide to take all this jabbering seriously, or you can hear your mind's drivel and dismiss it.

TIP

All minds generate a certain amount of negative chatter. You aren't unique in this respect. When you're depressed, you no doubt fall into the trap of listening to this jabbering as though it has true relevance to your worth as a human being. Understand that this chatter need not be taken seriously. Mastering this skill takes time; be patient.

Playing with your mind's thoughts

One of our favorite strategies for dealing with negative, self-downing thinking is to play with it. You can change the meaning of your thoughts and your response to them if you get playful. In the following sections, we have a number of ideas you may want to try.

Sing your thoughts

Write down all your negative thoughts for a day. Then sing those thoughts to yourself over and over again. That's right, sing them. You can use them as substitute lyrics to a popular tune or make up your own song. Somehow these negative thoughts don't have the same meaning when you sing. Or say them out loud in a highly distorted voice. We particularly like using a Donald Duck voice. Buying into negative chatter is more difficult when you hear it coming from Donald Duck!

Be sarcastic

If you have a truly trusted partner, you can do what we do with our mind chatter. We say our negative thoughts out loud and let the other one of us amplify the chatter. We speak in an obviously silly, sarcastic tone. The dialogue goes something like this:

> **Dr. Elliott:** What I wrote today felt like junk. Who will ever want to read this stuff?
>
> **Dr. Smith:** That's right! You never write anything interesting at all. You may as well quit right now!
>
> **Dr. Elliott:** You're right, I think I will quit! Perhaps I should find different work to do.
>
> **Dr. Smith:** Well, that would be a good idea, but who would ever hire you?

Obviously, this exchange is meant to be a good natured, lighthearted exercise. If you try it, and it doesn't feel that way, don't do it anymore! This technique *only* works if you and your partner fully trust each other and completely understand the nature of mind chatter as well as the value of approaching it whimsically. If you're so lucky, it can even be kind of fun.

Make a declaration

Next, consider making a demonstration for yourself about the impotence of your mind's thoughts. People so often act as though all thoughts have power and meaning, as though thoughts alone directly cause events. We have an exercise that you can use to convince yourself otherwise:

1. Declare out loud, "I can't read."

2. Say it louder, "I can't read!"

3. Now, shout, "I really can't read!"

4. One more time, "Truly, there is no way that I can read."

5. Now, realize that you read each of these statements in order to say them.

Thoughts have no power that you don't give to them.

Judge everything harshly

If you're still struggling to view your mind's stream of incessant judging thoughts as mere chatter, we have another idea for you to try. Wherever you are right now, survey your environment. If you're outside, look at the sky and the entire landscape. If inside, closely observe all the details of the room you're in. Now, evaluate every single aspect of what's around you negatively. Everything. It isn't that hard to do, is it?

The human mind is trained to evaluate everything. And it can do so negatively at the snap of a finger. But does that make the evaluation correct? Of course not! Especially when judging the self, the mind easily slips into automatic negativity.

Watch your thoughts float away

We have one more suggestion for dealing with your mind's thoughts and negative self-judgments. When you hear these thoughts, try imagining them written on a large leaf. Then see that leaf gently float down a stream. In other words, practice playing with these thoughts as something outside yourself. Observe them. Watch them float. See how they swirl and dance as they go by. Let them go. Meditate in this manner for 10 to 20 minutes. Simply sit and relax. Put each thought on a leaf and watch it float, one after another.

TIP

The bottom line: We suggest that you form a new relationship with your thoughts. Back away and just observe the thoughts (with the exception of occasional warnings of clear and present danger, which you'll want to act upon). At most, consider your thoughts as lightly held possibilities, rather than statements of fact.

Resisting what is

Everyone wants to feel good. And that's perfectly natural and human. In addition, some pop psychology books even make the claim that all you have to do is grab onto happiness and never let go. Never feel bad again!

So what does the mind do when it confronts a negative experience or thought? It resists. The mind tells you that you absolutely *must not* feel this way. Avoid, deny, and suppress all negativity! Refuse to accept what is.

TIP

Unfortunately, denying negativity causes a problem: The more you absolutely must not have or feel something, the more certainly you'll have it. Thus more often than not:

>> If you can't stand the idea of feeling anxious, you'll feel anxious.

>> If you can't tolerate any sadness, you're headed for depression.

>> The more you absolutely must not fail, the more likely you are to fail, at least in your own mind.

REMEMBER

There's nothing wrong with a few bad feelings and outcomes. It's often the struggle to suppress these feelings that intensifies and magnifies them to the point that they overwhelm. In fact, psychologists have studied what happens when people with depression attempt to suppress all negative thoughts. You guessed it; they experience more negative thoughts.

TIP

Depression is what you end up feeling when you desperately try not to feel anything unpleasant. Make a little room for bad feelings; open up a small space for them. Literally accept and invite the bad feelings to stay a while. By doing that, you take away some of their power.

Living anytime but now

Only humans have a deep appreciation of the past. Only humans can see far into the future. Sometimes that ability can be both useful and pleasant. But too often the mind keeps you waiting to live your life in the future or bogs you down in past regrets. This is unfortunate because some pretty unpleasant feelings can come from living in the past or the future. For example, dread, worry, concern, stress, anxiety, and hopelessness all bloom from focusing on thoughts about the future. On the other hand, guilt, resentment, revenge, self-hate, and sadness mushroom from dwelling on the past.

In this section, we show you how the mind messes you up with two kinds of illusions about the future; then we discuss what it does with the past to ruin your present. When you see how living in the past and the future mess you up, we hope you see the value of living in the present.

Waiting to be happy

How often have you thought that you'll be happy *when*

>> You finish writing the book you've been working on.

>> You can buy that dream home.

>> You retire.

>> You finish your degree.

>> You finally meet someone.

>> You can afford to buy that new car.

Thus, you find yourself continually engaged in a series of unsatisfying struggles to arrive at a happy spot. Perhaps you work excessive hours or choose a career that pays more, but that you find less agreeable than another lower-paying occupation. You set goals, but after you achieve them, the mind comes up with another goal promising even greater ultimate happiness. So you sacrifice again to seek this new objective. The repeated seduction of a promised future happiness manages to ruin present moment after present moment.

Projecting images of an intolerable future

The depressed mind has another trick to play on you regarding the future: The mind tells you that nothing but bleak, foreboding events lie ahead. And the mind makes you believe that these distant occurrences will prove intolerable.

> **Janet,** a PhD student in sociology, battles a low-level depression for more than a year. She's finished her coursework; only her dissertation stands in the way of completing her degree. Only? A dissertation is a very large body of work. She must exhaustively review a huge literature base. Then she must design a study, send the study for numerous reviews with her doctoral committee, obtain approval for her study proposal from the committee, conduct the study, analyze the results, and write the entire project up.
>
> Her mind focuses on horrific images of the mounds of work that lie ahead. These images cause a motivational meltdown. Janet has no idea how she'll move forward. But Janet eventually digs down deep and starts to work.
>
> When she finally completes her dissertation, Janet looks back and comes to a profound realization: She couldn't recall one single moment of working on her dissertation that actually felt horrible or insufferable. Not one. And quite a few times, the work felt surprisingly positive.

Janet's reaction is actually quite common. Like many, she predicted a horrible amount of burdensome work ahead, but found the actuality to be much less onerous and, at times, even enjoyable. People often predict negative futures that turn out either tolerable or gratifying.

Embracing victimhood from the past

We feel that understanding the origins of your negative thinking has a certain value. For example, you can appreciate that your responses to events often have more to do with events from the past than with what has just happened to you. Understanding that difference may help you to reinterpret the current reality in a more useful way.

However, don't allow your mind to become overly attached to tragedies from the past. If you do, your mind may focus on all the outrageous injustices that you encountered in your life. Soon you could find yourself turning into a victim that resents and blames others for all that has happened to you previously. In essence you could *define* yourself in terms of your past. Chapter 4 discusses the seductiveness of victim thinking as well as ways out of that mindset.

Finding guilt in the past

The mind also can lead you to judge yourself today based on your past. If you fall for this trick, you'll likely make these judgments harshly and immerse yourself in guilt and self-loathing. Do you know anyone who wouldn't love to redo many decisions and actions from the past?

TIP

Of course if you went back in time, knowing what you know today, you would do many things differently. But you didn't know then what you know now. Besides, you can't change the past. The past is useful for one thing and one thing only — as a guide for making changes. You make those changes *now* — in the present.

Our dogs don't live in the past, but they usually seem to learn from it. Eventually anyway. We came home a couple of months ago to an entire house of feathers. Feathers in the living room, feathers in the master bedroom, feathers in the bathrooms, feathers in the kitchen, feathers everywhere. A down-filled comforter no longer existed.

And our two dogs couldn't have looked guiltier if they tried. They truly appeared ashamed as we scolded them. But how long do you think it took them to recover from their transgression and guilt? About three minutes. We're pretty sure they felt bad about what they'd done. And we're equally sure they didn't spend the next few days berating themselves with self-loathing thoughts. In fact, only moments later they ran around happily as if nothing had happened.

TIP

The next time you mess up, try feeling guilty like a dog. Feel bad for a little while, and then drop the matter. Prolonged pounding on yourself will do nothing to enhance your life. It will merely ruin your present in addition to your past.

Living Mindfully

If you read the previous sections of this chapter, you'll be more prepared to live your life mindfully. Mindful living largely consists of two practices — acceptance and connecting with experience.

When life deals you a hand of cards, acceptance keeps you in the game. When you discover acceptance, you don't judge yourself as a good or bad player, you just play. And you view the dealer as neutral, neither good nor bad.

Connecting with experience also requires that you stay in the game. You don't spend time lamenting about previous hands or worrying about future games. If your hand is good, you play it out with pleasure. However, when you're dealt a poor hand, you do the best you can. You don't throw your cards down in disgust and walk away. Perhaps you may draw better cards, or not. Connecting embraces whatever deal you get.

Acquiring acceptance

Acceptance is a willingness to cope with whatever comes your way, including a certain degree of sadness. Acceptance is the opposite of rejection and resistance. In order to become accepting, you must give up judging and evaluating yourself, others, and events. That's because judgments and evaluations lead to rejection and unpleasantness.

Acceptance may be a rather strange concept for you. Your mind probably has been long trained to fight and resist anything and everything that feels unpleasant. To do the opposite seems downright illogical, self-defeating, and dangerous. Virtually unthinkable.

How could we possibly write an entire book about ridding yourself of depression and now suggest that you consider accepting depression? Do we *want* you to be depressed? Are we suggesting you *resign* yourself to depression? Quite the contrary.

Your mind may be telling you right now, "These ideas are crazy! You can't possibly accept feeling depressed! Don't listen to this garbage!" Try to hang with us a while.

TIP

Psychologists are discovering something that Buddhist monks have known for many centuries is apparently quite true: Acceptance actually provides a key toward peace and harmony. Accepting your current state of affairs may seem like the wrong thing to do, yet it has great value:

>> **Acceptance permits you to walk away from the struggle.** Imagine you're playing tug of war with your depression. You fight your depression with all your might and throw everything you have at it. Inexplicably, your depression only deepens. Yet, this tug of war is no game. Depression is like a 12-foot tall, 800-pound monster. And in-between the two of you lies a huge gaping canyon with no visible bottom. Every time you pull harder on your end of the rope, the depression monster pulls even harder. You feel yourself gradually being pulled into the hole. You feel hopeless. Then you have a novel idea. You drop your end of the rope. The monster falls on his butt. And you walk away from the struggle.

Acceptance involves walking away from the war. That's because, as we say earlier in this chapter in the "Resisting what is" section, the more you absolutely and totally must not have something like anxiety or depression, the more likely you'll end up with what you're trying to avoid.

>> **Acceptance of where you are now often helps you discover a better path.** Imagine that you're out driving in a blizzard at night. You're ten miles from home and your car slides into a snow bank. You push on the accelerator and the wheels spin. You accelerate more and they merely spin faster. You're completely and totally stuck. You fear you may die if not rescued soon. So, paralyzed with fear, you accelerate even more and the tires start to smoke.

Then you collect yourself for a few moments. You remember that the way out of such spots is not by stomping on the gas pedal. So you gently accelerate and when the wheels begin to spin, you let up. The car rocks back a little and then you apply a little pressure to the accelerator. You get into a rhythm. Slowly but surely the car makes bigger swings to and fro. Eventually you move on.

In essence, you escaped your predicament by *accepting* the idea of dealing with where you are for a little while (stuck), allowing yourself to rock backwards (not where you want to go), and only then gently moving forward a little. Working on depression is something like extricating yourself from a snow bank.

Now that you have a sense of what acceptance is about, we have more strategies in the next few sections for incorporating acceptance into your life.

Figuring out the skills of acceptance requires practice and time. *Any* gains you make can improve your life. Acceptance isn't about judging how accepting you manage to become. Accept where you are; move ahead gradually as you're able.

Accepting without judging

We suggest that you consider the value of nonjudgmental acceptance of yourself. If you want to evaluate or judge something, judge the consequences of your actions rather than your "self." By the way, this is the same advice psychologists give to parents about raising their kids. They tell parents to judge the child's behavior as bad or undesirable, but don't label the child as bad. For example, if a child pushes and taunts another child, you can tell the child that pushing and teasing is wrong, but don't tell the child that he is a bad boy.

If you don't like something you've done, appreciate the lesson you can gain by looking at the undesired consequences of your actions. Don't judge your entire self.

TIP

You probably don't judge others nearly as harshly as you do yourself. You enjoy your friends and acquaintances for who they are as a total package. Try to do the same for yourself.

Living as if no one will know

Imagine if no one would ever know about any of the important things you do in your life. No one would know about your achievements, your accomplishments, or failures. There is no one to judge you at all, not yourself or anyone else.

After you have this idea fixed in your head, ask yourself what you would do differently if no one would ever know about your successes or failures. Would you make any changes in the way you live your life? If so, you've been dancing to the tune played by the judgments of others. Try living for yourself.

Connecting with experience

As you begin to find acceptance, you'll be prepared to experience life grounded in the present. Connecting with present-moment experience is rather foreign to many people. Staying connected with now takes practice. However, even small steps in this direction can provide you with important respite and peace.

SELF-ABSORPTION

Research by psychologists has implicated the role of self-absorption in a range of emotional disorders, including depression. Researchers have found that the more one increases a focus on one's self, the more negative feelings intensify. Sometimes those with depression obsess about their thoughts and feelings in an understandable attempt to gain some kind of "insight." However, it appears that this practice may cause more harm than benefit. Furthermore, much of this self-focus involves judging and evaluating the self, often negatively. The techniques involved with both cognitive therapy discussed in Chapters 7 and 8 as well as mindfulness discussed in this chapter ultimately result in lessened self-focus. Although our exercises require you to look at aspects of yourself, the likely result at the end of the day is that you'll end up engaged in far less focus on self-evaluation.

Don't forget that few people in this world currently know how to mindfully accept what is. Today's world bombards you with countless pressures and distractions. In the face of all these distracters, give yourself time to acquire these skills. Be nonjudgmental about your attempts. Your mind will generate disrupting thoughts as inevitably as the sun rises and sets each day. You can acquire this skill more easily if you appreciate each accomplishment and accept each and every disruption.

Living like a dog

Relatively few moment-to-moment experiences feel terrible. Obviously, there are a few horrific events in life, but most of what upsets people is the small stuff. And thoughts can all too easily remove you from your actual experience and cause you to focus on *mind manufactured*, awful, horrible, or unpleasant feelings. The following example illustrates this concept.

> **Arturo** never feels as grounded and at peace as when he takes his dogs on a long jog three or four times each week. He heads out the door and in just a few minutes makes it to the West Mesa overlooking Albuquerque. You can view the entire city laid out at the footstep of a majestic mountain range. The view is stunning and you can see many miles out to the horizon.
>
> The mesa is laced with dirt roads and gullies created by occasional downpours that blow through the otherwise parched land. Rabbits routinely dart across the running path. And once in a while, you can spot a coyote in the distance. Arturo connects with the experience by noticing the rhythm of his running, the obvious joy the dogs exhibit, the quiet, and the (usually) gentle breezes.
>
> Because he runs a long way, sometimes predicting a sudden downpour is impossible. The first few times rain started to drizzle, Arturo cursed his fate and picked up the pace to return home as quickly as possible. But frequently Arturo got soaked before he arrived home, and he felt distressed at his soaked condition. After all, everyone knows it's awful to get drenched in the rain. Right?
>
> But he noticed that the dogs never seemed to mind the rain. They occasionally shook off the excess water and continued to enjoy the run as much as ever. Arturo wondered how they could continue to connect with their experience unfazed and undaunted. Then it hit him. Their minds are unfettered by thoughts of how awful it is to get soaked. They merely connect with their joyful experience, nothing else.
>
> And could he not do the same? Yes. He then realized that the sensation of the rain feels not much different from his usual morning shower. What does "getting soaked" matter? The experience of running in the beautiful setting, rain notwithstanding, felt wonderful if he let the thoughts go and simply existed.

Of course, you could wonder about lightning. Wouldn't that be dangerous and indicate a need for action? Yes, that's one way thoughts can be useful.

TIP

On the occasions that thoughts alert you to real, legitimate danger, you need to listen to them. However, all too often, thoughts send out false messages that don't involve realistic assessment of potential harm.

You can take the same approach that Arturo did with many of the activities in your life. When thoughts magnify the awfulness of what you're going through right now, try disengaging from your thoughts. Merely connect with the actual experience, not with what you're making the experience out to be in your mind.

Connecting with the present

When you find yourself dwelling on regrets from the past or worries about the future, try out the following exercise. We suggest you practice this exercise frequently — perhaps for 10 minutes per day for a couple of weeks. Over time, you'll discover that your ability to stay with the moment increases. This exercise teaches you how to observe your thoughts *mindfully*. Try not to get upset if troubling or distracting thoughts interfere with this exercise. But if those thoughts enter your mind, merely notice them without judging whether you're doing the exercise correctly.

>> Focus on each moment that comes to you.

>> Study all the sensations in your body, including touch, sights, sounds, and smell.

>> You'll probably notice thoughts coming into your mind. Notice if these concern the future or the past. If so, just notice the thoughts. Then return to your body's sensations. Focus on your breathing as it goes in your nose, into your lungs, and out again.

>> Notice the rhythm of your breathing.

>> No doubt more thoughts will enter your mind. Remember, *thoughts are just thoughts*.

>> Return to your breathing. Notice how good the air feels.

>> If you have sad or anxious feelings, notice where you feel them in your body. Does your chest feel tight or is your stomach churning? Stay with those sensations.

>> If you have thoughts about your feelings, notice how interesting it is that the mind tries to evaluate everything. Notice those thoughts and let them drift. Return to the present moment in your body.

>> If more thoughts come, notice the *you* observing those thoughts in the present moment.

>> Return to your breathing. Notice how nice and rhythmic it feels.

>> If you hear sounds, try not to judge them. For example, if you hear a loud boom box from the outside, just notice the sounds as sounds. Not good or bad. Pick out the rhythm or the notes and let yourself hear them. If the phone rings, do the same, but don't answer it right now.

>> Notice what you see at the back of your eyelids when you close your eyes. See the interesting patterns and forms that come and go.

>> Once again, notice your breathing for a while.

TIP

If you have trouble with this approach to dealing with your thoughts, you may wish to read or reread Chapters 7 and 8, which will help you appreciate how entrenched mind habits don't reflect reality. The techniques of cognitive therapy in those chapters have been shown to help people rework these thoughts in a useful way. After you've accomplished that task, the strategies in this chapter may help you further improve your relationship with your thoughts.

REMEMBER

As you start exploring the idea of viewing your thoughts as something to observe rather than statements of fact, you'll no doubt slip into old habits fairly frequently. Thus, you'll sometimes discover that you've been listening to your thoughts too seriously. At those times, be careful not to engage in negative thoughts about your negative thoughts. Realize that forming a new relationship with your thoughts takes time. The goal is a slow progression toward connecting more directly with experience rather than your thoughts.

Connecting mindfully even with the mundane

The mind has such an interesting way of turning everyday, mundane tasks into things to avoid. Perhaps you find yourself waiting in line at the local price club with 15 carts standing between you and the cashier. Do you ever hear thoughts rambling through your head such as:

>> This is terrible; I have so much to do today.

>> Why did I come here on such a crowded day, am I stupid or what?

>> I'll never get everything done today.

>> I can't stand waiting in line.

>> Why don't they have more lines?

>> This line isn't even moving.

>> I should have chosen that line; at least it's getting somewhere.

>> Oh no, the light is blinking; they have to get someone else to check a price. I'll *never* get through this line.

>> This line must have the slowest cashier in the world.

>> I hate this!

Sound familiar? Those are the sounds of a mind *resisting what is.* And what do you suppose all those thoughts do to the person hearing them? Most likely they stir up considerable tension, anxiety, and angst. And how futile, because what is, is. Simple as that.

As an alternative to resisting what is, consider *accepting what is* the next time you're somewhere or doing something that your mind tries to tell you is unacceptable. Take the often annoying task of waiting in a very long line, for example. It's a great chance to practice accepting what is:

>> Notice your breathing.

>> Feel the air go in your nostrils, down into your lungs, and out again.

>> Notice the rhythm of your breathing.

>> Notice how your feet feel in contact with the floor.

>> Notice the sounds around you. Try not to judge them. Rather, hear the loud, sharp noises, the soft sounds, the background hum, and the unexpected disruptions.

>> Notice the people around you without judgment. See what they look like. Notice what they do.

>> If thoughts start to enter your head about things you must do, notice how interesting those thoughts are and let them drift by. Then refocus on now.

>> Notice your breathing once more. Feel the air.

>> Notice any smells wafting by. Again, don't judge them as good or bad.

>> Don't suppress thoughts; just notice them as they may try to interfere with your attempt to experience and accept what is.

How many commonplace chores and tasks do you resist? Perhaps, doing the dishes, mowing the lawn, vacuuming, picking up the house, or shopping? You can probably come up with a pretty good list if you think about the things you put off.

The more you resist what is, the more you will store up negative feelings and tension.

Try approaching the tasks of life mindfully. At first, many thoughts expressing current irritation, future apprehensions, or past regrets will inevitably attempt to interrupt and disrupt your attempts to connect with what is. Slowly but surely, with practice, you'll begin to notice those interrupting thoughts as just passing thoughts. As you do, you'll find that most everyday tasks no longer elicit the same avoidance and upset in you.

Enhancing pleasure mindfully

The depressed mind manages also to rob you of small pleasures by generating thoughts about the future or the past. For example, how many times have you sat down to consume a meal and finished without even tasting your food? That happens when thoughts race through your mind. Generally, you're going over thoughts that dwell on the future or the past.

TIP

The next time you engage in what seems like ought to be a pleasurable activity (almost any activity will do), try to approach it mindfully. For example, if you sit down to eat a meal, do so with the *mindful eating* strategy as follows:

>> Notice your food sitting on your plate; observe the shapes, colors, smells, and textures.

>> Take a small bite of food and bring it to your nose.

>> Smell the food for a few moments.

>> Touch the food first with your lips and then your tongue.

>> Put the food in your mouth, but wait a moment before you chew.

>> Feel the texture of your food as it sits on your tongue.

>> Chew ever so slowly.

>> Notice how your food feels and tastes on different parts of your tongue.

>> Swallow your food and notice the taste and texture as it slides down your throat.

>> Continue consuming your meal in this manner.

Consider making a habit out of mindful eating. You're likely to experience enhanced pleasure if you do. If troubling thoughts start to interfere, deal with them in the same manner as we've suggested in several sections of this chapter — notice that these thoughts are just thoughts and return your focus to your eating when you're able to do so. You will likely experience an additional benefit by feeling more relaxed when you eat. You may even lose a little weight, because slower eating allows the brain to detect feelings of fullness.

REMEMBER

Thoughts are just thoughts.

Chapter **10**

Thinking the Worst: Suicide

O ver the last 20 years, the rates of suicide have been going up progressively. Suicides, before the viral outbreak of 2020, were at the highest levels since World War II. According to recent statistics, 1.4 million people in the United States attempted suicide, and more than 48,000 were successful in one year. Suicide is the tenth leading cause of deaths in adults and tragically the second leading cause of deaths among young people between the ages of 10 and 34.

Suicide rates have risen 30 percent in the last few decades. In women and girls, the rates have climbed by 50 percent, and in men and boys, by 21 percent. And this was before the pandemic. Since then, rates have continued to climb. Social isolation, financial stress, fear, and loss are contributing to an alarming rate of depression and suicide.

Suicide trends appear to be on the upswing since the beginning of the pandemic although it's too early to make definitive conclusions. Self-reports indicate that depression, a risk factor for suicide, has increased about four times when compared to rates in 2019. In addition, multiple indicators suggest that drug and alcohol use has also soared. Alcohol sales alone have risen by more than 25 percent. Finally, serious thoughts of suicide have been reported by over 10 percent of the population. Prior to the pandemic, such thoughts were hovering at less than 5 percent of the population.

In addition, the rate of opioid and drug use continues to rise at distressingly high rates. This increase in drug use has led to a sharp surge in drug overdoses leading to death (sometimes accidently; other times intentional). Some people with depression use drugs to self-medicate, often with deadly consequences.

Suicide is a topic all too frequently ignored or neglected. Suicide is a particularly painful subject for most people. They fear talking about suicide to depressed family or friends because they have an incorrect perception that talking about suicide may actually cause it to happen. Those who lose someone to suicide feel intense guilt, grief, and pain. They believe they should have done more to somehow prevent the tragedy and take on the blame for their loved one's death. They often experience a dark shroud of shame that follows them throughout their lives.

In this chapter, we discuss the warning signs and risk factors associated with suicide for adults as well as children and teens. We discuss ways to seek help and gain perspective. We give you information about where and how to get immediate support. Finally, we offer a bit of solace to those who have lost someone to suicide.

Warning Signs of Suicide in Adults

Mental health professionals have struggled over many years to reliably predict who might attempt or complete a suicide. Countless symptom scales, targeted lists of signs, psychological tests, and interview techniques have been developed and tested throughout the history of mental health treatment. Unfortunately, none have proven to be reliable in predicting who will or won't commit suicide. When these measures fail to predict a suicide, a tragedy occurs. When they over-predict suicide risk, they may result in needless psychiatric hospitalizations and intense emotional anxiety. Nevertheless, there are signs and risk factors that increase the likelihood of suicide, and those are considered carefully when people are assessed for suicidal potential.

We divide the following sections into two categories: symptoms and risk factors. These categories are not meant to be absolutely distinct from each other, but rather, they are generally descriptive of short-term symptoms versus longer-term risk factors. Both are generally considered when professionals assess suicide risk.

REMEMBER

Despite a lack of complete certainty, there are statistically relevant risk factors that experienced clinicians consider when assessing someone who may be suicidal. It's important to realize that although there are no absolute perfect ways to predict suicide, all people who are suffering should be evaluated. Most clinicians will err on the side of protecting the individual while respecting his or her autonomy to the greatest extent possible.

GRISLY STATS ABOUT SUICIDE AND DRUG OVERDOSES

The most common method of suicide in the United States is by firearm for both men and women. Over half of all completed suicides by men are by firearm and almost a third by suffocation (typically hanging). Finally, a small percentage of men use other methods such as drug overdoses. Women, like men, increasingly use firearms to kill themselves (about a third of all female suicides). The remaining two-thirds of completed female suicides are divided almost equally by poisoning or suffocation.

With close to 70,000 drug overdoses in the United States, drug abuse continues to be a public health emergency. With the introduction of synthetic drugs (such as fentanyl), that are much more deadly, the overdose rate will likely remain a serious problem. Drug overdoses are not counted as suicides unless there is evidence of an intent to end life (such as a statement to someone present or a suicide note). However, there are almost certainly overdoses that are misidentified as accidental and are actual suicides.

Troubling symptoms in adults

We want to emphasize, once again, that none of these symptoms in isolation indicate whether or not a person will or won't commit suicide. However, as a group, they can be considered red flags. So if someone you care about comes to you with some of these symptoms, make sure you provide ample opportunity for the one you care about to discuss these concerns. Ask if he or she is having thoughts of suicide, as it's a myth that raising the issue and asking the question raises the risk. Try to stay with the person until a professional or other source of help can be brought into the situation.

WARNING

If you personally experience thoughts, behaviors, symptoms, or chronic risk factors such as the ones we're about to list, you too should seek immediate help. They should not be ignored. Help is available. See the "Choosing Life and Getting Help" section later in this chapter.

The following list of symptoms typically raise the risk of suicide over the short term. Take these symptoms seriously and get professional help or advice for more clarification if you are concerned. Realize that even with symptoms, most people do not take their own lives; however, their symptoms certainly suggest the need for professional mental help. Suicidal people may do the following:

>> **Talk about the possibility of committing suicide.** For example, someone may indicate that she wishes she were dead. Others may openly discuss a suicidal plan. Someone else may say that the world would be a better place

without him. These cries for help represent warnings of a possible suicidal attempt.

>> **Express a current state of hopelessness.** Those with an increased risk of suicide often express a loss of hope. They feel trapped, helpless, and see no possible solution to their problems.

>> **Especially in someone with little or no history of aggressive acts, may start to demonstrate unexpected rage, anger, or desire for revenge.** Some suicides are attempts to get back at someone (usually a partner or spouse). A few suicides involve both murder and suicide.

>> **Have psychotic experiences, which involve a loss of contact with reality.** Psychotic experiences sometimes precede a suicidal attempt. People with psychosis may hear voices that tell them to end their lives. Those who suffer psychotic experiences are at greater risk for suicidal thoughts, attempts, and completions.

>> **Admit to conducting online searches for suicidal methods.** Like talking about suicide, online searching is almost always an indication of suicidal thoughts. However, some people may just be curious, so check it out by asking. Again, it's a common but erroneous myth that talking about or questioning someone about suicide will cause them to carry it out.

>> **Express symptoms of unbearable pain.** The pain is usually reported as unrelenting and excruciating. This pain could be either mental or physical. A suicidal person may see no possible end to their pain.

>> **Proclaim that they have no reason to live.** An outside observer may view this situation very differently, but suicidal people experience a profound loss of purpose and meaning in their lives.

>> **Believe that they are a great burden to others.** They see themselves as dependent, useless, and an excessive drain on those they care about.

>> **Isolate and withdraw from activities with others they care about.** They typically assume no one would want to engage with them.

>> **Experience a recent interpersonal conflict that ended badly.** The experience may include rejection, loss, or humiliation.

>> **Increase drug or alcohol use.** Over consumption of alcohol or other drugs often causes people to act impulsively. Excessive use may also exacerbate depression, agitation, and other health problems.

>> **Tell people they care about goodbye in a way laden with extra meaning suggestive of permanence.** For example, they may say, "You may not see me again for a long time" or "Hope to see you in a better place someday."

>> **Give away previously prized possessions such as valuable coin collec-tions, artwork, jewelry, or other meaningful keepsakes.** They may also talk about getting their affairs in order prior to a suicide attempt.

>> **Express new, unexpected sense of resolve and surprising peacefulness.** Once a decision to commit suicide has been made, some people feel emotion-ally stable and relieved. Unfortunately, they cannot see the better alternatives that almost always exist.

Even experienced professionals find the assessment of suicidal risk to be highly stressful because no one can make such a determination definitively with 100 percent accuracy. So you shouldn't have the expectation that, as a concerned friend or family member, you can make this determination yourself.

TIP

If you have serious concerns about someone you care about, seek help. Call a sui-cide hotline such as 1-800-273-8255 or text HELLO to 741741. Calls are confiden-tial and available 24/7.

TECHNICAL
STUFF

Medical aid in dying is a practice that allows a terminally ill patient, with less than six months or less to live, to request a prescription from a doctor to end his or her life. The person making the request must be able to demonstrate mental compe-tence. This practice allows a terminally ill person to ingest the medication and die peacefully while sleeping. This is not considered a suicide or assisted suicide and is legal in a growing number of states and countries.

Risk factors in adults

Many people have one or more risk factors for suicide, but that doesn't mean they are at risk for committing suicide any time soon, if ever. Lots of people live with chronic health conditions, come from impoverished backgrounds, or have experi-enced recent losses. Yet they may pose little or no suicidal risk. However, when you combine the symptoms discussed in the previous section with various chronic risk factors, concerns heighten.

Health issues

Health affects pretty much everything: moods, finances, mobility, earning capac-ity, and social relationships, just to name a few. Poor health and certain other health conditions such as substance abuse also increase the risk of suicide. The following list details particularly common, problematic health conditions that in some cases lead vulnerable individuals to consider suicide:

>> **Mental health conditions:** Depression is always a risk factor for suicide. Surprisingly, unrelenting anxiety, especially when it involves agitation is also a risk. People with attention deficit hyperactivity disorder (ADHD) are also at a higher risk for depression and suicide. Those with ADHD tend to be impulsive, which affects their decision-making ability, occasionally leading to impulsive suicide attempts.

>> **Substance abuse disorders:** People who struggle with problematic consumption of alcohol or drugs are at an increased risk of suicide. Multiple studies have shown that, prior to a suicide attempt, use of substances is typically increased.

>> **Physical health conditions:** People with chronic pain that is not well controlled are at a slightly higher risk for suicide as are people with chronic health conditions that cause physical or emotional suffering. Chronic, intractable insomnia is also a modest risk factor for suicide. When chronic or painful physical conditions also include depression, the risk is higher.

Social problems

Problems of living also contribute to suicidal risks. Once again, we want to stress that these issues are common in almost everyone's life from time to time. However, when social issues are combined with depression and other symptoms and risk factors, the concern about suicide climbs.

>> **Isolation:** Loneliness and isolation are risk factors for depression as well as suicide. When people are isolated, they may not seek help when feeling overwhelmed. Social isolation is of particular concern during the pandemic. Large portions of the work force are working from home with little contact with co-workers or friends. Others are unemployed and unable to enjoy their usual social activities. That may be one reason that rates of depression and anxiety have soared during the pandemic. In addition, seniors are at high risk for isolation because of loss of contact with friends and family because of stay-at-home recommendations that curtail their regular activities. In addition, seniors may be isolated because of loss of mobility, inability to master technology that could help them stay connected, and chronic health issues.

>> **Loss of important relationships:** Suicide risk rises after the loss of a relationship. However, for most people, that risk is very slight. Most people navigate the painful loss with grief and sadness, but not suicidal thoughts or actions. People who have extremely conflicted divorces or separations may experience more anger and depression that increases their chances of

suicide. In addition, the loss of a partner through death increases thoughts of suicide in both men and women. Some research suggests that although bereaved women experience more thoughts of suicide following the death of a spouse, men are more likely to complete a suicide. Social support from friends and families help to protect people suffering bereavement.

» **Financial problems or poverty:** The ability to provide food and shelter to you and your family is a goal shared by people all over the world. When there are obstacles to those basic needs, extreme stress and anxiety usually proceed depression. In addition to chronic poverty, suicides increase among those who face mounting debt. This risk is higher when there is a perception that the debt will be impossible to pay off. As long as there is hope, there is some protection from despair. But financial stressors are certainly a risk for depression and ultimately suicide.

» **Chronically poor relationships:** Social support is a protective factor against suicide. When adults have disruptive, upsetting, and particularly violent relationships with people they are in contact with, this conflict increases the risk for acting out and engaging in self-harm. Some suicides occur after major fights or disagreements with family or friends. On rare occasion, suicide attempts or threats may be successful cries for help when a threat or attempt results in meaningful relationship repair, but it's not a strategy that we recommend. The threat or attempt may also be an effort at punishing or getting revenge on the perceived perpetrator. If the suicide is completed, all of the survivors are likely to suffer long-lasting psychological trauma.

» **Poor access to healthcare:** For the millions of people who lack mental healthcare either through lack of insurance or lack of access, the risk of untreated mental illness is extremely high. Many areas in the United States have a shortage of trained mental health professionals or primary care providers. For too many, the cost of treatment is prohibitive. Lives are lost due to this heartbreaking situation.

» **Stigma attached to mental healthcare and suicide:** A stigma is a stain, disgrace, or negative evaluation associated with an act or circumstance. Mental health problems are ubiquitous in today's stressful world. Despite decades of attempts to normalize mental health problems and their treatment, it remains stigmatized for much of the population, which leads to a lack of treatment seeking. There is even more stigma associated with suicide. People who attempt suicide often feel embarrassed, ashamed, and stigmatized. They are likely to feel weak and unable to cope. Those who have suicidal thoughts often have similar, hopeless feelings. Therefore, they may try to hide these feelings from others. This shame can lead them to fail to reach out for help. In fact, the stigma attached to suicide may actually increase the risk of suicide.

>> **Fatal means:** The percentage of people who die from a suicide attempt is greatly influenced by the method of the attempt. It is important for family members to restrict access to potential deadly weapons from a suicidal person. However, it is impossible to prevent all suicide attempts. Firearms are the most lethal method of suicide and are usually fatal (about 80 or 90 percent of the time). This fact is especially concerning because about half of all suicide attempts by men and a third by women are by firearms.

REMEMBER

Suicidal thoughts are common. They may occur randomly in response to a stressful event and not taken very seriously. We don't want readers to become overly frightened by occasional thoughts of hopelessness or even suicide. However, we want you to know that communication with others about your concerns is imperative. Don't feel afraid of reaching out. There is nothing to be ashamed about. Help is available for you and your loved ones. Free consultation can be obtained through suicide helplines, and they can direct you to no-cost or low-cost options for help.

History

The risk of suicide is thought to be an interaction between mental and physical health factors, genetics, current stressors, and historical factors. When considering overall risk, all of these factors should be investigated and evaluated. Careful intake interviews by a mental health professional are crucial. The following risk factors involve prior experiences that add to the probability of a suicide attempt:

>> **Family history of disruption, abuse, and neglect:** Caring, supportive families are an important part of normal, healthy child development. When a family is distant, distracted, and chaotic, children can have developmental and psychological problems. These problems increase when there is significant abuse or neglect. Children in these circumstances are more likely to develop conduct disorders, anger issues, and depression. These issues often continue in adulthood and raise the risk of later suicide.

>> **Family history of suicide:** A suicide in the family, especially a close member, increases the odd of a suicide attempt or completion, which is thought to be caused by a variety of environmental and possibly genetic factors. Studies of fraternal and identical twins support the heritability of suicide. Identical twins are more likely than fraternal twins to attempt and complete suicide. A family like that of author Ernest Hemingway is a tragic example of the influence of family struggles with depression and suicide. Seven members of Hemingway's family completed suicide.

>> **Being a veteran:** Just about 20 veterans commit suicide every day in the United States. Overall, veterans are about 1.5 times more likely to die from suicide than non-veterans. Veterans with substance abuse problems are at even greater risk. Women veterans are 2.5 times more likely to commit suicide

than women non-veterans. Sadly, veterans older than 55 make up more than half of all veteran suicides.

>> **Previous history of suicide attempts:** Studies of completed suicides indicate that many people who die by suicide have attempted suicide in the past. This subject is obviously difficult to study. Some attempts to track hospitalized patients following an initial unsuccessful attempt indicate that many people attempt suicide again, and some complete the act. Specific rates are not known. However, most researchers and mental health professionals are certain that previous attempts increase overall risk and in fact may be one of the strongest predictors of suicide.

>> **Recent psychiatric hospitalizations:** People suffering from acute depression and who are evaluated to be a danger to themselves or others are often hospitalized for stabilization. This may actually increase their likelihood of a suicide attempt following discharge. A recent review published in *Harvard Review of Psychiatry* indicated that recently discharged patients from psychiatric hospitals were 20 times more likely to attempt suicide than those in the general population. They were also more likely to attempt suicide than similarly mentally ill patients who were not hospitalized. This review of research looked at the records of 1.7 million patients. These results obviously call for much closer outreach and care for those discharged from the hospital.

Medical school syndrome is a common problem among medical students who believe that they have symptoms of whatever disease they are studying. This also happens to armchair psychologists. We want you to know that it is always a good idea to be informed about conditions that you are concerned about, such as depression or suicide. However, it is never a good idea to try to diagnose yourself, your loved one, or a friend.

Recognizing Signs in Children and Teens

Suicide is always tragic. However, when young people kill themselves by suicide, the waves of grief spread across families, neighborhoods, schools, and the larger society. Young lives cut short by suicide leave everyone wishing that they could have intervened.

What makes suicides of children and teens especially painful is that for the most part, they typically do not actually seek to end their lives. Most suicide attempts by the young are attempts to gain acceptance, responsiveness, and empathy from close relationships (like parents or friends). These attempts are desperate means for finding solutions to problems of living. Although these problems may seem minor in the eyes of the survivors, they are painfully real to those young people who are struggling.

REMEMBER

The majority of young people with suicidal thoughts don't carry out attempt or complete suicide. However, all suicidal thoughts should be considered as cries for help.

Most children and teenagers commit suicide in their homes. The warning signs are as unreliable and unpredictable as with adults. Again, all threats and attempts should be taken seriously. The vast majority of suicides among youth occur in the home.

As in the prior section on adults, we divide the following sections into two categories: symptoms and risk factors. Generally, short-term factors are current symptoms, and risk factors are longer-term considerations. When assessing for suicide risk, both symptoms and risk factors should be considered.

Symptoms in children and teens

Children learn about suicide at a very early age. Most third graders know what the word suicide means. They are also able to describe ways to carry it out. Luckily, suicide in young children is very rare below the age of 12. Just a couple of years later, in adolescence, suicide emerges as the second leading cause of death. According to data collected in the United States, almost 12 percent of all adolescents contemplate suicide. All children and teens with the following symptoms should have access to mental healthcare:

>> Threats of suicide

>> Preoccupation with death

>> Self-harm (such as cutting, burning, and hitting themselves)

>> Intense depression, withdrawal from family, friends, and interests

>> Increased substance abuse

>> Declining grades

>> Severe sleep disturbance

>> Relationship crises and breakups

>> Irrational thoughts

>> Increases in risky behaviors (such as speeding, stealing, and fighting)

>> Giving away possessions for no clear reason

>> Suicidal social contagion (When classmates and friends attempt or commit suicide, it sometimes leads other vulnerable children to mimic the behavior.)

WARNING

Children and adolescents with suicidal risks are frequently prescribed antidepressants. Although these drugs can be lifesavers for depressed kids, there are significant dangers for this usage. The FDA has issued its strongest warning, the "Black Box Warning," to antidepressants being prescribed to suicidal young people. The FDA reports that antidepressants can actually increase suicidal thinking and behavior in children, adolescents, and young adults. Those prescribed antidepressants need to be monitored very closely for that possibility.

Risk factors in children and teens

In addition to current symptoms of suicide, longer-term risk factors also increase the likelihood of suicidal ideation and/or actions. Just because a child or teen has some of these factors does not mean that they will become suicidal. However, when combined with short-term symptoms, suicide risk should be evaluated by a mental health professional.

>> **Mental illness:** Depression increases the risk for suicide in all ages. Attention deficit hyperactivity disorder (ADHD) also increases risk, especially in younger adolescents and children. Impulsive decision-making, common in kids with ADHD, may increase suicidal behavior in disturbed children.

>> **Being the victim of physical or sexual abuse:** Child abuse increases the risk of most mental illness including depression, anxiety, and conduct disorders. These raise the risk of suicide.

>> **Severe family discord:** Children do not have to be physically or sexually abused to suffer from family conflict. Being a witness to violence and conflict may have negative lasting impacts on children. Psychological abuse can at times be as damaging as other types of abuse.

>> **Recent loss:** The loss of a close family member or friend is one factor that increases the risk of suicide in children and teens. In addition, painful anniversaries of a loss can be a risk factor.

>> **Social rejection or victim of bullying:** What sometimes seems like minor teasing to adults can cause excruciating pain to children and adolescents. Research has confirmed that victimization by peers increases suicidal thoughts and acts.

>> **Chronic illness and disability, especially when accompanied by pain and rejection by peers:** Children who are plagued by illness or handicaps such as spinal bifida, intellectual disabilities, and multiple sclerosis are especially vulnerable to depression and higher rates of suicide.

>> **Trauma:** Emotionally and physically traumatic events are also known to contribute to a slight increase in suicidal risks for young people.

>> **Family history of suicide:** Sadly, children and teens who experience a family member who commits suicide are also at increased risk for themselves.

>> **LGTBQ:** Problems with adjusting to sexual identity have been found to be another predictor of suicidal ideation and commission in youth. Part of this risk is due to bullying and rejection by peers, but those factors fail to fully account for the increased risk. Many LGTBQ youth struggle with accepting who they are. A study reported in *JAMA Pediatrics* noted that sexual minority youth were more than three times as likely to attempt suicide than their heterosexual peers. Transgender youth had an even greater risk (about six times higher).

WARNING Most kids experience one or more suicidal risk factors or symptoms from time to time. Although these do not usually pose a great risk, they should be talked about and help sought if the issues seem serious. If in doubt, it's best to err on the side of safety. Talk to a professional. Raising the issue will not instill the "idea" in a youth's mind.

Choosing Life and Getting Help

If you are faced with a suicidal crisis, whether it is your own or with someone you care about, the very first priority is to seek help. Often the quickest way to find help is through a suicide hotline, an emergency room, or by dialing 911.

First and foremost, realize that it is not up to you to intervene and prevent a suicide. However, here are some tips that you can do to help while waiting for professional intervention:

>> Stay calm and talk slowly and clearly.

>> Ask questions nonjudgmentally about suicidal thoughts.

>> Ask if there is a specific plan and access to means.

>> Offer hope and help.

>> Help the person focus on reasons for living; don't impose your reasons.

>> Don't leave the person alone.

>> Listen carefully without arguing.

>> Try to find out if he or she has taken an overdose.

>> Encourage the person to call a hotline.

>> If the person seems unable to make the call, offer to do it yourself.

>> Try to contact a family member or supportive friend.

>> Call 911 if you feel the act is imminent or that you are in danger.

REMEMBER

Most problems are solvable or at the very least improvable. Suicide, however, is a permanent solution to a typically temporary problem. You can make that point with the person in crisis, but don't argue or preach.

Suicide hotlines

Suicide hotlines are one of the fastest, best ways of soliciting help. If you live in the United States, call the toll-free number 800-273-8255 (available 24/7) or 800-273-TALK. If you speak Spanish or are a veteran, the staff will connect you with trained counselors with skills designed for you. They also have resources to find those who can speak 150 different languages.

You can call the lifeline simply for emotional social support. Some people call to talk about substance abuse, illness, relationship problems, domestic abuse, depression, or sexual identity issues. You can also call for support and information on resources if you are worried about someone you know who may be suicidal.

Calls are usually answered in less than a minute and are completely confidential. Trained volunteers and crisis workers will help develop safety plans and recommend local resources. In almost all cases, situations are de-escalated. When rare situations pose particular danger, the counselor may contact local authorities for additional help.

For people who prefer texting over phone conversations, you can text 741741. Just say "help" or "hello" and your text will receive a prompt response.

You should know that other hotline numbers exist. One in particular is called the Trevor Lifeline and is designed to help young people struggling with LBGTQ related issues: 866-488-7386.

For those living outside the United States, this site lists numbers throughout the world: www.suicide.org/international-suicide-hotlines.html.

Emergency departments

Most local hospitals have emergency departments that also serve suicidal patients. They are generally staffed with trained counselors and mental health workers. In rural areas, finding trained staff may be more challenging. However, emergency departments can keep suicidal patients safe during a crisis and help with finding appropriate follow-up care in the mental health community. Wait times can vary greatly. Emergency rooms can also be somewhat chaotic and loud. Consider bringing someone to help you communicate with staff about your concerns.

TIP

Staff will ask personal questions; be prepared to answer honestly and expect a nonjudgmental response. Communications are confidential.

DEALING WITH LOSING A LOVED ONE TO SUICIDE

The loss of a close friend or loved one is devastating under any condition. However, the loss of someone through suicide poses additional challenges to the natural grieving process. It is often difficult to talk about the death of a beloved, but when asked, most are fairly comfortable about briefly describing a death from illness or accident. However, when asked about the death of someone from suicide, most survivors feel stigmatized with shame and guilt. For many, suicide represents some failure on the part of friends or family to support the victim with adequate care. That guilt is almost always misplaced. Suicide is caused by multiple factors such as depression, substance abuse, and overwhelming problems. These issues are often unrelated to those left behind.

Self-blame is strong among those who lose a child through suicide. Any loss of a child is horrible, but when it is because of a suicide, parents feel that they failed in their responsibilities to give the child support and care.

Survivors are left wondering why. Suicide is sometimes totally unexpected, and reasons are often inexplicable. Complicated grief, depression, anger, suicidal thoughts, and impairment in functioning are common reactions to suicide. It is important that people left behind from suicide seek support through grief groups, spiritual counseling, or psychotherapy. For more about grief, loss, and mourning, see Chapter 15.

No matter how familiar you are with the symptoms and risk factors, no one can reliably predict who will or won't carry out suicidal intentions. Even highly experienced professionals struggle with this issue. It's never one person's fault.

3

Taking Action Against Depression

Chapter **11**

Getting Out of Bed

Depression robs its victims of confidence, energy, motivation, and desire. If you're seriously depressed, you likely feel that you truly lack the ability to perform even the basic tasks of daily living. The very act of getting out of bed seems like an ordeal.

In this chapter, we give you the tools for constructing a plan of action that works to get you moving again. First, we tell you how depression reduces motivation. Then we provide exercises and tools for overcoming inertia. At this moment, you may think that reading a few pages can't possibly help you deal with the overwhelming inertia you feel. But bear with us; what do you truly have to lose by reading what comes next?

> The clock chimes 1, 2, 3 . . . 10 a.m. Tears stream down **Paul's** face. He's still in bed. A new rush of shame floods over him. Another wasted day at home. He feels like a lazy failure since the pandemic stay-at-home orders kept him from going to work. He lacks the motivation for even simple day-to-day Zoom meetings. Laundry is piling up and his house is a mess. The crushing sadness paralyzes him. He's a prisoner of depression, unable to escape. The pain and boredom deepen, with each day being worse than the one before. "When will it end? I'm so lonely. I don't know if I can go on," he moans.

WARNING

If you've been virtually immobile for days and have thoughts of profound hopelessness or death, you need to consult a professional. Many health professionals have online or telehealth appointments available. And if making an appointment feels too difficult, ask a friend or family member to help you, or call a crisis line, such as 800-273-8255. You can also text HELLO to 741741 for confidential, immediate support. If you feel unable to quell your suicidal thoughts, call 911.

Taking Action

Doing the dishes, taking out the garbage, paying bills, and mowing the lawn — you probably don't look forward to these mundane chores, but when you're feeling pretty good, finding the necessary motivation isn't usually a major problem. Most days you just do what you need to do without giving it a second thought.

But when depression sets in, everyday living feels like walking in thick, gooey mud. A kitchen with a few dirty dishes may as well be a mess hall of an Army battalion, paying the monthly bills feels like doing three years of taxes, and taking out the garbage seems like scaling Mount Everest.

REMEMBER

When you're battling depression, you're likely to neglect important duties. And that's perfectly understandable. However, putting off necessary chores can set off a cascade of additional negative thinking and guilt, which further saps motivation and deepens depression. That's why it's so important to take action, even if the steps are very small.

We call these thoughts *action-blocking thoughts,* and they include any negative thought concerning your inability to act or the futility of doing so. These thoughts stop you dead in your tracks, preventing you from getting started and making you feel even worse when you fail to act.

If you find yourself thinking action-blocking thoughts, take some time to subject these action blockers to scrutiny. If you carefully consider the distortions within these thoughts, you'll find that they're built on fundamentally flawed foundations. This type of examination can help you escape their tenacious grip and break the cycle of inactivity.

In the following sections, we shine some light on four common action-blocking thoughts one at a time to uncover their central flaws. Later in this chapter, we provide tools for overcoming inactivity.

I don't feel motivated to do anything

When you're feeling okay, you don't usually lack motivation — and on those occasions when you don't feel particularly motivated, sometimes the desire to get started just seems to come to you from out of the blue.

Motivation rarely shows up spontaneously in the midst of depression. You simply can't wait for motivation. *When you're depressed, actions almost always have to precede motivation.* Taking action actually creates motivation.

I'm too tired and depressed to do anything

This thought, like the previous one about motivation, essentially puts the cart before the horse. When you're fatigued, believing that rest will recharge your batteries is easy. Some people spend more and more time in bed, continuing to think that if they just get enough rest, they'll be ready to tackle jobs they put off for a long time.

But the imagined flow of vigor never comes, because excessive rest causes muscles to weaken and fatigue to deepen. Humans, unlike batteries, stay charged only by a healthy balance of activity and rest.

Activity (unless it's unusually excessive and prolonged) actually recharges the body with more drive and energy. The only cure for fatigue and inactivity is to work on revving up your engine — one small step at a time.

If I try, I'll just fail

Of course you'll fail! Everyone fails. We can't think of anyone we know who doesn't fail from time to time. So, where's the flaw in this thought? No one, not a single person, fails at everything, every time. Depression invites negative predictions and failure is one of those predictions. But by starting small and breaking tasks into doable steps, you can minimize failure.

I'm just a lazy person

Assigning yourself the *lazy* label only makes getting started more difficult. The problem with labels is that they grossly overgeneralize and assign judgments about your character. When you're depressed, you truly feel tired and have far less enthusiasm for accomplishing necessary tasks.

Psychologists know that people don't fall into depression as a result of laziness. Out of the thousands of studies we've seen on depression, we can't think of a single one that implicated laziness as a cause. Getting started on tasks when you're feeling down is hard enough; don't add the burden of guilt and shame by sticking the *lazy* label on yourself.

Putting One Foot in Front of the Other: Activity Logs

TIP

Keeping an Activity Log is one of the best first steps you can take if you have severe depression and you're neglecting important responsibilities or chores. The technique is straightforward and fairly simple. (Check out Table 11-1 for a sample Activity Log.)

1. Get out your notebook and write down each day in a column on the left side of a page. (You can also use the calendar app on your phone or device if you prefer.)

2. Schedule one neglected activity for each day. *Make it a small activity at first!* And we mean very small. Get out some glass cleaner and wipe down your bathroom mirror. Or respond to one single text message. Don't try to do too much.

3. After you complete the activity, write down how it went and how you feel about accomplishing it.

Will simply tracking your activities increase motivation? Surprisingly, yes. We find that it focuses attention and typically helps get you moving.

Karlene's story gives you an example of how to keep an Activity Log. **Karlene** is sinking into depression slowly. For the past month, she's been spending most of her weekends in bed. Her mind fills with self-loathing. Although she makes it to work most days, the minute she gets home, she collapses. Her diet now consists of cold cereal and crackers because she doesn't have the energy to prepare anything or drive to the grocery store.

Karlene's best friend, Becky, notices her deteriorating mood and weight loss. Becky is worried about Karlene, so she stops by for a visit. She asks Karlene what she's been eating, because she sees that the refrigerator is almost bare. Karlene tells her, "Mostly just dry cereal." "So what will you do when you run out of cereal?" Becky inquires. Karlene shrugs her shoulders and replies, "I guess I'll just stop eating. I don't really care."

Her friend suggests that Karlene start an Activity Log and briefly explains how to do it. Becky says, "I'm going to check back with you in a couple of days. I want to see food in the refrigerator. If you don't start moving a little and feeling better pretty soon, I'm taking you to your doctor."

Karlene reluctantly agrees, because she knows that Becky means business. At first, Karlene thinks that she can't muster the motivation to start an Activity Log. She also thinks that she's too lazy, and that if she tries, she'll probably fail. However, Karlene trusts Becky so she figures that she has little to lose by trying the exercise.

Table 11-1 shows Karlene's Activity Log for the first week. Notice that the Activity Log in Table 11-1 doesn't feature huge projects.

TABLE 11-1   Activity Log

Day	Activity	Outcome
M	Go to a fast-food place and pick up something from the drive-through window.	Well, I did it. I didn't feel like eating, but I spoiled myself with a chocolate malt. That tasted pretty good.
T	Stop at the convenience store and pick up a couple of things for dinner, and some cereal just in case I don't feel like cooking.	This was a lot harder. I didn't want to get out of the car, but at least the line was short. When I got home, I didn't cook the food; I just ate cereal.
W	Drop off some clothes at the cleaners.	That felt surprisingly good to get off my agenda. I even decided to microwave what I picked up yesterday. It wasn't too bad.
Th	Make an appointment for my yearly checkup.	This wasn't as hard as I thought it would be. I had to force myself to do it, but I guess that's okay.
F	Pay my bills online.	I was just too tired; I couldn't get myself to do it. Maybe tomorrow.
Sa	Pay my bills. Shop for food at the grocery store.	I actually paid my bills on time this month! What a relief. I really get down on myself for accumulating late fees because of my procrastination. I felt so good. I actually went to the grocery store and shopped.
Su	Call my friend Becky with a report.	I have to admit I felt pretty good telling her I did a few things. I have a long way to go, but it's a start.

TIP

When you develop your Activity Log, select small, manageable goals. None of them should take more than 20 to 30 minutes at first. After you get started, you can consider taking on slightly larger tasks.

Karlene didn't do everything she set out to do each day. And don't worry if you don't complete everything. Celebrate your successes and forgive your failures. If you don't complete an item, consider putting it on the list for the next day. If you don't get to it the next day, the item may be more than you can handle right now. Try to hold that activity off for another week or so.

REMEMBER

If you find yourself unable to get started on your Activity Log or don't feel a little better after using the log for a couple of weeks, consult a professional for assistance.

Conquering Can'ts

The human mind produces an almost constant stream of thoughts about the individual, other people, and the future. Whether you're depressed or not, many of these thoughts have about as much to do with reality as the idea that you're about to sprout wings and fly. In the following section, we review specific "can't" thoughts and ways to defeat them. Throughout this book, and especially in Chapters 6, 7, and 8, you can find more information about the myriad of other ways that thoughts warp everyone's vision from time to time and what you can do to change them.

Depression substantially magnifies the negativity of the mind's chatter. One of the most common thoughts we hear from our clients when discussing the idea of taking action is, "Well, I would, but I just can't." If you've ever had that thought, you most likely truly believe that you're incapable — whether due to basic inadequacy, incompetence, or depression itself — and the contemplated action lies beyond your ability.

Reviewing your thoughts

When you routinely tell yourself that you're incapable of accomplishing given tasks, we call this type of thinking "can't do-itis." Although this diagnosis may sound a bit whimsical, we assure you that its effects aren't. Through repetition alone, "can't do-itis" can become a mantra that you eventually view as a fundamental truth. Review the following common thoughts:

>> I can't think clearly.

>> I can't possibly clean out the garage; it's just too overwhelming.

>> I can't concentrate on anything.

>> I can't motivate myself to do anything.

>> I can't even function anymore.

Do these thoughts sound familiar? They do to us! On some days, thoughts like these bellow through our minds. For example, although we've written over a dozen books, some days we think, "We just can't write today!" Although we *choose* not to write on certain days, it simply isn't true that we absolutely *can't* sit down and write a little when that thought pops into our heads.

So when "can't thoughts" appear out of nowhere on our scheduled writing days, we usually try using a strategy for conquering them. Specifically, we put the "can't thoughts" to the test. We sit down at the computer for 30 minutes and see if we can write something — anything at all. Even a single sentence typed on the computer can disprove the we-can't-write-today thought. A sentence or two usually leads us to feeling like writing more. On rare occasions, the desire to write more doesn't increase, and we make a decision to take the day off. Nothing wrong with that: By writing just a sentence or two, we still refute the "can't thoughts."

Perhaps you're thinking that putting "can't thoughts" to the test may work for productive authors, but it won't work for you when you're terribly depressed. If so, you may want to know that the vast majority of our depressed patients also think that the strategy won't help. Nevertheless, when they try it, they almost always discover that testing out these "can't thoughts" helps.

Testing the waters

TIP

Try putting your "can't thoughts" to the test. You can prove each of these thoughts to be false with a single piece of disconfirming evidence. And after you find one contradiction, you can work on accumulating more. Here are some ideas you can use to test a few of the "can't thoughts" we list in the "Reviewing your thoughts" section, earlier in this chapter.

>> **I can't even function anymore.** Breathing is practically all you have to do to refute this idea! You can test the idea by getting out of bed, pouring yourself a glass of water, and just picking up and actually doing a couple of small activities. If your "can't thoughts" start to interfere, ignore the thoughts by focusing only on moving your body to perform the task. Make a daily habit of refuting this kind of thinking: Construct an Activity Log that lists a new task each day.

>> **I can't remember anything nowadays.** We have our colleague, Dr. Steve Hayes, to thank for this idea. Try remembering this number sequence — 1, 2, 3. Now pretend that we offer you one million dollars (don't forget that we said "pretend!") if you can remember "1, 2, 3." That's right, we're going to give you a million dollars if you can remember "1, 2, 3."

We're willing to bet that if a million dollars were on the line, you'd remember that sequence a few minutes from now. (If not, we suggest that you see your doctor, because something other than depression may be going on.) If you can pass this test, you can probably find many more examples of things you can remember. If you can remember something — anything — you can refute your "can't thought." At the same time, please realize that depression does cause some difficulty with memory. If you want more help with your memory, please see Chapter 20.

>> **I can't possibly clean out the garage; it's just too overwhelming.** Clean out one very small item or space in your garage. After you accomplish that, consider cleaning another small area the next day. Perhaps in a few more days you can tackle two or three small spaces. Believe it or not, that's how insurmountable projects get done — a single piece at a time.

When you're depressed, your mind tricks you into focusing on the entire project that confronts you — as though you must accomplish it all at once. For example, if you picture all the miles you're going to walk in the coming year, and you believe that you must walk the entire distance today, you probably won't even feel like starting.

REMEMBER

Break tasks down into very small, achievable chunks. You can conquer "can't do-itis" by choosing a small piece of what you think you can't do and then going ahead and doing it.

Charting Your Course through Negative Predictions

The mind maintains inaction in another clever way — by providing petrifying predictions for you to ponder. When depression sets in, these negative predictions usually seem more believable and monumental than ever. You may feel as though your horoscope consistently says, "Today is a horrible day for trying new things. Retreat, withdraw, and maintain a passive stance. Wait to take on any action." But the message never wavers; every day delivers the same forecast.

If you're hearing similar dire predictions from your mind's fortune-teller, perhaps the time has come to test out whether you should continue to pay for this "splendid" advice.

TIP

If you stall when it comes to tackling important tasks, try using our Negating Negative Predictions technique. Start off using it for one week. You just may find that it helps you get moving. We're not saying that this strategy will cure your depression, but it can help get the improvement process rolling. Follow these steps and check out the sample chart in Table 11-2.

1. **For each day of the week, write down one or two tasks you've been avoiding.**

Try to think of relatively small, doable projects. If you choose something larger, break it down into small pieces and then tackle one piece at a time.

2. **Make a stress prediction for each task.**

   Predict (on a 0 to 100 point scale) how much stress the task is going to cause you. For example, do you envision that paying the bills is going to feel ponderously difficult? If so, you may want to predict the stress factor as 70 or above.

3. **Make a "boost" prediction for each task.**

   Rate (on a 0 to 100 point scale) how much of a boost in satisfaction, confidence, and mood you predict you're going to feel by completing the task. For example, if you think that paying bills is going to give you a mild to modest boost in feelings of satisfaction, mood, or confidence, you may want to rate the expected boost as 25 or so.

4. **Record the outcome (or your actual experience) on your chart for both the stress and "boost" categories.**

5. **After you complete the chore, write down how much stress and aggravation you** *actually experienced* **from doing the project, plus how much of a boost in satisfaction, confidence, and mood you actually felt.**

The following story shows how using the Negating Negative Predictions technique can pay off.

> **Anise,** a college professor, has been depressed for the past month. She starts arriving to work late and collapsing the moment she gets home. She drags herself to bed after watching mindless television all night. Important tasks such as preparing lectures, grading exams, paying bills, and shopping for groceries start piling up. Anise decides to try the Negating Negative Predictions Technique. Table 11-2 shows you her chart.

As you can see in Table 11-2, Anise consistently predicted that activities would involve more stress and hassle than she actually experienced. The stress was as great as she anticipated in only one case — and that was because her lawnmower kept stalling. Although not every task gave her a huge boost in satisfaction, confidence, and mood, the boost that she actually experienced was always far greater than she imagined it would be. After one week, Anise still felt depressed, but she at least felt a little lift from the exercise. And that lift made it easier to take on new tasks.

If you're like most folks with depression, you'll likely experience results similar to Anise's. You'll predict activities to be more stressful and less rewarding than you actually find them to be. Try this simple strategy for a couple of weeks.

TABLE 11-2   **Negating Negative Predictions Chart**

Day	Task	Predicted Stress	Experienced Stress	Predicted Boost	Experienced Boost
M	Grocery shopping	50	25	10	20
T	Grade one exam	70	20	10	30
W	Do the dishes	45	10	5	20
Th	Finally call Thomas to talk	50	5	20	60
F	Pay bills	75	30	25	70
Sa	Mow lawn	50	50	15	50
Su	Plant flowers	40	10	25	60

We didn't include any items that involve especially pleasurable, fun activities in the preceding exercise. Did we exclude these items because we think that you shouldn't or can't enjoy yourself if you're depressed? No. We excluded these items because we think that finding renewed pleasures is so important that we devote all of Chapter 13 to the topic.

Giving Yourself Credit

Depressed minds can pull another cruel trick that can easily stop you dead in your tracks. What's the trick? Glad you asked. Consider this scenario:

You eventually manage to get yourself to accomplish something you put off for quite a while. Then your mind trashes the success with the thought, "Well, sure I did that, but so what? Any moron could have done that!" As this thought demonstrates, depression not only spoils quality of life but it also disrupts efforts you make on your own behalf to venture forward.

When you hear thoughts from your mind telling you to discredit your accomplishments, consider an alternative perspective. If you went grocery shopping in a normal mood, perhaps you wouldn't think too much of your achievement. But if you went grocery shopping with a broken leg, wouldn't you value the deed more highly?

Okay, you don't have a broken leg. But the effect of depression is rather similar. Depression makes everything harder to do than when you're in a good frame of mind. As we discuss in Chapter 2, depression depletes the body of energy; it saps enthusiasm, steals sleep, and creates mental confusion.

TIP

Given the wide array of physical and mental maladies that depression inflicts, accomplishing any task in this condition is a remarkable feat. Therefore, don't forget to give yourself a substantially greater amount of credit for getting things done when you're depressed. You give yourself credit by congratulating yourself for each effort you carry out.

Chapter **12**

Working Out to Lift Depression

When you feel depressed, the last thing you probably want to do is go to the gym or take a jog. Depression usually drains energy and pushes you to go back to bed with the covers over your head. However, as you probably know, that's really not a great idea.

In this chapter, we tell you how jumping jacks, jogging, and gymnastics soar above anything else you can do to improve the quality of your life and health. Exercise exorcises depression. When depression tells you that you can't get going, we explain how to talk back to your depression and establish a plan for overcoming inertia. And we help you choose the type of exercise that's just right for you.

At 4 a.m., **Patricia** wakes up and can't get back to sleep. She knows that a lack of sleep affects her performance at work, which makes her even more upset and makes getting back to sleep even more difficult. This early awakening has got to stop. Yesterday, her boss even commented that she looked tired. Patricia tosses and turns for the next two hours and then finally gets up at 6 a.m. What a miserable start to the day.

Depression runs throughout Patricia's family. She has been treated with medication off and on for about five years. Her physician tells her that she will likely need to take antidepressant medication for the rest of her life. But lately, medication alone just doesn't seem to work. Her depression intensifies. First, her doctor increases the dose; when that doesn't work, he suggests adding another drug to improve her response to the medication. Patricia, worried about both short- and long-term side effects, asks her doctor about other alternatives to consider instead of the additional medication. He suggests regular exercise. (And we agree!)

REMEMBER

As much as we advocate exercise, it represents just one piece of the puzzle. If you try and try, and you just can't get into exercise, don't beat yourself up. This book is filled with other ways to defeat depression.

Why Exercise?

Extensive research has shown that exercise does as much good for you as the combined contents of most medicine cabinets. Doctors regularly encourage exercise as a critical part of healthy living. That goes for 8-year-olds as well as 80-year-olds. Unfortunately, their recommendations often go unheeded. In general, for many people, exercise is a luxury afforded to those with the time to do it. In today's busy world, it doesn't always fit into already overflowing schedules. So doctors recommend exercise, but they know that most of their patients will ignore their advice.

Mental health benefits: Endorphins

Who doesn't want to feel good? All kinds of ways to feel good exist: laughter, a great meal, sex, or a walk on the beach are a just a few examples. But what about these activities actually make people feel good?

The answer lies, in part, in the brain. The brain has special receptacles that receive *opiates,* drugs such as heroin and cocaine that relieve pain and induce a heightened sense of well-being. The human body produces natural substances, called *endorphins,* that function like opiates in the brain. They produce the same sort of "high" that heroin and cocaine do. Except endorphins are legal. You can generate endorphins through exercise and pleasurable activities. Endorphins induce a feeling of pleasure and well-being that may counteract depression.

You can increase endorphins by having sex, eating chocolate, consuming spicy foods, and, you guessed it, engaging in exercise. You can try to increase your endorphin level by sitting around eating chocolate all day or having nonstop sex, but obvious factors make these approaches a bit difficult or unadvisable. So you're left with exercise.

ENDORPHINS: A MIRACLE CURE?

Science is very sure that endorphins reduce pain. Stories abound about soldiers who, after being injured in battle, manage to carry on heroically for hours, seemingly oblivious to the pain from wounds that would normally be incapacitating. Endorphins, released by the body in response to the demands of the battlefield, temporarily stop pain signals from getting through to the brain.

In addition, many have speculated that endorphins play a role in enhancing the immune system by activating natural killer cells that attack diseases. Endorphins may improve circulation and even keep brain cells young and healthy by neutralizing toxic substances. The endorphin system may provide a buffer against stress. And some have suggested that the body fails to produce sufficient endorphin levels during depression. In time, science is bound to clarify how and to what extent endorphins influence our body in beneficial ways. But we can be sure that endorphins at least provide a temporary boost in mood and well-being.

TIP

A growing body of research suggests that exercise alleviates depression. Of the various types of exercise, it isn't yet clear whether one form may be best at decreasing depression (or if they all work equally well). Although we don't recommend exercise as your sole answer to major depression, you will benefit enormously from regular workouts.

Physical health benefits

Regular exercise not only stimulates endorphin production but it also tunes up your entire body. Exercise improves physical health in the following ways:

- » Strengthens your heart
- » Increases lung capacity
- » Reduces the risk of various cancers
- » Decreases the risk of diabetes
- » Balances your cholesterol ratio
- » Strengthens your bones
- » Keeps muscles toned and healthy
- » Helps with weight management
- » Fights insomnia

>> Rids your body of excessive adrenaline that causes anxiety and other problems

>> Improves physical range of motion and pain management

>> Keeps skin looking healthier and younger

>> Boosts energy

>> Helps you retain good cognitive functioning

Who would ever ignore benefits as extensive as these? Only a fool! Actually, most humans fail to incorporate enough exercise into their lives. Few can claim that they get an ideal amount of exercise most days. In fact, it's been estimated that 80 percent of United States citizens fail to exercise an optimal amount. That's too bad because, flat out, exercise makes you healthier.

TIP

Most experts recommend either 150 minutes of moderate exercise or 75 minutes of high-intensity exercise each week. You can accomplish that with a few brisk walks.

WARNING

Always check with your doctor before beginning an exercise program — especially if you're overweight, over the age of 40, or have health problems. You also need to see your doctor if you experience serious pain, dizziness, nausea, or other troubling symptoms after exercising, because these symptoms don't normally occur after moderate exercise.

Conquering Couch Potato-itis

Exercise can help you feel better emotionally and physically, but there's just one problem: Depression tells you to withdraw, retreat, and hibernate. When you're depressed, paralysis can set in. Simple, everyday living takes extraordinary effort, and you may feel like staying in bed with the cover over your head.

Thus, the mere thought of exercising may sound utterly impossible to you in the midst of depression. You can hardly put one foot in front of the other; how can we possibly suggest that you start working out? The depressed mind spins out thoughts that stifle initiative and motivation. These thoughts may be telling you that you can't possibly succeed in implementing an exercise regimen. We know you may feel this way. Please understand that we don't underestimate the difficulty of overcoming the inertia of depression. Nevertheless, we believe you'll find that the benefits of exercise outweigh the costs.

REMEMBER

You *can* talk back to these dark thoughts that stifle activity. You don't have to allow them to take over your will. You can start by subjecting them to scrutiny and analysis. Ask yourself if there's an alternative perspective to your depressed mind's view. Is your mind exaggerating, distorting, or making negative predictions without any real basis? If so, try to replace the negativity with realistic alternatives. You need to short circuit any negative thoughts that come into your mind and start moving your body.

TIP

In the first column of Table 12-1, we list the five thoughts that most frequently get in the way of reasonable, alternative viewpoints and prevent you from getting going. If you find yourself thinking any of these demotivating thoughts, argue back with motivating thoughts like the ones in the second column. (See Chapter 8 for other ideas on how to overcome action-blocking thoughts.)

TABLE 12-1   **Defeating Demotivating Thoughts**

Demotivating Thoughts	Motivating Thoughts
I'm too depressed to exercise.	Yes, that's how I "feel," but it doesn't mean that it's true. I can test this thought out by walking for ten minutes.
I can hardly get out of bed; I can't possibly exercise.	Another interesting thought. But I do get out of bed every day. And, if I can get out of bed, I can push myself to do a small amount of exercise.
Exercise isn't worth doing.	That's how it feels, but the evidence says otherwise. Exercise helps people feel better.
I don't like to exercise.	True. But I don't have to turn into a fitness buff. I can profit from even a small amount of exercise.
I don't have time to exercise.	I take time to brush my teeth every day. If something is really important, I can find a way to work it in a few days a week.

After you identify your demotivating thoughts and dispute them, you may still feel unmotivated. And a few demotivating thoughts will likely linger. Realize that thoughts are just thoughts — they're not necessarily true.

TIP

To show how thoughts aren't gospel, we have a brief exercise for you. (If you have a physical problem that prevents you from comfortably getting out of a chair, construct a similar scenario that affirms your ability to conquer demotivating thoughts.)

1. **Sit down in a comfortable chair.**

2. **Say out loud, "I can't stand up!"**

3. **Forcefully say out loud, "I can't stand up!" ten more times.**

4. **Now stand up.**

Did you manage to stand up? Your mind said you couldn't stand up, but you did (or at least, we assume you did). The point of this admittedly silly exercise is to demonstrate that the negative thoughts people listen to aren't always inherently true.

People often think things that aren't true, and then act as though they are. For example, we bet that you've heard more than a few people say, "I can't stop smoking." Indeed, stopping smoking is incredibly difficult; at times, it may seem impossible. Yet *millions* of people who make that pronouncement eventually manage to quit. Of course, when smokers have the thought that they can't stop, they truly believe it. And when you're depressed, you fully believe the thought that says you just can't exercise.

REMEMBER

Thoughts are just thoughts — many thoughts generated by a depressed mind have no more reality than "I can't stand up," or "I can't stop smoking."

TIP

If your mind is telling you that you can't stop smoking (or vaping), consider taking a look at our recent book *Quitting Smoking & Vaping For Dummies* (Wiley).

Easing into Exercise

With any luck, you can convince yourself that you can start exercising. But that doesn't mean exercising will be easy. Depression truly saps your body of energy, so we suggest that you start your exercise program gently and ever so slowly.

TIP

Most exercise gurus preach the importance of exercising for at least 30 minutes, five times per week. Research shows that almost any exercise is far better than none, so even 10 minutes, three or four times a week, can help. And you can ease your way into the world of exercise with activities that barely seem like exercise at all:

>> Park a little farther from your workplace.

>> Take the stairs rather than the elevator.

>> Do a few brief exercises during work breaks.

>> If you use a cordless phone, walk while you talk.

>> The next time you shop, walk a couple of laps around the mall.

Walking a little farther, taking the stairs, and moving around more make a good start for your exercise program. Then, if you want, you can add a little more motion to your daily routine. To obtain the maximum benefit from exercise, work your body a little harder each day.

TIP

The following list shows you three decisions you have to make when designing your exercise program. For each, start small and build up slowly. And remember that you're not competing with anyone, so don't compare yourself to others at the gym or on the track.

>> **Frequency:** "How often am I going to work exercise into my life?" For starters, consider committing to twice a week.

>> **Intensity:** "How fast am I going to walk or run? How heavy are the weights I'm going to use?" For starters, we suggest not very fast and not very heavy!

>> **Time:** "How long do I want to exercise each time?" Again, try starting with ten minutes.

But what type of exercise is going to work best for you? We can honestly say that we have no idea. And you may not know either. So in the following section, we briefly discuss a few types of exercise that you can consider. If you want even more info on all the possibilities that are out there, check out a local health club or pick up a copy of *Fitness For Dummies*, by Suzanne Schlosberg and Liz Neporent (Wiley).

VACUUMING AWAY DEPRESSION?

Research has shown that exercise can help alleviate depression, but how about aerobic housework? Your spouse or roommate may urge you to increase your exercise by washing the dishes, sweeping floors, or dusting the furniture. Of course, their motives may not be all that altruistic — especially if it's their turn to tackle one of these chores.

But does housework alleviate depression the same way that exercise does? Apparently not. According to researchers at the University of Glasgow, domestic chores, unlike almost any other type of exercise, actually lowers mood. And the more housework you do, the lower your mood drops. So if you're depressed, start exercising, but it's okay to let the housework go for a little while until your mood improves.

On the other hand, we're not suggesting you totally let the house go. Doing a little housework may even provide you with a sense of accomplishment. But if you do get a small lift from doing housework, the lift comes from a sense of accomplishment, not the aerobic benefits.

Weighing Your Exercise Options

TIP

We recommend that you review the various exercise options and pick one that holds the most initial appeal to you — or at least the one that looks the least awful.

No matter what type of exercise you settle on, try it out for a couple of weeks. If you don't find yourself starting to like the exercise you chose, try another type of exercise. You may have to experiment a little, but you'll likely find an exercise that works well for you. In this section, we review strength training, aerobic exercise, and yoga — three of the most popular exercise options.

EXERCISE DURING A PANDEMIC

When the COVID-19 pandemic caused many gyms to close or operate at reduced capacity, exercise became a bit more challenging for house-bound people. Depending upon local regulations and mandates, some people struggled to find adequate locations and methods for exercising. People miss their gym friends, variety of workouts available, and equipment. Of course, most folks are able to walk, bike, and jog outside with masks on (when required) if they live in an area where it's safe to do so. But often, parks, bike paths, and outdoor facilities are overly crowded, and weather sometimes interferes. Here are some tips when attempting to exercise under less than optimal conditions:

- If you don't have to commute any longer, use the time you're saving to prioritize exercise.

- Find space for an indoor bike, rowing machine, or stair stepper. (You can put it in your living room, as you're probably not having company during a pandemic.)

- If you don't have room for equipment, get a few hand weights, kettle bells, or some resistance bands.

- Follow exercise routines available online (often for free or a small subscription price). YouTube is full of them.

- Change up your routines to keep from getting bored.

- Do squats or jumping jacks during television commercials.

- Stand up during meetings.

It's normal to feel a bit lazy and frustrated when you can't keep your regular routines going. But with the added stress during stay-at-home orders, exercise is a great way to keep your spirits up as much as possible.

The goal isn't to become an accomplished triathlete; you only need to increase the intensity of your exercise slightly to start deriving benefits.

Pumping iron

Strength training involves building muscle. You can accomplish this build up through weightlifting with barbells, weight machines, or dumbbells. However, you don't actually need to use machines or weights at all. You can try the following strength-enhancing exercises that don't require any special equipment:

>> Chin-ups

>> Crunches

>> Lunges

>> Push-ups

>> Squats

You may think that strength training is only for body builders or the younger set. Not so. Numerous studies have demonstrated that strength training provides incredible benefits at almost any age, perhaps even more so in older populations. Strength training appears to improve mood, reduce the risk of falls, enhance memory and thinking ability, and prolong life.

We've previously hired a personal trainer to show us what strength training is all about. After the first week, we weren't so sure about our decision to work out. We discovered aching muscles that we didn't even know we had. But by the end of a month, we picked up a new, healthy habit. Consider doing what we did and hire your own personal trainer to introduce you to the myriad of benefits that strength training can bring to your life. For those of you working from home, you can hire personal trainers through Zoom.

Strength training can easily lead to injury if you aren't careful and don't know what you're doing. We recommend that you first either consult a trainer at a gym or pick up a book on the subject, such as *Weight Training For Dummies*, by Liz Neporent and Suzanne Schlosberg (Wiley).

Revving up your heart and lungs

Aerobic exercise (or *cardiovascular exercise*) is one of the easiest exercise programs to start. This type of exercise increases your oxygen intake and speeds up your heart rate. (*Aerobic* means "with oxygen.")

Walking is the most basic form of aerobic exercise. To participate in aerobic exercise, all you have to do is increase the pace of your walking so that your heart rate increases. Of course, you can also perform other aerobic activities, such as jogging, skating, bicycling, and — hold onto your hat — aerobics. Basically, an activity qualifies as aerobic if it revs you up to the point where you feel a little winded, but you can still say a short sentence without gasping for air.

TECHNICAL STUFF

Healthcare professionals often recommend that you establish a *target heart rate* for your aerobic exercise. You can determine your target heart rate zone by first subtracting your age from 220. That number represents your absolute maximum heart rate, a rate you want to avoid exceeding. Your ideal zone lies between 0.5 and 0.8 of your maximum heart rate, depending on your fitness level.

For example, a 45-year-old would subtract 45 from 220, which is 175 beats per minute. Depending on fitness level, the target would be anywhere between about 85 beats per minute to about 150. However, this method may not be appropriate for your body and health condition. Your physician can help you determine your fitness level and thus your ideal zone.

Yikes! Yoga?

When you think of yoga, you may conjure up images of bodies twisted up like pretzels. Or maybe you visualize rows of robed monks seated cross-legged on mats, chanting "Ommmm. . . ."

But today, you're more likely to find practitioners of yoga dressed in the latest gym attire, straining and sweating at a local health club. And although some people with highly advanced yoga skills may twist their bodies like pretzels, most yoga exercises don't require such awesome flexibility. We started practicing yoga some time ago, and we can guarantee you that we're not that limber.

You can take yoga classes at your local health club or YMCA. You can also learn yoga by reading a book, such as *Yoga For Dummies*, by Georg Feuerstein, PhD, and Larry Payne, PhD (Wiley). As with many exercise routines, you won't know how you feel about yoga unless you try it.

Chapter **13**

Rediscovering Healthy Pleasures

When you're depressed, nothing sounds appealing. Food doesn't taste as good, music doesn't soothe you, and comedy doesn't strike you as funny. Even the activities you used to enjoy seem flat, dull, and uninteresting. So, what can you do to bring back pleasure into your life?

In this chapter, we tell you about the surprising effects of pleasure on both your mood and body. Next, we help you rediscover a few of your favorite pleasures or find some new ones. We explain why pleasure is something you deserve, even if you don't think so. And you may not believe that you're capable of having fun, but we show you how to defeat your negative predictions.

Taking Fun Seriously

When depression sets in, you can hardly get through the demands of the day. You may not even feel like getting out of bed. Having fun feels both inconceivable and frivolous.

Nevertheless, we propose that you take a serious look at pleasure. Why? First, because pleasure lifts mood. The boost may be temporary and slight in the beginning. But with time and persistence, pleasurable activities can help defeat depression.

Striking the right balance

Some people are lucky enough to enjoy and get significant pleasure from their work. A few are so happy at work that they rarely take time off to spend time with family or do something special for themselves. However, for most people, finding a way to give enough to their jobs or careers while balancing their home life is a struggle. Research has found that working families with children have the most difficult time juggling responsibilities. Here are a few tips for keeping in mind when you attempt to live a balanced life:

>> Be realistic about how much you can accomplish in one day.

>> Watch out for procrastination, and don't waste time on useless gossip.

>> Communicate honestly when you need extra time off; most bosses are flexible.

>> Find time to turn off devices and unplug when you are at home.

>> Try to keep a schedule that includes time for relaxing.

>> Don't overschedule either for yourself or your family.

>> Stay as healthy as you can with good food and exercise.

>> Find something that the whole family can enjoy and do it!

REMEMBER

Okay, we get it. Sometimes life is so busy that you just can't get everything done. These are aspirational goals. Strive to simplify your life and do the best you can. Your family and you deserve to be happy.

Understanding the need for fun

In addition to its positive effects on your emotional and mental state of affairs, pleasure may provide physical benefits, such as

>> Alleviation of chronic pain

>> Decreased risk of heart attacks

>> Improved overall health

>> Increased immune function

>> Prolonged life expectancy

Pleasure also combats everyday stress. People who pursue enjoyable activities typically feel happier, more relaxed, and calmer. When you take all these factors into account, the pursuit of pleasure isn't a frivolous endeavor.

Making a List and Checking It Twice

When you're depressed, you may not even be able to remember what pleasure feels like. And generating a list of possible pleasurable activities may seem unimaginably difficult. Don't worry — we're here to help you get started.

If you're depressed, review the pleasurable activity lists in this section. Obviously, not all of these activities will appeal to you. However, we suggest that you circle each of the items that you either currently *or have ever* found enjoyable. Then think about which ones seem doable. For example, if you currently live alone, and you don't have a willing sex partner, having sex may not be a reasonable choice for you at this time. Try to start bringing as many of the doable items into your life as possible.

TIP

The following list contains the results of an international survey of what people find enjoyable. Simple pleasures provide the most enjoyment. These activities include

>> Drinking a glass of wine

>> Drinking tea or coffee

>> Eating chocolate

>> Entertaining friends

>> Exercising

>> Going out for a meal

>> Having sex

>> Playing with children

>> Reading

>> Shopping

>> Spending time with family

>> Taking a hot bath or shower

>> Watching television

PAIN OR PLEASURE? SOME LIKE IT HOT

In our great state of New Mexico, we consider pain a flavor! The pain comes from the hot chili sauce that chefs pour over just about everything. The hotter the better. A common question asked at a New Mexican restaurant is, "Red or green?" which refers to the color of the pepper used to make the sauce. The sophisticated diner often replies, "Which one is hotter?"

Newcomers and visitors don't understand this ritual. In fact, many plates remain almost untouched after the first bite or two. These visitors frantically search for something to quell the pain (which can be accomplished with sour cream or honey). They sit bewildered, watching other, more experienced chili enthusiasts wolf down huge quantities of fiery foods. But if they're willing to try the food again, many of these neophytes soon find themselves craving chilies as much as the natives do.

Science has discovered a cause for the strange eating habits of New Mexicans and others who crave hot, spicy foods. Chilies are actually addictive. Here's why: When you bite into something peppery, *capsaicin* (the portion of the chili that makes it hot) is released into your mouth. When capsaicin contacts the nerves in your mouth, pain signals rush to your brain. The brain responds by releasing a flood of *endorphins* (covered in Chapter 12), which kill pain and induce a state of well-being and pleasure. The brain also releases endorphins when you engage in any of a variety of highly pleasurable activities, such as the ones we detail in this chapter.

If you've ever been to a French bakery, it probably won't surprise you to discover that the French have a particular fondness for indulging in pastries. Italians rank sex high on their pleasures list. The British apparently enjoy drinking tea as well as alcohol.

TIP

Perhaps the previous list doesn't capture your interests. If so, realize that you have many other sources of enjoyment to consider. Many of these other pleasures involve the senses, such as:

>> Eating spicy foods

>> Getting a massage

>> Listening to music

>> Looking at beauty in nature or art

>> Sitting by a lake or ocean

>> Smelling fresh flowers

» Spending time in a sauna

» Taking a long, warm bath

TIP

You can seek pleasure through entertaining activities as well, such as

» Camping

» Dancing

» Hiking or walking

» Hobbies

» Live plays, concerts, or comedy

» Movies

» Participating in sports

» Playing board games

» Playing with pets

» Playing cards

» Binge-watching shows

» Cooking

» Taking an afternoon nap

» Volunteering

» Spectator sports

» Travel and vacations

TIP

A great game for anyone with a GPS device is geocaching. You take a walk, just about anywhere in the world, and basically go on a treasure hunt. A geocache is a hidden container with special items inside. Sometimes you leave a few coins, pretty rocks, or other interesting items. You sign your name and the date you found the cache. Then you return it so that another seeker can find it. The game is great during a pandemic because you can play by yourself or with your house-mates. (Of course, wear masks if called for under current guidelines.) For more information about this type of entertainment, go to www.geocaching.com.

Fighting the Pleasure Busters

When you're wrestling with depression, reincorporating pleasurable activities into your life isn't always as easy as it sounds. In fact, you may have the following negative reactions when trying to incorporate pleasurable activities back into your life.

>> **Guilt tripping:** Guilt tripping occurs when you believe that pleasure is wasteful, frivolous, undeserved, inappropriate, unproductive, or even downright sinful. We explain more about guilt tripping in the next section.

>> **Negative predicting:** Depression increases the likelihood that future events will be seen as bleak and joyless. See more about negative predictions in the "Expecting the worst" section later in the chapter.

You aren't going to get very far in your attempt to bring pleasure back into your life if either guilt or negative predicting is blocking the doorway to happiness. Therefore, we address each of these killjoys separately.

Guilt busters

Guilt can be a good thing. When you do something truly wrong, guilt tells you not to do it again. And knowing that you may feel guilty can prevent you from acting in ways that are either unhealthy or morally wrong. Guilt gives you a moral compass *when it's working right.*

REMEMBER

When you wave a magnet around a compass, the needle spins every which way. In the same manner, too much guilt causes the needle on your moral compass to point you in the wrong direction. Out-of-control guilt grossly exaggerates the significance of any real or imagined transgressions. For example, excessive guilt may tell you that a single bar of chocolate represents uncontrolled gluttony. Furthermore, guilt may make you feel undeserving of any pleasure.

Excessive guilt is a prime feature of depression. So you get to feel down and blue, and guilty to boot. Guilt and depression make the pursuit of happiness excruciatingly difficult, because depression drains you of energy for pursuing pleasure, and guilt tells you that you don't deserve to feel good in the first place.

Increasing your awareness

Increasing your awareness of how guilt may influence your decision to undertake healthy pleasures is critical. We find that when guilt gets in the way of taking on the task of searching for enjoyment, certain thoughts may repeatedly run through your mind. See if any of these thoughts sound familiar:

>> I'm not good enough; I don't deserve to be happy.

>> I feel like pleasure is a frivolous waste of time.

>> If I beat up on myself enough, I just may get motivated to do something more productive.

>> I *should* have done things differently (there are about a million or so variants of this thought).

>> I'm just a loser; pleasure is for winners.

Thoughts such as these induce powerful feelings of guilt. But how can you tell if your guilt indicates an appropriate, healthy response based on a well-functioning moral compass, or an out-of-control response, misdirecting you toward self-abuse and self-defeating thoughts and actions? Actually, identifying the type of guilt you're experiencing isn't that difficult.

REMEMBER

Guilt is appropriate and reasonable only when it occurs following intentional, unnecessary acts that cause harm to you or someone else. And appropriate guilt has a time limit; it doesn't go on and on, because prolonging the bad feelings merely harms you by intensifying your depression. Holding on to guilt simply leads to unproductive rumination and self-abuse.

Breaking guilt's pleasure-denying power

TIP

Ask yourself if your pleasurable indulgences truly reflect conscious, maliciously motivated behaviors. If they do, perhaps a little short-term guilt will remind you to put on the "brakes" in the future. But before you reach that conclusion, be sure to ask yourself these Guilt-Quelling Questions:

>> Was my indulgence primarily intended to harm myself?

>> Is it possible that a little enjoyment can be a good thing rather than a bad thing?

>> Is it possible that I'm magnifying the "awfulness" of my indulgences?

>> Am I excessively blaming myself for something that actually has many causes?

>> Am I berating myself merely for having human imperfections?

>> Where is it written that I *should* have done something different?

Here's an example of how you can put these questions to use.

> **Connie** works as a nurse practitioner at a busy hospital clinic. The stress of working long hours (which are filled with handling the urgent needs of patients) piles up on her. The shortage of healthcare workers in her community pushes her to accept

extra work shifts on a regular basis. She has little time for friends or fun. Her fatigue and loneliness gradually meld into depression.

A few co-workers notice Connie's deteriorating mood. They tell Connie that she needs to do something for herself once in a while. Their suggestions include

- Eating chocolate

- Going shopping for herself

- Getting a massage

- Going to a comedy show

As Connie contemplates her possible pleasures, negative thoughts churn in her mind. She thinks, "Great, I'm already ten pounds overweight, just think of how fat I'll get eating chocolate. And I'd feel horribly guilty spending my hard earned money on something so self-indulgent as a shopping for myself or a massage. Massages are for the rich. So that leaves going to a comedy. In my mood? Not a chance I'd like that."

Connie feels guilt *in advance* of indulging in a few simple pleasures such as eating a couple of chocolates, drinking an occasional glass of wine, or getting a massage. After she answers the Guilt–Quelling Questions we list earlier in this section, her feelings may change:

>> **Was my indulgence primarily intended to harm myself?** Connie's response: "Well, actually I haven't even done it yet. But my intent is to enjoy something, not to harm myself."

>> **Is it possible that a little enjoyment can be a good thing rather than bad?** Connie's response: "I guess I rarely give myself latitude to indulge in much of anything. What's so horrible about a little pleasure? I'm starting to sound like my mother! I've read that pleasure actually is good for the body and mind."

>> **Is it possible that I'm magnifying the "awfulness" of my indulgences?** Connie's response: "I suppose an occasional chocolate, glass of wine, or massage doesn't exactly equate with being a mass murderer. Ben Franklin had a point when he advocated the benefits of taking all things in moderation."

>> **Am I excessively blaming myself for something that actually has many causes?** Connie's response: "Well, in the case of my weight, I realize it's caused by so many things: genetics (most of my relatives are overweight), too little exercise, food dropped off by the pharmaceutical sales reps almost every day, processed foods, too much fast food, and on and on. A few carefully selected candies or a glass of wine has relatively little to do with the problem."

>> **Am I berating myself merely for having human imperfections?** Connie's response: "Hey, at least I'm good at beating up on myself! I guess if I think about it, everyone has their flaws. Ten pounds of extra weight isn't exactly the worst thing I could imagine."

>> **Where is it written that I *should* have done something different?** Connie's response: "I use that word *should* on myself a lot. Maybe I *should*, oops, I mean maybe it *would be better if* I rethought that word. Although diet books don't exactly promote eating chocolate and drinking wine, most of them advise modest indulgences and recommend that almost no foods should fall under an 'absolutely never' category."

We hope that you can seriously review these Guilt-Quelling Questions and come to Connie's conclusions about healthy pleasures. We believe that you deserve a reasonable balance of pleasure in your life. You don't need to earn the right to pursue happiness — indulging in a few joys can be a powerful tool in fighting depression if you give yourself the right to do so.

TIP

If you answer the Guilt-Quelling Questions we list earlier in this section, and guilt still blocks you from seeking enjoyment, please read Chapters 4, 6, 7, and 8 for more information about tackling the guilt that rides along with your depression and robs you of a basic human right: the right to experience pleasure.

GUILT: THE WORLD TOUR

An international survey looked at the relationship between guilt and enjoyment. They found that guilt destroys the experience of enjoyment. Apparently, the Dutch like to have fun, and they don't feel guilty when they indulge in pleasurable activities. On the other hand, Germans feel more guilty about having fun than other Europeans, and thus they land at the bottom of the pile in terms of their overall enjoyment.

Although the researchers didn't conduct a survey on enjoyment and guilt in the United States, had they done so, we surmise that they would have discovered high levels of guilt and relatively low levels of enjoyment. We believe that the so-called work ethic that is so heavily promoted in the United States may lead to these feelings of guilt. For example, most American companies dole out vacation time with all the generosity of Ebenezer Scrooge. We also believe that guilt thrives in the United States because of the constant stream of contradictory, yet sensational headlines that admonish the citizenry to stop drinking as well as to drink moderately, to eat low fat diets as well as eat high fat diets, or to eat carbohydrates as well as avoid carbohydrates. You may get the impression that, no matter what you do, it's the wrong thing.

Expecting the worst

You select a variety of potentially pleasurable activities to try, and then as you contemplate actually doing them, your mind fills with dread. You begin to picture the so-called pleasurable activities as distasteful, dreary duties. Depression forms a cloud of dismal thoughts that obscure your ability to think about the future clearly.

Lucas graduates with a degree in architecture and immediately finds work he loves with a small firm in Seattle. However, when the economy tanks, his firm downsizes and lays him off. Around that same time, Lucas breaks up with his girlfriend of the past four years. Understandably, he finds his mood miserable, his energy low, and his sleep disturbed. Lucas's counselor suggests that Lucas make a list of activities that he has found pleasurable in the past. He comes up with:

- Spending time with friends
- Camping
- Joining a softball league
- Going to clubs

But his mind immediately floods with negative thoughts. He predicts that his friends are going to find him boring because of his bad mood. He envisions having a miserable time camping because of all the hassle involved, and he believes that he has no spare money for going to a club.

WARNING

If you're experiencing even a mild depression, beware. Your predictions of the future are likely to be as unreliable as a cheap used car from a sleazy car lot. Because pleasure seems impossible when you're down, anticipating enjoyment is particularly difficult to do. Press on and try to ignore your mind's pessimism.

TIP

If you find it difficult to simply ignore dire mental predictions concerning activities that are meant to be fun, you can combat your mind's gloomy forecasting with an activity we call Firing Your Mind's Faulty Forecaster. Put down your umbrella, pick up a pen and some paper, read the following steps, and construct a chart similar to the sample in Table 13-1. You may be surprised how helpful this activity can be.

1. Pick three or four small, potentially pleasurable activities.

You don't have to view these activities as truly pleasurable yet. However, you should choose items that either seem relatively "unawful," or that you enjoyed in the past.

REMEMBER

If you have solid reasons for not engaging in a particular activity (other than low expectations of pleasure), don't select that item.

2. **On a point scale of 0 to 10, rate the amount of pleasure or fun you anticipate feeling from the activity.**

Zero indicates that you expect absolutely no fun, five means that you anticipate a moderate amount of enjoyment, and ten suggests that you anticipate total ecstasy. We doubt that you're going to have many nines or tens if you're depressed.

3. **Perform the activity.**

This is the hard part. Even if you rate an item as zero or one, push yourself to do it anyway. Your mind may resist with negative thoughts. Short circuit those thoughts and move your body.

4. **After you complete the activity, rate how much pleasure you actually experienced and briefly describe your reaction in words.**

If you complete this exercise, you're likely to find that you experience more fun and enjoyment from activities than you predicted. Discovering that your predictions were inaccurate may spur you on to try more pleasurable activities. And the more pleasure you experience, the less depressed you will be.

Checking back in with Lucas from earlier in this section, he has four items on his pleasure list. None of them sound satisfying to him, so he tries the Firing Your Mind's Faulty Forecaster exercise. Table 13-1 provides his results.

TABLE 13-1 **Firing Your Mind's Faulty Forecaster**

Activity	Forecasted Fun	Experienced Fun
Spending time with friends	3	6 — I had a surprisingly good experience.
Camping	2	4 — It was a hassle, but I did like getting away.
Softball	3	5 — I was pretty rusty, but it was nice to be with the guys.
Going to a club	4	2 — I felt horrible about spending the money.

Notice that in three out of four cases, Lucas experienced significantly more fun and pleasure than he anticipated. In one case, however, he actually had a pretty rotten time. Experiencing less pleasure than you originally anticipate can result for any number of reasons. For Lucas, his concerns about finances actually were somewhat realistic.

Also notice that Lucas didn't have the greatest time in the world with any of the activities; this is normal, because depression mutes joy. However, if Lucas continues to pursue pleasurable activities, the amount of fun he feels will very likely increase slowly over time.

Like Lucas, you may have less pleasure than you anticipate occasionally. For example, you could go camping on a rainy weekend. Or going to a club, you could feel uncomfortable or awkward. But realize that the more pleasurable activities you attempt, the more your odds go up of experiencing pleasure.

REMEMBER

Depression is a formidable foe. Adding pleasure to your life is but one small step in the fight. Give fun a chance, and realize that rediscovering healthy pleasures takes time and patience.

Chapter **14**

Solving Life's Headaches

D epression pours sludge into your brain's problem-solving machinery. The resulting diminished capacity for finding solutions causes every difficulty you face to grow in size and complexity. Problems that may look like minor molehills to someone in a normal mood suddenly loom larger than mountains. And when you're depressed, big problems induce a state of paralysis and hopelessness. This bleak discouragement in turn increases your depression and further clouds your ability to see a way out.

Nevertheless, we have some good news for you. Learning more effective problem-solving strategies helps defeat depression. This approach has continued to be supported by research over the last few decades. A large number of studies have validated that problem solving works. This technique works for people with and without depression. You'll find that our take on problem solving is easy to get the hang of; you can readily find ways to apply it to your real-life problems.

In this chapter, we present a comprehensive game plan for unraveling dilemmas that come in a wide variety of shapes, colors, and sizes. Adele's story is just one of the numerous types of problems that people with depression face. But getting the hang of something new is always easier if you have examples, so we use her story throughout this chapter to provide further insight into how to follow our formula to solve your problems.

We use the example of Adele and her husband Eddie throughout this chapter to give you an idea on how problem solving works. First, we introduce Adele and her slowly growing realization that she has some difficulties to solve if she and Eddie will be able to have a happy marriage.

> **Adele** married her husband **Eddie,** a self-described computer geek, at the age of 19. On their 25th wedding anniversary, Adele realizes that she's fallen into an oppressive boredom. She and Eddie don't seem to talk to each other anymore, and their life together feels stale and boring. Her children are mostly off living their own lives, and her job seems less interesting than it used to be. She tries to discuss her feelings with Eddie, but he's uninterested and distant. As the months go on, Adele slowly slides into a deepening depression. She contemplates getting a divorce or having an affair, although neither option appeals to her. She feels stuck, and she's unable to see a way out.

Drawing Up the Problem-Solving Game Plan — S.O.C.C.E.R.

In recent years, the problem-solving approach to combating depression has gained wider popularity due to increased research efforts that have demonstrated its effectiveness. The primary goals of this approach, when applied to depression, are to

>> Uncover life problems that may be contributing to depression

>> Figure out how depression decreases coping

>> Teach effective problem-solving techniques

>> Prevent relapse as a result of improved skills

TIP

To make our problem-solving plan easy to remember, we base it on the acronym S.O.C.C.E.R. S.O.C.C.E.R. guides you through a series of steps. These steps will help you find effective solutions to your problems and help you implement these solutions.

> >> **S** stands for the *situation,* or the problem itself. The situation includes the nature and cause(s) of the problem, your feelings about the problem, and your beliefs about trying to solve it. For example, you may believe that the problem is insurmountable. That belief is part of the situation or problem.

>> **O** stands for any and all possible *options* for approaching the problem creatively.

>> **C** stands for the likely *consequences* that carrying out each option entails.

>> **C** involves making a final *choice* about which option you want to try.

>> **E** stands for your *emotional plan* for carrying out your option, because some choices require a bit of courage.

>> **R** stands for *run it* and *review*. This step calls for you to implement your plan and then review the outcome in terms of whether your solution worked. It also includes figuring out what to do next if your plan doesn't work.

TIP

S.O.C.C.E.R. problem-solving game plans don't guarantee success. But the approach does give you a better way to think through your problems. A thorough analysis helps improve your chances of discovering and implementing the best possible solutions. S.O.C.C.E.R. helps alleviate depression by increasing your confidence and competence.

In the following sections, we explore each of the steps in the S.O.C.C.E.R game plan individually. Like many of the exercises throughout this book, most of the steps involve putting pen to paper (or fingers to keyboard), so get out a notebook (or turn on your computer).

WARNING

If you currently view the problems in your life as utterly hopeless, and you can't imagine even attempting to tackle them, please seek professional help prior to using our problem-solving plan. Getting help is especially important if you have feelings that life is not worth living or you're experiencing suicidal thoughts. The plan may still help you, but you'll need professional assistance to carry it out.

Assessing Your Problem Situation (S)

The first step in our S.O.C.C.E.R problem-solving approach entails a careful observation of the ins and outs of the current conundrum. You need to consider a number of issues, which we cover in the following sections.

Come up with a description of the problem

Carefully consider what the problem actually involves. If a problem seems to entail a variety of issues, try to zero in on one important aspect first. After you zero in on a key issue, write down as much about the nature of the problem as you can.

> Adele (who we describe at the beginning of the chapter) reflects and decides that the quality of her marriage is a larger problem than boredom — although the latter still plays an unwelcome role. She decides to zero in on her marriage. She also realizes that she and her husband don't share any common interests; they rarely have sex anymore, and their evenings usually consist of her watching mindless television for several hours while he works on the computer. She wants a change, but she doesn't know what to do.

Reflect on your feelings about the problem

Reflecting on all the feelings you have regarding a given problem is important. Doing so helps you understand the impact of the problem on your life.

> Adele realizes that boredom is one of the feelings she is experiencing. She has to work hard to figure out the rest of her feelings, because she has a habit of thinking that she doesn't deserve much from life and that she has no right to have certain types of feelings, such as anger. However, Adele eventually concludes that, in addition to boredom, she feels resentment and anger toward her husband and anxiety about the possibility of leaving her marriage.

Consider the causes of the problem

Depression may mislead you when it comes to figuring out the causes of your problem. Depressed minds often make the assumption that the person who has the problem is also the cause of the entire problem. Although you may be partially responsible for the problem, considering any and all causes of the problem is important. Sometimes an understanding of all the causes can point the way toward certain solutions.

> In Adele's case, she first blames herself for being an inadequate, unexciting wife. As she ponders the situation further, she realizes that she has made attempts to improve things and her husband Eddie has rebuffed her. She concludes that another cause may lie in the emptiness they've both felt since their second and last child chose to attend an out-of-state college six months ago. Finally, she speculates that she and Eddie were left feeling like they have no social outlets after their close friends moved away last year.

Search for information about the problem

Odds are, you're not the first person to ever experience a problem like the one you're having. Look around for websites, books, and articles on the subject. Whether the problem lies in the area of finance, relationships, career, sex, in-law troubles, difficulties with your kids, or whatever, articles on the subject probably exist in abundance. Read. In addition, consider talking to an expert in the area for further advice.

> Adele, who prefers to listen to podcasts and watch YouTube videos to get her information, learns about a well known researcher in marriage and relationships, Dr. John Gottman. She watches several of his short videos and picks up some good tips that she hopes will help her marriage.

Consider the importance of the problem

Ask yourself how much this problem matters to you and your life. Will solving it help you? If so, how much? You can rate the problem on a scale of 0 (no importance to you whatsoever) to 100 (nothing in the world could be more important). This rating may tell you how much effort to put into the project.

> Adele realizes that the quality of her marriage matters a great deal to her. She rates the issue as 75 on a 0 to 100 point scale. She decides that it's worth putting some work into.

Check out solution-interfering beliefs

After you've described the preceding aspects of the problem, a crucial step remains. You need to ask yourself if you have any beliefs that may interfere with your attempts to solve the problem. These beliefs can stop you from even attempting to do something about your problem. Therefore, they form part of the problem itself.

> Adele realizes that she has five major beliefs that may put up a barrier to her problem-solving attempts. Her interfering beliefs happen to be the ones we encounter most often when we teach problem solving to our patients.

TIP

Table 14-1 lists the five beliefs that most commonly interfere with problem solving (in our experiences) and provides positive alternative ways of looking at those beliefs to facilitate solutions.

TABLE 14-1

Common Solution-Interfering Beliefs and Some Facilitating Views

Solution-Interfering Belief	Facilitating View
My problems are too big to solve.	Sure my problems are large, but they don't have to be solved all at once. People solve big problems all the time. It just takes persistence.
I don't think my problem is solvable.	Of course, it's always possible that my problem isn't solvable, in which case I'll have to work on figuring out how to cope with it. However, I won't know if it's solvable unless I try everything I can first.
I'm not a good problem solver.	Well, I haven't always tackled big problems easily in the past, but that doesn't mean I can't learn. The S.O.C.C.E.R. problem-solving plan looks pretty straightforward. Besides, what do I have to lose by trying?
I prefer to let problems solve themselves.	Oh sure, I guess that could happen — probably when pigs fly. My experience has been that problems usually just stick around or get worse if I don't do something about them.
If I try and fail to solve my problem, I'll just feel like an even bigger failure. It's better not to try.	And of course if I don't try, I'll ensure failure. Besides, if my attempts fail, I just may learn something from the failure and make another run at the problem, armed with additional information.

TIP

If you discover that you have beliefs standing in the way of your attempt to solve the problems in your life, put them in a table like Table 14-1 and see if you can come up with facilitating views that counter those interfering beliefs. If you attempt this strategy and come up short on alternative views, consider reading Chapters 6, 7, and 8 for more information on dealing with problematic thoughts and beliefs.

Foraging for Options (O)

Step two in our S.O.C.C.E.R. problem-solving plan helps you find possible solutions for your problem. At this point, you need to suspend all judgment while searching far and wide for these solutions. Write down anything your mind comes up with; don't listen to your internal critic saying, "That's a really stupid idea!" We ask you to evaluate your ideas later, not now. Sometimes the most absurd solution leads to another idea that's more grounded in reality.

Creative solution searching without judgment is also known as *brainstorming*. We've found three ways to improve your brainstorming ability — "letting go," "thinking visually," and "permitting playfulness." After your brainstorming session, you can review all the options you come up with.

Letting go

Believe it or not, if you try too hard to solve a problem, you're likely to hit a wall. Too much intensity can stifle creativity. You need to give the process time; don't push yourself. You've probably been working on the problem for quite a while, so taking a little more time to solve it isn't going to hurt anything — in fact, it just may help.

TIP

First, we suggest relaxing your mind and body as a means for unleashing your creative potential. We have a quick relaxation technique you can use for this purpose:

1. Place your hand on your abdomen.

2. Take a slow, deep breath, and watch your abdomen expand.

3. Hold that breath momentarily.

4. Slowly breathe out and let your shoulders droop.

5. As you exhale, say the word *relax.*

6. Repeat this exercise ten times.

If you practice this relaxation technique several times a day for five days in a row, you may find it helps to calm your mind and body. If it doesn't work for you, or even if it makes your tension worse, you may want to read Chapter 21 for more ideas on how to let go. Also, if you suffer from anxiety in addition to your depression, you may want to also read another book of ours, *Anxiety For Dummies* (Wiley).

You may profit from other letting-go strategies when attempting to search for options to your problem. We often find our best ideas for writing or other problems when we take our two dogs out for a long walk or jog. Somehow the obvious pleasure the dogs experience helps distract us from any worries or concerns. Thus, our minds feel free to wander and consider new possibilities without pressure.

Feel free to experiment with exercise. Other activities like walking, weight lifting, or yoga (see Chapter 12) are also good ideas. Or you can try a recreational activity that you enjoy as a means to let go (which we cover in Chapter 13). Of course, hot tubs aren't bad either.

REMEMBER

Letting go as a way of finding creative solutions works best if you don't force your mind to find answers.

Thinking visually

Many people find that their creative juices start flowing more easily when they get into a visual mode. You can start by relaxing and picturing your problem in your mind. Picture, in your imagination, the various ways you can tackle the problem; do so without the expectation of necessarily carrying any particular idea out.

TIP

Some people find that flow charts and diagrams help them find better options for solving their problems. Try picturing all the components of your problem in separate boxes. Draw possible solutions to each component in these separate boxes, and then draw arrows to the relevant component of the problem.

Adele put her marital problems on a flow chart. She put each component of her problematic marriage in a box, and then she developed solutions for each one. Take a look at Figure 14-1 to get your juices flowing. It contains one of the components of Adele's situation as well as ideas for attacking the problem.

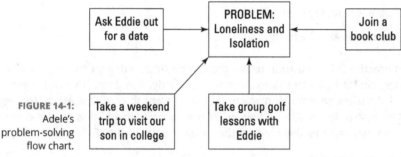

FIGURE 14-1: Adele's problem-solving flow chart.

© John Wiley and Sons, Inc.

Permitting playfulness

Yes, we realize the seriousness of your problem. However, allowing yourself to play with ideas is important. Realize that rigidity merely keeps you stuck. Play with the most absurd solutions imaginable. Play allows you to forget about the usual rules and break out of the box.

One way to play around is to consider solutions that appear to be the total opposite of your first ideas. For example, Adele (who we describe at the beginning of this chapter) has a difficult marriage. One solution she considers is having an affair. Then she thinks of the opposite — having an affair with her husband. "How absurd," she initially thinks to herself.

But then she realizes that it just may be worth a try. She can imagine that he's a man who she just met and finds attractive (after all, she did find him very attractive years ago, and he hasn't changed all that much). Then she can plot how to seduce him.

Reviewing your options

As you brainstorm options for dealing with your problem, list everything that you come up with. Don't leave any ideas out at this point. After you finish writing your list down, review it and see if a little pondering leads to more ideas.

Adele lists options for handling her marital problems. As you can see, Adele's options list contains possibilities that range from probably productive to downright destructive:

- Have an affair.

- Have an affair with my husband.

- Get a divorce.

- Ask for a temporary separation so that I can clear my head.

- Seek marital counseling if I can convince Eddie to go.

- Simply work on my own to improve our marriage by showing more caring and affection, as well as by working on being non-defensive (which we cover in Chapter 16).

- Go on an exotic trip to Asia and not tell anyone.

- Focus on making myself happy in ways that aren't related to my marriage, such as developing new hobbies, looking for a more interesting career, expanding my social circle, finding volunteer work, and so on.

- Drink more.

- Quit my whining and try to forget about this issue!

TIP

We expect that your list of possible solutions may contain options ranging from really helpful to pretty destructive. Good brainstorming avoids judgment of even the wildest options. The evaluation phase comes next. In this phase, you don't evaluate yourself for having good or bad ideas; instead, you merely evaluate the likely consequences of your ideas.

Contemplating Consequences (C)

TIP

Take the options you cook up in the earlier "Foraging for Options" section of this chapter and list them in the "Options" column of a two-column table, as shown in Table 14-2. Next, label the second column "Likely Consequences." Then contemplate each option, one at a time. For each option, list possible outcomes or consequences. Think about the probability of each outcome when you begin to consider what option might work the best.

Table 14-2 lists Adele's options and the outcomes she deemed most likely for each one. This example can give you an idea of how to begin your table.

TABLE 14-2   **Likely Consequences of Adele's Options**

Options	Likely Consequences
Have an affair.	Fun and excitement; guilt and regret; sexually transmitted disease; eventual ruination of my marriage
Have an affair with my husband.	Fun and excitement; possible enhancement of my marriage; utter rejection from my husband
Get a divorce.	Some relief from the struggle; sadness and loss; eventually, a new and better relationship; possible loss of close relationships with my kids
Temporary separation.	Clear my head to see what I really want to do; increased distance from my husband; increased chance my husband will have an affair or just decide to leave me
Seek marital counseling if Eddie will go.	Improvement in the marriage if he agrees; anger and rage from Eddie because he's always opposed this idea; rejection from Eddie; divorce if it doesn't work
Work on my own to improve marriage.	Improve marriage; harm marriage in some way; get more frustrated
Go on an exotic trip and not tell anyone.	Fun and excitement; guilt; end my marriage when Eddie finds out
Increase my own happiness through a new career.	Be happier; become more distant from my husband; not be so dependent on his attention
Drink more.	Temporary decrease in pain; become addicted to alcohol; increase pain in the long run
Quit whining and forget the problem.	Increased dissatisfaction; marriage will unlikely improve on its own

Sometimes this exercise points the way to a single, simple solution that stands out as the obvious option. But all too frequently, the best options aren't so obvious. So, in the next section, we help you dive in and make a choice.

Choosing Your Plan (C)

After you go through the first three steps of the S.O.C.C.E.R. problem-solving plan, you can choose your option(s). Make a commitment to yourself.

Even when you decide not to choose an option for dealing with your problem, you're still making a choice — you're choosing to live with your problem "as is."

The fourth step in the S.O.C.C.E.R. problem-solving plan requires you to carefully reflect on each and every option. You may be able to quickly zero in on the one, two, three, or perhaps four best possibilities simply by reviewing the likely consequences of each. Tune into your feelings about each option. Does the option make you feel hopeful, distressed, anxious, calm, angry, sad, relieved, eager, or some combination of these feelings? Your feelings may provide you with additional information.

Please realize that the option you choose for dealing with your problem can entail a combination of several options; they don't have to be mutually exclusive.

Adele picks three options that look like they have the best chance of helping her distressed marriage:

- Do everything I can on my own to improve the marriage.
- Increase my own happiness by exploring a new career.
- Seek marital counseling.

After further reflection, Adele decides not to choose the option of having an affair with her husband — he has seriously rebuffed her sexual advances in the past, and she doesn't want to risk rejection again. She decides that the first two options from the previous list could improve her happiness without incurring great risk. Even though she initially believed that exploring a new career could create distance from her husband, she believes that it won't do so if she combines it with the first two ideas.

Adele has just one problem. She greatly fears that she'll incur Eddie's wrath if she brings up marital counseling one more time. And if it doesn't work, she fears an increased chance of a gut-wrenching divorce. Is this the choice she really wants to make?

If you find yourself stuck with indecision about one or more of the options you've chosen, we have two more strategies that may help: Consulting the Friend Within and Choosing Sides. You'll need a couple of chairs for both of them. Yes, chairs — just go with us on this one.

Consulting the friend within

You have a friend that you can call on for another perspective. That friend resides in you! This technique may be one of the simplest you find in this book. But don't be fooled by the simplicity.

TIP

We find the Consulting the Friend Within strategy to be surprisingly useful. To use this strategy, sit down in a chair and place an empty chair opposite from you. Imagine a close friend of yours is sitting in that chair. Your friend happens to have pretty much the same problem you do; she came up with the same choice for a solution, but dreads carrying it out. Start talking to your friend. Talk out loud. When you're done, ask if the advice sounds good for you, too.

You may not only think that this idea sounds simplistic, but you may also wonder how it could possibly help you when you failed to choose an option up to now. Well, frankly, we aren't entirely sure why it works, but it does. We suspect that it's because the procedure helps give you a little emotional distance from the issue, which frees up your stuck mindset.

Adele tries this strategy. Here's her imaginary monologue with her friend:

> "Well, you know, as much as working on your marriage on your own sounds like a great idea, I doubt it will work unless you combine it with marital therapy. Sure you're scared! But do you really have anything to lose by trying? What are the odds that your marriage will work out on its own if marital therapy fails? Pretty low, I would guess. Your husband gets angry, but he's never beaten you. If he gets angry, so what? It happened plenty of times before, and you lived through it. If he totally rejects the idea, try again. Then again, if he still won't go at the end of the day, maybe you need to listen to that information and consider other options. Stop avoiding the issue!"

Adele finds this exercise helpful, but she doesn't quite feel ready to implement her decision to ask Eddie to go to marital counseling. She needs one more technique: Choosing Sides. You can give it a shot too.

Choosing sides

TIP

The Choosing Sides strategy, like the preceding Consulting the Friend Within technique, requires you to place two chairs facing each other. Label the first chair as representing one side of your argument and the second chair as representing the other position. Sit in Chair No. 1 and imagine the other side of your argument is sitting in Chair No. 2. Argue with the other side out loud and as forcefully as you can. When you run out of steam, switch chairs and argue the other side of your argument.

Are you going to feel a little silly? Maybe. But do this technique by yourself and have a go at it. You may be surprised at how useful you find it to be. Psychologists have recommended this approach for many decades, and clients continue to report that it helps them reach difficult decisions.

Here's what Adele's dialogue sounds like when she tries the Choosing Sides strategy to help her determine if her option of marital counseling truly is the best option for her. She labels Chair No. 1 "Get Counseling" and Chair No. 2 "Don't Do It."

Get Counseling chair (Speaking to the Don't Do It chair): "Look, you know that counseling has the best chance of succeeding. You made a few attempts on your own, but they didn't work. You reviewed the likely consequences, and you know that getting help looks better than anything else."

Don't Do It chair: "Okay, sure. I thought about it carefully, but the bottom line is that I don't think I could stand it if therapy failed and I ended up divorced. The loneliness and sense of loss would feel overwhelming to me."

Get Counseling chair: "Oh, so that's what's holding you back! First, who says marital therapy will fail? The odds aren't that bad if you combine it with your own efforts. You already found those ideas in the books you've read encouraging. With the help of a trained professional, it just may work."

Don't Do It chair: "Sure, but if Eddie rejects it, I'll just feel more frustrated and angry. That would increase the odds of divorce. Bottom line is — I don't think I could stand it."

Get Counseling chair: "So you think that ignoring the problem has a better chance? I doubt it! If your marriage is headed for divorce, it's better you find out now than later. And who says you couldn't stand it? People get divorced every day, and most manage to get through it."

Don't Do It chair: "But I'd hate it."

Get Counseling chair: "Of course you wouldn't like to get divorced! I don't know many people who do. But stop saying you couldn't stand it. You were okay on your own before you met Eddie, and you could do it again. Furthermore, dating may not sound too great right now, but other men are out there you know."

Don't Do It chair: "Okay, I get your point. I wouldn't like it, but life would probably go on. Somehow I'll find the courage to carry this option out . . . I think, anyway."

Adele feels more resolute in her decision to seek marital counseling after trying the Choosing Sides technique. Nevertheless, she quivers and trembles at the thought of approaching Eddie. She's still not sure she has the courage to do this.

Some options for solving problems can cause unexpected reactions. You can be quite certain that your decision is the right one but still feel fearful. If that's the case for you, you may need an emotional plan for helping you proceed. And we just happen to have one for you in the section that follows.

Handling Your Emotions (E)

Assuming that you chose the option or options that look as though they have the best possible chance of helping to solve your problem, troublesome emotions may sabotage your best intentions. This step in the problem-solving process is best viewed as a crutch for helping you implement your choice.

TIP

If you feel great uncertainty about your selection, go back through the suggestions on the topics of foraging for options, contemplating consequences, and choosing your plan in the earlier sections of this chapter. If you come up with the same solution and still feel uneasy, rest assured that your uneasiness represents normal feelings that can be handled with this problem-solving step.

REMEMBER

Most solutions to difficult problems require a little courage to carry out. If that weren't so, the solutions would probably pop into your mind more easily. After all, we did say "difficult" problems.

Two fairly simple techniques can help quell the queasiness that lies in the pit of your stomach as you anticipate acting on your solution: rehearsal and self-talk.

Holding the dress rehearsal

Imagine the quality of a Broadway musical if the musicians, actors, and actresses never attended rehearsals. The performers' stage fright would then make good sense, because no one would know what to do. The production would likely result in disaster. And it probably wouldn't take long for the audience to start throwing tomatoes. Rehearsals not only enhance performance, they also help to decrease stage fright.

TIP

If your problem-solving option involves a confrontation with someone or stirs up anxiety, rehearsal may help. You can rehearse your plan

>> In your mind

>> In front of a mirror

>> Through role-playing with a trusted friend

>> By writing out a script

Talking to yourself

You may be thinking, "Talk to myself? Do you guys think I'm crazy?" Actually, most people talk to themselves. However, people don't often try to control the content of their self-talk; they merely go on autopilot. And if they feel anxious or depressed, their self-talk usually contains negative predictions and self-defeating statements.

REMEMBER

The short positive self-statements in the following paragraphs are no cure for depression, nor do they work for long-term issues and problems. However, they can serve as a temporary band-aid for getting you through difficult moments.

You can decide to select new, more productive content for your self-talk. In order to push out negative thinking, you may first need to rehearse the script out loud. Write down short, simple, positive statements. Possibilities include the following:

>> What I'm about to do is the right thing to do.

>> This is really hard, but I can do it.

>> I considered all the options.

>> I have the right to do this.

>> Just do it.

Returning to Adele's situation, here's what she decides to do:

> Good ol' Adele decides to ask her husband Eddie to see a marital counselor as a means for solving her problem — the state of her marriage. She makes an appointment on an evening that's free on both of their calendars. First, she rehearses how she's going to approach Eddie with the idea. Then she chooses the self-talk coping phrase, "I can handle whatever reaction he has." She uses this phrase like a mantra, repeating it over and over in her mind as she approaches her husband.

Running and Reviewing (R)

Okay, at this point, you've gone through all the problem-solving steps but the final one. You've described the problem situation, chosen an option, and you're ready to roll. The time has come to take a run at your problem and execute your plan.

The chances of your problem working out are higher because you've done your homework. Nevertheless, S.O.C.C.E.R. doesn't come with an unconditional guarantee. After you implement your solution, review how it worked. Carefully consider what worked and what may not have. Perhaps all went well and the problem has been resolved. But if the problem or a remnant remains, go back to the drawing board and start a new S.O.C.C.E.R. game plan.

Here's how Adele's S.O.C.C.E.R. plan works out:

> Adele repeats, "I can handle whatever reaction he has," in her mind repeatedly as she enters the study where Eddie is sitting at the computer. "Eddie, could we talk for a couple of minutes?"
>
> Eddie swivels to face her and replies, "Okay, but not too long, I'm in the middle of something."
>
> "This won't take long. I've been concerned about our marriage; neither of us seems very happy," Adele begins.
>
> Eddie interrupts her, "Speak for yourself. I'm not unhappy. Women, they're never satisfied. What more could you want? This isn't paradise; it's real life."
>
> Adele, who is now close to tears, continues, "I'm not asking for the moon, Eddie. I want us to be closer. And I've made an appointment with a marriage counselor. It's for next Thursday at 6 p.m. I want you to come with me."

"Forget it. I'm not going to some touchy-feely, nosey therapist," Eddie's voice rises, "Here's another way you've found to throw my hard-earned money away. I'm not going to waste my time talking about this!" Eddie turns back to his computer and ignores Adele.

Ugh. Adele went through all the steps and received a lousy outcome. It takes her a couple of days to recoup, but she goes through a new S.O.C.C.E.R. game plan. This time she decides to go to counseling by herself and explore other options with the counselor. After several sessions, the counselor helps Adele find a better way to ask Eddie to attend at least a few sessions with her.

Over a period of months, Eddie realizes how much he values Adele. Both commit to making their marriage stronger.

TIP

We confess, sometimes we like to have a happy ending. In some cases, especially with long-term marital problems, things don't work out so smoothly. But hard work and therapy can help many of the most difficult relationships get stronger. In addition, therapy can help someone with depression get through a difficult breakup and find contentment in other ways. So even when problems seem insurmountable, it's worth stepping back and taking a logical, problem-solving approach. And don't hesitate to get help when you feel stuck.

REMEMBER

If you or someone you care about is depressed, problems loom larger than life. And solutions seem amazingly elusive. Take the time to prepare a game plan. See how S.O.C.C.E.R. works for you.

4 Rebuilding Connections

IN THIS PART . . .

Cope with losses from life transitions and work through grief.

Communicate more clearly.

Plan positive interactions.

Chapter **15**

Working Through Loss, Grief, and Mourning

H ave you ever stood at the kitchen counter with tears welling up in your eyes as you quickly cut onions? If so, you've experienced your body's response to irritants. Tears help clear out the noxious molecules released by the sliced onion. However, after tearing up over onions, you probably don't feel any change in your emotional state. In fact you just might feel a bit annoyed by the pain you're experiencing in your irritated eyes.

As you're also probably aware, your body produces tears in response to another stimulus — strong emotions. The two types of tears have different chemical compositions. Given the nearly universal reports of relief following emotional crying, scientists speculate that crying somehow cleanses the body of emotional toxins and brings it back to a more relaxed state.

Grief and crying are normal reactions to loss. However, sometimes grief lingers and disrupts life in major ways. Mourning can trigger depression (see Chapter 2 for a description of the types of depression). Loss may cause depressed feelings without your awareness. Sometimes events in the past continue to plague you far longer than you realize. Even if you haven't experienced a major loss in decades, looking at unresolved grief as a possible cause of your current depression may yield fruitful insight.

In this chapter, we explore the uniquely human response to loss. We discuss the various types of losses people experience and how they react to them. If you're depressed, consider whether any of your problematic feelings stem from one of these losses. Working through your grief may help relieve your depression, so we give you a variety of ways for working through grief, whether it's a normal, uncomplicated grief or a profound, traumatic experience.

Losing What You Care About

All people experience loss of one kind or another during their lives. People grieve about all different types of losses. Yet the response to each particular loss varies from person to person. We don't have any easy way to tell how someone will react when something bad happens. And there's no right or wrong way to handle loss. Some people seem to bounce back quickly, while others remain in a prolonged state of intense grief.

WARNING

If your grief stretches over many months without letup, if you're overwhelmed by thoughts of yearning and loss, if you have thoughts about the futility of the future, or if you feel worthless and excessively guilty, you may have a complicated grief and/or a major depressive disorder (see Chapter 2 for more information about grief and various types of depression). If you have any of these symptoms, seek professional assistance. Both of these conditions require prompt treatment.

We can't possibly give you a complete list of the types of losses that lead to grief, but the three major categories are

>> Death

>> Life transitions

>> Relationship loss

In the following sections, we discuss these categories of loss at length. There's no right or wrong way to deal with such losses. Understanding how each event affects you is what's important. With awareness, you can draw on your resources for coping. In the "Working Through Grief" section, later in this chapter, we give you ideas for handling these losses effectively.

ARE THERE STAGES OF GRIEF?

Elisabeth Kubler-Ross, MD, is a psychiatrist who devoted the majority of her professional career to the care of the dying. Her widely cited book, *On Death and Dying* (Scribner), proposed that people go through a series of stages when they face terminal illness:

- **Denial:** No way, I'm not sick; it can't be me!
- **Anger:** Damn it! Why me?
- **Bargaining:** God, help me! I'll do anything to get out of this.
- **Depression:** I just can't go on, I can't stand it. I give up.
- **Acceptance:** This is the end; I'll try to go in peace with dignity.

These stages have been extended to include reactions to other types of loss, such as death of a loved one, loss of physical health, or relationship breakups. However, each person is a unique individual, and it appears that not everyone goes through all the stages reported by Kubler-Ross. Research indicates that people may bounce from one stage to another, skipping some or even returning to an earlier stage. In that sense, they really aren't best thought of as stages so much as states of emotional reactions that people frequently experience when grieving a loss.

Yet some mental health counselors erroneously believe that resolution of grief only comes about after experiencing all these stages of grief in sequence. But no single, healthy way of going through the grief process exists. Each person grieves in a unique way. Kubler-Ross's work has helped people around the world handle difficult transitions. However, grief is complicated, diverse, and not easily categorized.

Losing someone

Death is never easy to deal with. Even people with strong religious convictions feel great sadness upon the loss of a loved one. Unexpected death generally is more difficult to accept than death following a prolonged illness. But the period of anticipation before the loss isn't the only factor that affects the response to death. For example, the person's age, the difficulty of the dying process, whether there was an opportunity to say goodbye, and the remaining resources and connections available to the griever all contribute to the reaction in complicated ways.

REMEMBER

Your relationship to the individual also plays a large role in how the loss affects you:

>> **Death of a life partner:** This type of loss is often thought to be one of the most difficult to get through. It requires major adjustments.

>> **Death of a child:** Most experts believe that this loss probably involves the most painful, lengthy recovery. Somehow it feels as though it's against the laws of nature for a child to precede a parent in death.

>> **Death of a parent:** The difficulty of this loss hinges on many factors, such as the age of the parent and child at the time of the death, the nature of the relationship, and unresolved issues. Sometimes the grief is actually intensified if the relationship was stormy and conflicted.

>> **Death of friends and relatives:** Again, the difficulty of dealing with departed friends and relatives varies considerably.

>> **Death of someone you care about through suicide:** As we discuss in Chapter 10, the loss of someone through suicide may involve more difficult emotions such as guilt and regret.

>> **Death of a pet:** The attachments people form with their animals can be very strong. Pets become special family members. Sometimes other people don't fully appreciate or understand the intensity of the bereavement that the loss of a pet can evoke. Such a lack of understanding by others can compound the sense of isolation.

>> **Death of others:** Sometimes a traumatic event witnessed by uninvolved parties can cause grief reactions. For example, when a drunk driver kills a child, it may re-traumatize a family that lost a child years before. Or witnessing a violent crime or combat death may also cause the observer to mourn.

CAN DOGS EXPERIENCE GRIEF?

We recently lost one of our dogs. Although she was an elderly dog, we both mourned the loss and still miss her most days. Our younger dog also seemed lost without his sister. Normally, he would go for his daily walk with tail high and wagging while enthusiastically sniffing every bush. After her death, we noticed him listlessly walking, tail straight down, seemingly searching for her.

Veterinarians report that dogs experience loss in many ways similar to people. They often show a loss of energy, loss of appetite, and loss of interest. Luckily for us, our younger dog appears to have rebounded and actually seems to be enjoying his new status as "only dog." We'll see how long that lasts!

Transitioning through life

Nothing ever remains completely the same. People have a variety of roles to play in life. For example, people are parents, employees, employers, students, husbands, wives, or partners. Much of the way people define themselves comes from such roles.

People also define themselves according to their self-visions, such as seeing yourself as a person who is consistently healthy, safe, prestigious, attractive, and so on. Yet, roles and self-visions frequently change due to unavoidable circumstances. When these changes take place, the transition can be smooth or rocky.

People routinely fail to appreciate the impact that transitioning from one role or self-vision to another can have on their sense of self and well-being. When the transition involves a loss (and many transitions do), grieving or depression can result. Sometimes the transition is obvious, such as when you lose a job; other times the transition is more subtle, such as losing a feeling of safety because of an increase in the crime rate where you live.

TIP

No one responds in exactly the same way to these life transitions. As with death, no right or wrong answer exists. The types of transitions that frequently cause trouble include

>> **Leaving home:** Adolescents and young adults often look forward to the day when they can leave home. However, when they actually do leave, they experience loss, as well, and they're generally quite surprised. No longer can they turn to their parents for instant advice and support. They may feel a loss of connection, and they may sense a loss of the free, irresponsible aspects of childhood. Another related loss comes at graduation time. The young person must move on from the familiar routines and friendships of high school or college and onto new, unexplored responsibilities.

>> **Getting married:** You may wonder why we include marriage as a troubling transition. For most people, marriage is a joyous but nerve-wracking time in life. Yet marriage includes losses, which occasionally lead to unexpected feelings of depression. When you get married, you give up your identity as a single person. You may lose contact with single friends. Like leaving home, marriage requires giving up the irresponsibility of childhood.

>> **Having a baby:** Another joyous occasion! But along with considerable love and joy, bringing a newborn into your life causes a loss of freedom and ushers in new stress. When you have a baby, you find yourself having to spend more money, and you lose the opportunity to sleep in on Saturday mornings.

WARNING

Experiencing some minor distress after having a baby is normal for both parents. However, depression in women after childbirth can become serious: This condition is referred to as *postpartum depression*. See Chapter 2 for details about this disturbing condition that requires prompt treatment.

- » **Changing jobs:** Whether you're starting your first job, getting a promotion or demotion, or going through a layoff or firing, changing what you do everyday entails stress and loss. A first job leads to a loss of free time. A promotion can lead to overwhelming responsibilities. Demotions, layoffs, and firings cause a loss of both money and status.

- » **Going to jail:** Being convicted of a crime and subsequently incarcerated entails numerous losses. Duh.

- » **Experiencing major economic and political changes in society:** All stock markets decline. Most people know a few people who had to postpone retirement or had problems sending their kids to college when stocks plummeted. Most of the time, no one feels enduring disappointment when political leadership changes hands. However, in some countries, new regimes can bring on the loss of freedom, economic hardship, or possibly war. These changes can disrupt families and lives in devastating ways.

- » **Loss of feeling safe:** The 2020 COVID-19 pandemic changed the world in many ways. Most people felt a loss in the confidence of a predictable world. In addition, other losses included loss of freedom of movement, of social connections, financial security, and health. Rates of anxiety and depression soared across the globe.

- » **Moving:** Moving to a new home, whether in the same city or somewhere else, is exciting, but it comes with losses. You may lose connections with friends, the simplicity of your former residence, or the sense of history with a place you cared about for a long time.

- » **Dealing with an empty nest:** Parenting is the only loving relationship in which the goal is to foster independence and eventual departure. Do your job well and your children leave you. You may feel not only the loss of the kids but your role as a mother or father, as well.

- » **Going through a chronic illness:** The diagnosis of a chronic illness shakes up your world. You lose a measure of control over your life; suddenly the health-care system takes charge of significant aspects of your daily living. You encounter the loss of invincibility. In addition, your financial situation, freedom, and status may suffer.

- » **Aging:** You'd probably rather be old than the alternative. Nevertheless, aging inevitably illuminates the certainty of death. Along with the threat of loss of life itself comes the loss of function, loved ones, independence, appearance, status, and good health.

TIP

These changes are expected over the course of a lifetime. But depression may be an unexpected consequence. If you feel intense sadness or depression, and you can't figure out why, review the recent transitions in your life. Ask yourself if any of the issues we discuss in the previous list may be part of the problem.

ANTICIPATORY GRIEF

Millions of people throughout the world are caregivers to family members with chronic illness. As the illness progresses, there can be changes in the needs and abilities of the person with the disease. Both the person who is ill and the caregiver experience what is called *anticipatory grief,* which is when people mourn what is currently lost and the loss of the once-hoped-for future.

The person who is receiving care may mourn the loss of health, role in the family, self-esteem, and possibly mental abilities. The person with illness may feel guilty for new dependence on others and be very frightened by the potential of future disabilities. The caregiver is also likely to experience grief — from the loss of the previous relationship, the anticipated loss due to illness, and from loss of freedom. Caregivers often assume added responsibilities in the home and are at a high risk for depression. Since the health of the caregiver can prevent unnecessary hospitalizations and long-term care, it is imperative that they receive needed support from other family members, friends, and, when necessary, healthcare professionals.

With adequate support, this challenging time of loss can lead to stronger family relationships, deeper communications, and appreciation for the life already lived. The anticipation can lead to precious times of care and love that make the loss a part of life to cherish.

Facing the challenges of isolation

The COVID-19 pandemic highlighted the stress of isolation among large groups of the population. Stay-at-home orders sent many workers home to put together a semblance of a home office. Social distancing, mask wearing, and the restrictions on crowd size have increased a sense of isolation for many. These public health actions were ordered to reduce the spread of the virus. Many people experienced a rise in anxiety and depression; however, most people were able to cope with the disruption of normal life.

Sadly, many senior citizens have fared less well with the imposed isolation. Millions of seniors lacked social connections prior to the pandemic, and loneliness is a serious second pandemic for an already isolated population. Seniors may feel invisible in isolated rural neighborhoods or high-rise apartments. Loneliness in senior citizens have been associated with premature death and illness. One study indicated that isolation is a greater health risk to seniors than obesity, air pollution, smoking, and physical inactivity.

So the next time you are out and meet up with senior neighbors, be sure to check on how they are doing. Reach out to seniors when you can, and consider volunteering to pick up prescriptions or groceries. If you have a senior member in your family, for heaven's sake, give them a call or teach them how to use Zoom, FaceTime, or Skype.

Breaking up is so hard to do

Losing someone through a breakup or divorce can also lead to severe mourning. Unfortunately, society tends to provide much more support to those who lost a loved one through death than to those who lost someone through the end of a relationship. The typical expectation is that people will regroup and get on with their lives in a fairly short period of time. The intensity of grief that is felt after a breakup may catch people by surprise and overwhelm them. After a relationship ends, feelings of loneliness and isolation take hold.

Yet, when people consider breaking up, they too often fail to comprehend the magnitude of the disruption and loss. Thus, they make cavalier decisions about leaving loved ones. Anger, lust, or boredom may drive the choice to end the relationship.

When you break up with your partner, you potentially incur many types of losses:

>> **The relationship:** Companionship, affection, mutual goals, support, a sense of history accumulated with the partner, love, and sex.

>> **A vision:** Most people who begin a serious relationship together have an expectation concerning the future of the relationship. In the case of partners with children, the vision of an intact family disintegrates when the relationship ends.

>> **Family and friends:** Bonds with the family of the lost partner often vanish. Mutual friends sometimes choose sides.

>> **Finances:** Whether the money is spent on lawyers, therapists, or establishing two households, divorce or the breakup of live-in partners costs major dollars.

>> **Status:** Sometimes people derive prestige from the connection with their partner.

>> **Ego:** Your ego may suffer, especially when you feel like you are being rejected. However, even the person making the decision to leave is sometimes surprised by feelings of failure and guilt, and by the other losses we cover in this list.

There's not a right or wrong way to handle grief after a breakup or divorce. Giving yourself permission to feel whatever feelings come up can help you deal with the loss. If those feelings engulf you or endure, we provide strategies for helping you deal with your distress in the remaining pages of this chapter.

Working Through Grief

The loss of people, roles, and self-visions, as we describe earlier in this chapter, usually leads to feelings of grief. That's to be expected. However, such grief sometimes digs in and continues to disrupt happiness and well being well beyond the typical 6 to 12 months. When grief endures far longer, people often fail to realize the source of their unhappiness.

TIP

So if you're currently depressed, we suggest you consider if any losses in your life, whether recent or old, may be contributing to your melancholy. (And see Chapter 2 for more information on the differences between simple bereavement and depression.)

REMEMBER

Long-standing or complicated bereavement frequently requires professional assistance. Seek professional help if your efforts at self-help like the ones in this book don't bring substantial relief or if you have severe depressive symptoms.

If you determine that unresolved grief is part of your life, you need to think about how you can lighten your load. Explain your situation to trusted friends and family. Let them know that you'll need some extra consideration during this period of time by asking for their support and help. Consider delegating or even letting go of a few responsibilities for a while. Even if you're not physically ill or sick, you should give yourself the same considerations you'd give someone who is.

TIP

When you're ready to approach friends and family for their assistance and understanding, you may wonder how they're going to give you a break if your grief involves a loss from long ago. You may want to explain that your grief work is a temporary project, and that if you don't improve, you intend to seek professional help. Tell them you realize that it's been a very long time, and that you too were surprised by the discovery that grief was still causing you trouble.

Bereavement saps you of energy. Getting better takes effort and time — you can't push the process. While you're at it, don't forget to take care of your body:

>> Eat healthy foods.

>> Exercise on a regular basis.

>> Make sure that you're getting enough rest.

REMEMBER

Before you tackle the job of untangling your grief, you should understand that the goal of this work isn't to make you forget about your painful losses. Nor is it designed to make you give up caring about the absent person or other losses. Rather, the goal is to help you get back to the business of living a productive, happy life.

People sometimes say that they would feel consumed by guilt if they got over their grief. Again, working through grief isn't about "getting over it" *per se*. You'll always feel the loss, but you can refocus and renew your spirit. You deserve to love and laugh again.

WARNING

Working through grief may actually lead to an increase of negative feelings for a short time. These feelings are natural. If you experience significantly increased depression with feelings of hopelessness or thoughts of suicide, you need to get an immediate evaluation from a professional.

In the following sections, we discuss ways of coping with the loss of people, roles, and self-visions discussed in the "Losing What You Care About" section earlier in this chapter. The next section deals with the loss of important people in your life, whether from divorce, death, or separation.

Reconstructing the relationship

When grief endures or involves complex issues, people often focus on only the details of the loss they endured. In other cases, they fixate on some specific aspect of grief, such as the emptiness they feel. Having such a narrow focus can block your ability to process all the effects of the loss. It can also prevent you from experiencing difficult feelings.

TIP

We suggest broadening your field of vision to help you reconstruct all aspects of the lost relationship and what it meant to you. Appreciate the fact that no person consists of all positive or negative qualities. Then ask yourself the following Grief Exploration Questions. You may want to write down your answers to these questions in a notebook or notes app:

>> What was my life like with this person?

>> What difference did this person make in my life?

>> What did I value in this person, and what did I struggle with?

>> What did I learn from this person (both good and bad)?

>> How has my life changed as a result of this loss?

>> What do I feel resentful for with respect to this person?

>> What things do I feel grateful for with respect to my relationship?

Take your time answering these questions. They may require some careful pondering. And they may evoke unexpected pain. After you thoroughly exhaust your review, you may want to discuss and possibly compare your feelings with someone you fully trust who knew this person well.

When you complete this portion of the task, you may want to compose a letter to the person you lost. This letter can help you more fully process the meaning of the relationship and the nature of your loss.

REMEMBER

When you avoid feelings, you keep them stirring inside you. Expressing your feelings can help with healing.

Bruce's mother died when he was a child. Now, many years later, Bruce is a father. He discovers himself having sad feelings. Bruce concludes that he has unresolved grief. Bruce answers the Grief Exploration Questions, and then he processes his grief in the letter to his deceased mother in Figure 15-1.

Dear Mom,

Guess what? My wife and I have a baby. A girl — we named her after you. I've got a job and a house. And I'm doing pretty good. But after the baby, I started having some really sad times. I did some reading and I think it's about never really dealing with your death. I know it happened a long time ago, but I guess I never got over it.

I was only 12 years old when you left me. I was outside playing and a police car drove up. I ran up to the porch. Dad was standing there, already crying. I never saw him cry before. Mom, things changed so much after you died. Dad never got over it; he was sad or drunk most of the time. I started getting into more and more trouble. My life was pretty hard. I even spent some time in jail. I never talked about you to anyone. I wouldn't even let myself think about you. It hurt.

I knew I was sad, but I didn't realize until now how mad I am. I'm mad because I remember when you were home, you'd usually be in the bedroom. Somehow, I thought it was my fault you were always crying. I was lonely and scared. I'm mad, Mom, because you were so depressed but you didn't get help. I'm mad because Dad didn't get you help. Mom, if you cared about me, you wouldn't have killed yourself.

Now, I've said it. I am mad. But over the years I've learned that depression is an illness. And that you and Dad probably didn't realize that people could get help and get better. So, Mom, I forgive you for leaving me. And I promise to not let my own sad feelings hurt my little girl.

Love,
Your son, Bruce

FIGURE 15-1: Bruce's attempt to process his grief.

After you complete your reconstruction of the relationship, you'll be more prepared to deal with the next issue.

> **Eileen** left her husband two years ago. She experienced unexplained sadness, guilt, and anger. Her therapist helped her connect unresolved feelings about her divorce as the cause of these emotions. She first answers the Grief Exploration Questions we list earlier in this section. Then she constructs the letter in Figure 15-2.

> Dear Henry,
>
> Why did I leave you? I was afraid. Your rage was carefully hidden at times, but I never knew when it would surface. Henry, you never hit me, but the punishment was worse than being beaten. You tortured me with silence — silence that seemed to last forever. Silence for the holidays, on trips, for birthdays and graduations. Silence at the dinner table and after we made love.
>
> We never played with ideas or worked on compromise. You were always right; you knew the truth. I feared expressing my thoughts, feelings, or emotions, because if they differed from what you wanted to hear, you were angry. When you got angry, I was punished. The more critical you were with me, the more I withdrew from you. I couldn't properly plant tomatoes or fold the laundry. After losing self-confidence, self-worth, and self-control, I got help. And I became more independent and more ambitious — so that I could stand alone, and so that I wouldn't need you.
>
> I know you were deeply hurt as a child. I understand how my own overreactions to your criticism stemmed from my childhood issues. Now, from a distance, I remember the good times. You are a brilliant man and generous to a fault. You care about people. I hope you are happy.
>
> Take care,
> Eileen

FIGURE 15-2:
Eileen's letter to
her ex-husband.

TIP

When you're ready, ask yourself how you can begin the process of replacing as much of what you've lost as possible. You may want to think about active alternatives, such as:

>> **Dating:** This can feel scary, but ultimately you can learn to love again.

>> **Grief support groups:** You may find comfort in commiserating with others who've experienced similar losses. You can find support groups for bereavement as well as for the loss of a relationship.

>> **Recreation:** People who are filled with grief typically pull away from pleasurable activities and then fail to pick them back up again when their grief subsides. (See Chapter 13 for more information on rediscovering pleasure.)

>> **Religious congregation groups:** These groups can provide support, connections, and spiritual guidance.

>> **Volunteer work:** This can be a great way to reestablish connections and obtain a sense of renewed purpose.

Rolling through roles

As we discuss in the "Transitioning through life" section earlier in this chapter, circumstances can compel you to give up one or more of the roles you occupy in life, such as the role of parent, employee, student, or child. Because these roles encompass much of how people define themselves, the loss can feel devastating.

TIP

Society hasn't clearly defined the transition type of loss. But at times, the grief involved feels almost as intense as the grief you feel after a death or divorce. It can also leave you feeling bewildered by what to do next. If a role transition seems to be causing you trouble, we recommend that you ask yourself Role Exploration Questions. Again, consider writing your answers down in your notes app or a notebook.

>> What did I enjoy about my old role?

>> What did my old role allow me to do?

>> What did I dislike about my old role?

>> What freedoms and limitations did I feel in my old role?

>> What were the negative and positive feelings I experienced when I gave up my old role?

>> What did I resent about my old role?

>> Do I feel grateful for having had my old role?

Your answers to these questions will help you more fully appreciate and understand the nature of your loss. If you've been idealizing the position you used to occupy, answering these questions should help you see your old role in a more realistic light. And when you review exactly what you feel was important in the loss, you can start to search for alternatives. The alternatives may lie in finding a new role, looking for new ways to meet your needs, or even exploring new interests and meanings. See Chapter 21 for information on using findings from the field of positive psychology to facilitate this exploration.

Mike retires from his position as a high school English teacher. He was counting the days until his retirement. He plans to travel, read books he never had the time to read, and go fishing. Four months into his retirement, he starts waking up at 4 a.m., unable to go back to sleep. He puts off his travel plans and fishing trips. Those books he was going to read remain on the shelf. Mike is suffering from the consequences of his role change. His wife suggests that he answer the Role Exploration Questions. Here's what Mike came up with:

- **What did I enjoy about my old role?** "I liked the interaction with the kids. I loved getting through to an unmotivated student."

- **What did my old role allow me to do?** "I could make a difference in a few kids' lives. That was fantastic."

- **What did I dislike about my old role?** "I hated the endless paperwork. And the boring meetings drove me crazy."

- **What freedoms and limitations did I feel in my old role?** "I loved the freedom to develop new ways to teach. But as the years wore on, there were more and more requirements. We lost most of the freedom to choose materials."

- **What were the negative and positive feelings I experienced when I gave up my old role?** "I couldn't wait to start fishing! And seeing new places excited me. I felt relief from the day-to-day grind. And I felt happy and joyous. Later I felt a deep sense of loss. I miss working with the kids. And I miss thinking of myself as a teacher."

- **What did I resent about my old role?** "The salary, of course. I also resented the increasing pressure from administration to dole out passing grades even when undeserved. I resented the lack of respect from some parents — that seemed to get worse over the years."

- **Do I feel grateful for having had my old role?** "Not many people get a chance to make a difference in other people's lives. I know I did that. And despite the pathetic salary, I feel quite grateful for the excellent retirement benefits."

After he reviews his answers, Mike more fully appreciates where his grief has been coming from. And he realizes that he can replace some of what he's lost by volunteering at an adult reading clinic near his home. He can use his skills as a teacher to make a huge difference in the lives of illiterate but enthusiastic students.

REMEMBER

Your depression could be coming from a change in your life. Remember, sometimes the change can be good, such as getting married, starting a new career, or having a baby. Nevertheless, all adjustments take a little time, energy, and planning.

Chapter **16**

Relationship Enhancement

D epression extracts a heavy toll on friendships and intimate relationships. But all isn't lost! You can do much to improve the quality of your relationships whether you're depressed or not. That's the purpose of this chapter — to show you how to outwit the deviousness of depression's handiwork when it starts to harm your relationships.

In this chapter, we discuss the ways that depression insidiously affects important relationships. But don't despair — we wouldn't present that information without giving you ideas for what you can do to turn things around. We offer some good tools for improving your relationship skills.

TIP

If your relationship is suffering, you may want to ask your friend or partner to read this chapter, too. But if your partner refuses, you can still do a lot to improve your relationship.

You can use the tools we present in this chapter to enhance the way you relate with friends, co-workers, family members, and intimate partners. However, we focus our discussion and techniques on intimate relationships here because problems in these relationships create more distress than difficulties with friends and acquaintances. Depression can cause problems in close relationships, and those problems can deepen depression.

WARNING

Abusive relationships sometimes cause depression. If you believe that your partner has been emotionally or physically abusive, you may need to terminate the relationship. However, when you're depressed, making that decision can be especially difficult. Seek professional guidance if you have any doubts. If you have questions about abuse or want to talk to a trained counselor, call The National Domestic Violence Hotline at 1-800-799-7233 (SAFE).

The Depression-Rejection Connection

Depression feels terrible — you experience sadness, fatigue, pessimism, and feelings of worthlessness. These feelings can be difficult to deal with in their own right. Yet one of the cruel tricks that depression inflicts on its sufferers is an increased likelihood of rejection. Rejection hurts, and it can intensify your depression.

When people get depressed, friends and family initially respond with offerings of empathy and support. But after awhile, and as much as they want to help, friends and family struggle to sustain their support — for a number of reasons:

» Spending lots of time with someone in the throes of depression can be difficult.

» Depressed people don't have the energy to respond positively to others, so they typically retreat from interaction. Friends and family, who may begin to feel rejected themselves, eventually decrease their support and show less caring and engagement.

And to add to this increased likelihood of facing rejection, depression causes people to deal with communications from others in three self-defeating ways. First, they magnify the negative intentions of others. Second, they look for negative feedback even if it doesn't exist. And finally, they tend to get angry and defensive in response to legitimate criticism. All these tendencies lead to more interpersonal trouble.

Exaggerating the negative

REMEMBER

When depressed people receive negative feedback, they usually see more negativity than there actually is. In other words, they magnify the degree of any rejection they receive.

Keith's story illustrates how depression clouds the vision of its victims. **Keith,** who is from Southern California, chooses a college in Upstate New York. His freshman year begins unremarkably. However, as fall draws to a close and the days shorten,

Keith's mood deteriorates. He has trouble getting out of bed and starts missing his morning classes. His roommate makes a number of efforts to help him — offering to wake him up, suggesting that he talk to a counselor, and inviting him to social events.

But Keith responds with sullen withdrawal. One morning, feeling at his wit's end, his roommate snaps, "Look, I've done what I can for you. Stop feeling so sorry for yourself and get out of bed, or at least get help."

Rather than understand his roommate's frustration, Keith concludes that his roommate despises him. His roommate's remark was negative, but it came from concern and worry. Keith magnified and personalized the message into total rejection.

See Chapters 6, 7, and 8 for more information about how depression insidiously distorts peoples' perspectives about events in their lives.

TIP

Looking for negative feedback

REMEMBER

Depressed people actually ask for disapproval and disparagement from other people. A series of studies conducted by Dr. William B. Swann and other colleagues demonstrated that depression leads people to seek negative feedback from others. And when they get that poor feedback, they feel even worse.

Do these findings mean that depressed people may actually *desire* feeling bad? We don't think so. Considerable evidence exists that says most humans are highly motivated to *self-verify*; in other words, people actively seek information that confirms whatever it is that they believe about themselves and reject information that runs counter to those self-beliefs. Thus, people with positive self-views work to maintain their rosy outlook, while people with negative self-views labor just as diligently to sustain a sinister, dark take on themselves.

Sometimes depressed people seek positive reassurance from their partners. If they receive a dose of support, more often than not they find a reason to reject and deny their partners' positive efforts (due to the drive to self-verify). Not surprisingly, their partners then feel rejected. And a rejected partner typically withdraws and provides less support. This pattern can evolve into a vicious cycle of rejection and increased depression.

Billy has a chronic, low-level depression known as persistent depressive disorder. He complains to his wife that he's a failure at work, expecting reassurance. When his wife tells him that he's very successful, his depression causes him to reject her support by saying, "You don't know what you're talking about." His wife feels hurt and withdraws.

Fighting off constructive criticism

Seemingly contrary to the info we present in the preceding sections, some people with depression occasionally attempt to fend off criticism. However, their depression rarely allows them to do so constructively. Instead, depressed minds sometimes dictate a defensive response that either denies the feedback or counterattacks.

When offered constructive criticism, they may become angry and accuse the person who is attempting to offer feedback of attacking them personally. They may also deny the veracity of the information, refuse to accept responsibility, and blame others. Again, a cycle of negativity and rejection ensues.

Pursuing Positives

Depression encourages withdrawal, avoidance, and isolation. The depressed mind tells you to not only expect negative reactions, it also guides you to elicit them. Therefore, many of your relationships may suffer. Overcoming those dark messages from your mind requires considerable effort. And mustering effort isn't easy when you're depressed. But you can ignore your mind's chatter and start reaching out to the ones you love, one step at a time.

If you've been depressed for quite awhile, you've probably fallen into some bad habits in your relationships. Even if you don't seek negative feedback, you probably don't feel like building positive interactions. And your depressed mind may be telling you that if you do something positive, others will only reject you.

REMEMBER

Repeating the same old behaviors isn't going to improve your relationship. You have to do something different. What do you have to lose? Infusing positive interactions into a relationship rarely causes trouble! If you don't get an overwhelmingly positive initial response from your partner, keep at it. Persistence is the key.

Everyone likes an occasional pat on the back. When you're depressed, you don't pat yourself on the back, and you don't pat anyone else on the back either. After a while, no one wants to pat you on the back, either. But the glue that holds relationships together is based on positive interactions.

We think that pats are a way to improve relationships. When you infuse your relationships with pats, they inevitably improve. And improving your relationships will help decrease your depression.

Pats come in four forms: giving compliments, doing nice things, planning positive times together, and introducing "nice" into your daily routine. If you're depressed, we fully realize that you probably don't feel like putting forth the effort to perform these good deeds. That's why we make them simple for you.

Giving compliments

TIP

Receiving appreciation, thanks, gratitude, and compliments feels good. Make a goal of giving your partner one or more of these expressions of your feelings each day. Find a way to remind yourself to do so. Perhaps you can write a note in your day planner or put a sticky note on your mirror. Don't forget that, when you're depressed, your memory can defeat your best intentions. (See Chapter 20 for more information on depression and memory.)

Keep just a few things in mind when giving compliments and appreciation:

>> **Be specific.** Don't merely say, "I appreciate you." (Although it's okay to say that sometimes.) Try to single out reasons why you feel appreciative, such as your partner's help with cooking, childcare, cleaning, shopping, or finances. Or compliment your partner about specific aspects of his or her appearance, friendliness, problem-solving ability, or special talents.

>> **Avoid "buts."** Avoid the temptation to give a compliment and then take it back. Don't tell your partner, "I appreciate your attempt to balance the checkbook, but you made an error."

>> **Be sincere.** Don't give false flattery. Only say things you really mean. You can find something positive to appreciate. If you can't, don't make something up. However, if you can't think of anything positive to say, you want to consider getting expert help.

Doing nice things

TIP

Compliments can be very useful, but actions speak louder than words. Again, depression may make doing nice things difficult, so here's a list to get you started. Having a list can inspire you to take action even if you don't feel like it. (See Chapter 11 for information about how action creates more motivation.) So circle the items you think your partner will like, and feel free to add some of your own. Make a goal of doing one positive action two or three times a week. We call this plan Making Nice.

>> Bring home flowers.

>> Cook a romantic meal.

>> Express how much you care.

>> Give a hug.

>> Hold hands.

>> Send a text to express caring.

>> Offer your partner a backrub.

>> Prepare a breakfast in bed.

>> Put a love note in your partner's lunch.

>> Run an errand.

>> Send an e-card for no specific reason.

>> Take over a task your partner usually does, such as the laundry.

>> Tell your partner to take a hot bath while you do the dishes.

>> Wash your partner's car.

REMEMBER

Making Nice isn't a quick fix. Don't expect instant returns, and don't keep score. Over a period of weeks, the exercise will likely improve the emotional tone of your relationship. If it doesn't, consider seeking relationship counseling.

Planning positive times together

Many busy couples devote time to pleasing others — they shuttle their kids to and from after-school activities, they take care of their elderly parents, and they work long hours to impress their bosses. But they neglect devoting time to their relationship. If one member is depressed, this neglect almost always increases.

TIP

You can improve your relationship by planning positive times together. These activities don't have to involve elaborate vacations or expensive outings. Rather, simple pleasures can work wonders. The key is to sit down to plan pleasures and then make sure that they happen. Be creative; make sure the activity is something you'll both enjoy. Here are some suggestions to help you get started:

>> Buy a couple's massage at a day spa.

>> Get an ice cream sundae.

>> Go dancing.

>> Go for a scenic drive.

>> Plan a date.

>> Plant a garden.

>> See a movie and hold hands.

>> Spend the night together in a motel.

>> Take a walk together.

REMEMBER

If you're depressed, these outings may not sound very appealing. However, depression causes you to have a bleak outlook on future activities. See Chapters 11 and 13 for more info about this process of negative predicting and how to overcome it.

Introducing nice into your everyday routine

TIP

One of the best ideas for doing something nice is to suggest having a conversation with your partner at the end of every workday. And if your schedule just won't permit a daily talk, try to at least schedule it in three times a week. We call this exercise The Daily News. The purpose of The Daily News is to build closeness with your partner. The Daily News consists of a number of important components:

>> **Set aside 20 to 30 minutes of uninterrupted time.** Unplug the phones.

>> **Talk one at a time.** Let your partner talk for 10 to 20 minutes, and then you take a similar amount of time.

>> **Allow any topic.** Each of you can discuss your day, your worries, or whatever you want to discuss.

>> **Avoid conflict.** Only discuss items that don't involve conflict between the two of you. In other words, discuss things that occur outside of your relationship.

>> **Express empathy.** Tell your partner that you understand how he feels. Try to endorse or validate his emotions. You can say, "I think I'd be stressed by that too," or, "I can see why you'd be upset." Stay focused on your partner's perspective; don't find fault. For example, if your partner is complaining about someone else's behavior, it's not a good time to point out that the other person may be right.

>> **Listen.** Listening means asking questions for elaboration and better understanding. It means focusing on your partner and showing interest through head nods, light touches on the arm, and brief comments such as, "I see," "Oh," "Uh huh," and "Wow." You can also enhance listening by demonstrating affection and approval. For example, you can say, "I really like your thinking on that," or offer a hug if you see distress.

>> **Stay away from advice.** Don't give advice unless your partner specifically asks for help with an issue. Even if your partner asks you for advice, give it sparingly and merely as a possible option to consider.

You may be surprised by how much The Daily News can enhance your relationship — sometimes in a matter of days.

> **April** and **Tasha** have been together for eight years. Their relationship starts to suffer from April's depression. April is in the midst of a difficult menopause complicated by a prolonged depression. Tasha, her partner, is years away from menopause. Although she sympathizes with April, Tasha's patience wears thin after months of withdrawal, moodiness, and irritability. The women, who were once almost inseparable, find themselves becoming more and more distant.
>
> April begins to talk to a counselor and realizes that her withdrawal from Tasha is a normal response to her depressed feelings. The counselor tells April about a technique similar to The Daily News that she can use as a tool to combat depression and improve her relationship. April values her relationship and vows to make it better. Despite feeling momentarily unenthused, she explains, "Tasha, depression has tried to come between us. I can't promise an instant recovery, but having positive time together every day could help. Let's sit down with a cup of tea and talk."
>
> Tasha, feeling relieved that her partner is making an effort, responds with renewed empathy and compassion. Their daily conversation becomes a ritual that helps close the gap between them.

Defeating Defensiveness

When relationships begin heading downhill, people start making what we call *malicious assumptions* about their partners. In other words, they reflexively interpret potentially ambiguous or even caring statements as coming from someone who has malicious, hostile motives. Depression, with its inevitable gloomy outlook, can increase the frequency of malicious assumptions.

After the malicious assumption takes over, people typically do something that is especially self-defeating — they get defensive in response to the perceived attack. And defensiveness pretty much assures that the other party will become hostile, even if hostility wasn't originally intended!

> **Ed** notices that his wife, **Sheila,** has been lethargic and depressed for the past few weeks. The bills that she normally pays begin to stack up, unopened on her desk. Sheila, who is usually meticulous about her appearance, recently stopped wearing makeup. Ed cares deeply about her and worries that she may be ill. One Saturday morning, he approaches her and asks, "Sweetheart, I'm worried about you. You haven't been taking care of things like you always do. Are you feeling all right?"

Sheila erupts sarcastically, "So great, you think I'm not measuring up. Thanks for being so supportive. I do the best I can; I work ridiculous hours; all I ever do is work. On top of everything else, I don't need your criticism."

"But Sheila, I'm not being critical. It's just, you've changed, and you don't seem to be your old self. I'm not trying to start an argument, I just want to help," Ed pleads.

"If you want to help, just leave me alone. Can't you tell that I work myself to the bone already? Of course some things aren't getting done! I'm not a machine after all." Sheila stomps away in tears.

TIP

So just what constitutes a defensive response? Basically anything you may say to absolve yourself of any blame or responsibility for a perceived criticism. And you may wonder what could possibly be wrong with that; after all, you may have done nothing wrong whatsoever. Well, defensiveness is a problem for two reasons:

>> It absolutely assumes that your partner intended to be hostile in the first place.

>> Adding spice to your defensiveness in the form of criticism and hostility is all too easy to do.

So what can you do to keep from falling into a defensive, critical mode when you feel that your partner may have said something scornful to you? The following sections discuss two particularly useful strategies: Checking It Out and Depersonalizing.

Trying the Checking It Out strategy

TIP

The best way to counteract malicious assumptions that lead to defensiveness is to use the Checking It Out strategy. This two-step technique is basically what it sounds like:

1. Stifle your urge to get defensive or attack.

2. Make a gentle inquiry about your partner's meaning and intent.

In the previous section, Ed says to Sheila, "Sweetheart, I'm worried about you. You haven't been taking care of things like you always do. Are you feeling alright?" Sheila responds defensively and sarcastically, "Great, you think I'm not measuring up. Thanks for being so supportive. I do the best I can; I work ridiculous hours; all I ever do is work. On top of everything else, I don't need your criticism."

Sheila obviously interpreted Ed's comment as critical and malicious. But she could have checked out her assumption by saying, "Ed, are you upset that I'm not doing enough? If you are, I'm willing to talk about it."

Likely, Ed would have replied with something like, "No, not at all. I've just been worried that you look a little run-down lately. Is anything wrong?"

Generally speaking, if you take the time to check out the meaning of what you perceive as critical, you'll find that the intent wasn't as vicious as you had thought. Feeling a bit defensive when you "think" that you've been criticized is perfectly natural. But take the time to take a deep breath and check it out.

On the other hand, sometimes you may discover your partner has a real complaint. If so, try to maintain a non-defensive posture. Keep asking questions and consider using the buffering and defusing techniques that we discuss later in this chapter.

Don't attempt to use Checking It Out, or even the other communication techniques we discuss later in this chapter, if you're feeling hostile and significantly upset. If you rate your upset as higher than 50 on a 100 point scale, the odds of you thinking of anything useful or productive to say are about one in ten billion. Ask for a timeout and come back to discuss the issue when you feel relatively calm — perhaps in 30 minutes, a few hours, or even a day or two. But don't put off talking for much longer than that, because resentments may build. And taking time to get into a better frame of mind on your own isn't a license for avoiding communication altogether.

The Checking It Out technique requires you to block out your malicious assumption while you inquire gently about your partner's meaning and intentions.

Depersonalizing

Personalizing occurs when you attribute your partner's tantrums, tirades, and upset remarks as being about you.

> For example, **Patrick** spills a glass of water on the computer keyboard. And his partner **Beth** explodes. Patrick, already deeply embarrassed by the accident, feels even worse about himself after hearing Beth explode. Patrick, perhaps naturally, assumes that Beth's explosion is all about him and his clumsiness. Not so.

In actuality, Beth came from a highly abusive family in which accidents were treated as catastrophes. Yelling at Patrick was a habit learned long ago. Someone else may have responded with a little annoyance or even empathic concern.

Depersonalizing means figuring out when your partner's reactions have less to do with you and more to do with previous upbringing or learning that formed core beliefs about the meaning of certain types of events.

Everyone has core beliefs, instilled during childhood, that continue to exert a huge influence on how they perceive and feel about events. Core beliefs lie behind your hopes, dreams, and fears — in other words, all the issues you have strong feelings about. And you don't have to be depressed for one or more of these core beliefs to generate a lot of emotion. Table 16-1 shows a few of the common core beliefs, or hot buttons, that interfere with relationships.

TABLE 16-1   **Relationship Hot Buttons (Core Beliefs)**

Hot Button	What It Means	Common Origins
Vulnerable	Expecting the worst and having intense worries about issues such as health, money, or safety.	An impoverished childhood, pessimistic parents, and traumatic events during childhood.
Abandonment fearful	Fearing that anyone close to you will eventually leave.	A parent who was emotionally unavailable, parents that divorced at an early age, and other serious losses of people close to you.
Inadequate	Thinking that you need more help than you really do.	A parent who stepped in to help whenever things got frustrating, or critical parents who gave messages that you were incapable.
Perfectionistic	A driven need to make everything you do perfect, or believing that something just isn't good enough.	Highly critical parents, or parents who excessively focused on accomplishments.

When people are in a relationship and they have different core beliefs, communication can be difficult. Stan and Norma's story illustrates the point:

> **Stan** grew up in a very unstable and poor family. He developed a core belief of pessimism and vulnerability. **Norma's** father abandoned her when she was 6. After he left, Norma's mother became seriously depressed and withdrew from her. Norma developed the core belief that people who love her will eventually abandon her.
>
> Stan and Norma are now married. Stan opens a credit card bill and discovers that Norma spent slightly more money this month than their paychecks can cover. He confronts his wife. "Norma, we can't afford to pay the credit card bill this month. We're getting deeper and deeper into debt. If you keep this up, we'll end up having to declare bankruptcy! Stop this wild spending at once!" Norma starts to cry and says, "Fine, if you want a divorce, just do it now. I knew this marriage would never work out."

Are Stan and Norma crazy, or just irrational? Neither. Stan's exaggerated response comes from his childhood, when his family often had to scramble to put food on the table. Stan's hot buttons concerned vulnerability and pessimism. And Norma's abandonment hot button comes from the physical loss of her father and the emotional loss of her mother. Both reactions may be excessive, but they make sense if you understand their backgrounds.

If your partner consistently gets upset, distraught, or passionate about an issue in a way that seems either excessive or possibly irrational, odds are that one or more core beliefs is at work. Doing some detective work can help you find out which core belief may be affecting your partner's perspective. You can start by determining your own core beliefs. One of *your* core beliefs may help explain why your partner's feelings seem excessive or irrational to you. The following core beliefs are common; however, there are endless possibilities.

>> **Abandonment fearful:** Worry that people you care about will eventually leave you.

>> **Entitled:** A pervasive perspective that you always deserve the best and feel outraged when your needs go unmet.

>> **Guilty and blameworthy:** A pervasive sense that you must always do the right thing or else.

>> **Guiltless:** Shameless disregard for ethics and morality.

>> **Inadequate:** A sense that you lack important skills, abilities, or other qualities.

>> **Inferior:** Viewing yourself as insignificant and less important than others.

>> **Intimacy avoidant:** A sense that you don't like getting close to people.

>> **Invulnerable:** No sense that you need to take even reasonable precautions because everything will be fine.

>> **Perfectionistic:** A compulsion to believe that you can and should do everything perfectly. See Chapter 7 for more information about the destructive influence of "shoulds."

>> **Superior:** A view that you stand far above others.

>> **Unworthy:** A sense that you don't deserve good things or have good things happen to you.

>> **Vulnerable:** A belief that the world is a dangerous place and horrible things are about to happen.

TIP

After you figure out what your hot buttons (and those of your partner) are about, you may still disagree. However, you can at least appreciate that much of the emotional charge isn't about you. Step back and depersonalize. Realize that the conflict has more to do with either your own or your partner's early upbringing than it does with you. Doing so can help reduce your own negative feelings.

Getting Your Message Across

Poor communication can rip your relationship apart. On the other hand, using the right communication style can help keep your relationship together. Communication matters most when you're talking about difficult issues and conflicts. And improved communication techniques aren't that difficult to master.

We've found that certain people resist using these techniques. For some depressed people, asserting their concerns may seem too difficult to accomplish. But the alternative of stuffing their concerns and avoiding the expression of their views only leads to resentment and hostility.

Other folks always want to express themselves with brutal honesty. Yet doing so frequently leads to hostile rejection. We urge you to give these techniques a try; they can improve your communication with friends, family, co-workers, and loved ones.

TIP

Three strategies are particularly helpful for improving communication whether you're depressed or not: I Messages, Buffering, and Defusing. These techniques are particularly designed to help you communicate about difficult issues while preventing the discussion from deteriorating into conflict.

Using the I Messages technique

When two people disagree, the language they use to express themselves can do much to add fuel to the fire. A simple technique called I Messages can help prevent the disagreement from getting out of control. The idea is to state how you're feeling rather than accuse or criticize your partner. This technique is an alternative to using blaming messages. Table 16-2 shows some examples of blaming messages and their more productive I-message equivalents. Read the examples of both types of messages. Then, when you feel tempted to blame your partner, try rephrasing your concerns in terms of I Messages.

TABLE 16-2   The I Messages Technique

Blaming Messages	I Messages
You never show affection.	I wish you would hug me more often.
You spend too much money.	I feel worried about our finances, can we talk about it?
You are so critical about everything I do.	I feel like I'm not pleasing you.
You make me so mad.	I'm feeling a little upset right now.
You never do the things you say you're going to do.	I feel unhappy when you don't follow through on something you promised.

Creating buffers

Buffering gives you a way to add a spoonful of sugar to distasteful messages. This technique involves finding ways to soften any criticism you want to communicate. You add a phrase to acknowledge the possibility that your position may not be entirely correct. After all, can anyone ever truly be 100 percent certain that they are correct in their views about a particular event? Not often.

TIP

Buffering offers the opportunity to discuss your concerns and opens the door to compromise. The following list provides some good buffering phrases:

>> "I could be wrong here, although I have a concern that . . ."

>> "I may be making too much out of this, . . ."

>> "Please correct me if I'm off base; I feel a little upset that . . ."

>> "Help me understand your take on what I have to say."

If you use such phrases prior to talking about your concern or criticism, your partner will be less likely to go into a defensive or attacking mode. The technique increases the likelihood that you'll be heard rather than dismissed.

Defusing criticism

The Defusing technique helps prevent a criticism from escalating into a full-blown argument. This technique helps you deal with criticism from your partner (instead of defending or fighting). In a sense, it's the opposite of Buffering. With the Defusing technique, you find *something* about the criticism to validate or agree with. And apologizing for any valid portion of the agreement doesn't hurt, either. Here are some examples of responses you can use to help defuse an argument:

>> "I'm sorry, you could have a point about that."

>> "Sometimes what you're saying is probably true."

>> "I can see why you think that."

>> "I can agree with part of what you're saying."

TIP

Excuses actually convey the idea that you care more about saving face than you do about your partner's concerns. When you provide a partial agreement and a sincere apology (Defusing), you indicate that your interest lies in repairing your partner's hurt feelings. When you make excuses, you demonstrate that you're more interested in repairing your own ego.

TIP

When you're depressed and your self-esteem is low, you may feel like making excuses in order to prevent further erosion of your self-esteem. If you work hard to avoid that temptation, you'll be rewarded in the long-run.

Putting the techniques to work

Now that you've seen what Buffering, Defusing, and I Messages look like, you may want to see how they look in action. That way, you're more likely to appreciate the value of these communication strategies. But first, we show you how gruesome communications can sound when you don't use these techniques. **Aretha and Dennis** are having a disagreement about housework. Here's their conversation without the Buffering, Defusing, and I Messages techniques.

> **Aretha:** You never help me with any of the housework. I'm really getting sick and tired of it.
>
> **Dennis:** Yes I do. I mowed the lawn last week. Just what do you want out of me?
>
> **Aretha:** Mowing the lawn is your job. I'm talking about laundry, cooking, shopping, dishes. You don't do any of those things. If it weren't for me, this place would look like a pigsty.
>
> **Dennis:** Look, I make more money than you, and I'm beat when I get home. When we got married, you said if I was the main bread winner, you'd take care of the house. This isn't fair!
>
> **Aretha:** Fair? What are you talking about? I work too, you know. You can't even talk about a simple thing like housework without shouting!

Not a very productive discussion, is it? Both Dennis and Aretha resort to criticism, defensiveness, and anger. Nothing is solved, and bad feelings escalate. Now we're going to take the same conversation and insert the Buffering, Defusing, and I Messages strategies.

> **Aretha:** Help me understand your viewpoint (Buffering). I feel a little overwhelmed with the housework (I Message), and it kind of seems like you're not pitching in as much as I'd like.
>
> **Dennis:** Well, I agree that you do more of the housework (Defusing). I'm sorry that I've made you feel so overwhelmed. I guess I come home so tired that I often don't think about housework, but maybe I should (I Messages). What do you need?
>
> **Aretha:** Sometimes I feel like I do everything (I Messages). And maybe I'm overreacting (Buffering). Still, if you could help with the dishes after dinner, that would feel better.

Dennis: (Defusing) I can see why you'd like that; after all, we do have a large family and a whole lot of dishes (Defusing). I'm just so tired after dinner (I Message). How about I take on the laundry on the weekends instead? And maybe we can start getting the kids more involved with the dishes. They're getting old enough.

Aretha: Well, that's not a bad compromise I suppose. Thanks for listening to my concern.

That turned out a little better, didn't it? When you use the Defusing technique, you focus more on finding something to agree with (or even apologize for some aspect of the complaint), and you pay less attention to conjuring up defensive excuses. Buffering allows you to express concerns in a gentle, non-confrontational manner. I Messages keep the focus on your concerns and prevent you from blaming your partner. All three of these techniques can be applied to communicating with intimate partners as well as other important relationships.

TIP

After you've read the dialogs between Aretha and Dennis, consider writing out a dialog that you have with someone that doesn't go too well. Then rewrite the conversation inserting as many Defusing, Buffering, and I Messages as you can. With a little work and practice, you'll find yourself gradually communicating better over time.

WHO TO TURN TO: PEOPLE OR PETS?

Many studies suggest that improving the quality of your relationships and social support can help you cope better, decrease the severity of your depression, and even prevent future bouts with depression. That's why we devote this chapter to giving you advice on enhancing the quality of your important relationships. Of course, we now realize that we left out one important type of relationship: the relationship you have with your pet.

A study by Karen Allen, PhD, and colleagues at the State University of New York found that pet owners have lower blood pressure, slower heart rates, and appear to handle stress better than people who don't have pets. We know that chronic stress leads to a host of problems, including depression. So if you currently have no one else to turn to, it actually makes sense to find a furry friend. By the way, the researchers found that dogs and cats work equally well for reducing stress and battling depression.

5

Fighting the Physical Foe: Biological Therapies

Chapter **17**

Prescribing Pleasure

U ntil modern times, many people believed that depression resulted from a character flaw or weakness. Because of that belief, those suffering from depression often didn't seek treatment. Feeling embarrassed, guilty, and worthless, they suffered in horrible silence; or worse, ended their pain with suicide.

Medication for depression has alleviated suffering for millions. And maybe even more importantly, it encourages treatment. If a pill indeed can change your mood, then it would seem there really must be a physical cause for depression. Those afflicted can declare, "Depression isn't our fault."

Depression is an illness of the body and mind. Left untreated, it not only robs you of happiness, but also takes a lasting, physical toll as well. Please get help if you're depressed. Toughing it out is not an option. Take a look at this chapter to help select the best treatment for you — therapy, medication, or a combination.

In this chapter, we help you decide for yourself whether medication is a good choice for you. We provide a guide for making that important decision. Then we tell you about where to get help, how long you may have to take medication, and when mixing talk therapy with drugs may give you even more relief. Finally, we provide some guidance to the most popularly prescribed pills.

Hammering Depression: Choosing the Right Tool

You've probably heard the saying that if the only tool you have in your toolbox is a hammer, you're likely to treat everything like a nail. Well, physicians and psychiatrists have prescription drugs in their toolboxes, and psychologists and therapists hammer away with talk therapy. So it's no wonder that each group tends to recommend their treatment as the best treatment for depression.

We've spent the vast majority of this book giving you methods to improve your mood and defeat depression. Most of these tips are based on techniques borrowed from the fields of cognitive-behavioral therapy (a combination of cognitive therapy reviewed in Part 2 and behavior therapy discussed in Part 3). Honestly, we want to encourage readers to adopt healthy thinking and behavior to battle the blues as their first line of defense against depression. Is that because the only tool is therapy? Certainly not!

TIP

We've reviewed the latest research. And a huge body of studies pits prescription medications against psychotherapy for the treatment of depression. Most studies concur: Cognitive-behavioral therapy is at least as effective as medication for the treatment of depression. Better still, psychotherapy may help prevent relapse.

And just in case you're skeptical, a study completed at the University of Pennsylvania and Vanderbilt University looked at people with severe depression and compared how they reacted to treatment with cognitive therapy and medication. This study included both physicians and psychologists and was funded through the National Institute of Mental Health and a major pharmaceutical company.

The results were impressive. Cognitive therapy worked at least as well as medication for the long-term treatment of severe depression (in this study, *severe* didn't include people with psychotic symptoms). Realizing that relapse in depression is a serious problem, scientists looked at what happened to these folks a year later. They found two groups less likely to have relapsed. The first group still took their antidepressant medication and the other group had completed cognitive therapy. In fact, 25 percent of those who completed therapy relapsed compared to 40 percent of those who took medication. Remember that cognitive therapy adds an additional boost to any treatment of depression. (See Part 2 for more information about cognitive therapy.)

TIP

For some people with depression, the combination of medication and therapy appears to give them a slight edge over using just one or the other. Sometimes antidepressant medication may help a person make better use of therapy.

Ultimately, the decision as to whether or not to take medication is up to you. If you choose to stick with self-help or therapy, work seriously through the exercises provided in this book or preferably, with your therapist. Don't expect to get better without considerable effort. With work, you can expect that the skills you pick up can help inoculate you against future struggles with depression. But for many folks, medication is part of the solution — and for good reason.

Exploring the Medication Option

TIP

Given all of the evidence that therapy works, why would anyone take medication? Well, for many depressed people, a single medication or a combination of medicines can be found that will decrease symptoms of depression. Opting for the medication route is often advisable when

>> **You have serious suicidal thoughts or plans.** You need help now. First, get checked out by a mental health professional to determine the best treatment for you. Sometimes antidepressant medication can work a few important weeks faster than cognitive therapy.

>> **You have bipolar disorder or depression with psychotic features.** Usually medication is the best answer for folks with bipolar disorder or people whose depression is so severe that they hear voices or see things that aren't really there. However, therapy often helps stabilize and keep people from discontinuing medication and suffering relapses.

>> **You've given cognitive therapy or interpersonal therapy a good try and your depression keeps reoccurring.** Evidence indicates that untreated depression becomes more severe, frequent, and resistant to treatment. If your depression keeps returning, you should probably consider adding long-term use of medication to your other efforts.

>> **Your symptoms of depression are mostly physiological.** For example, you have problems with your appetite or sleep, you feel overwhelming fatigue, forgetfulness, and poor concentration. *Caution:* Not everyone with the physical symptoms of depression will respond better to medication, and some of those with physical symptoms may be trying to stuff feelings and thoughts inside. So, if medication doesn't work, a visit to a therapist may be a very good idea.

>> **Depression takes control of your life.** If severe symptoms cause you to neglect the important tasks of everyday living, you may need medication to get you going again. But, after you're feeling a little bit better, consider psychotherapy to keep you healthy.

>> **Medical conditions cause your depression.** Sometimes people with other illnesses become depressed. (See Chapter 2 for more on causes of depression). Doctors aren't sure how that works, but many believe that one disease sometimes causes the other (for example, a heart attack may trigger a depressive episode). Medication may be the quickest way to overcome this type of depression.

>> **Panic or anxiety accompanies depression.** You may have too much on your plate to wait for the benefits of therapy. Again, when the medication starts taking effect, you may have more mental energy available to tackle anxiety and depression in or with the help of books like this one or another of our titles, *Anxiety For Dummies* (Wiley).

>> **Therapy doesn't work.** A few people just don't seem to benefit from therapy. Or they may need long-term therapy because of complicated issues. In this case, medication may be a good adjunctive choice.

>> **Your depression has lasted most of your life.** Some evidence suggests that extremely chronic depression (such as persistent depressive disorder) may benefit from medication in addition to therapy.

>> **You don't have time for therapy.** For a few folks, therapy is too time consuming. If your schedule is already too full, we hope you at least take a few minutes out of your busy day to read through this book.

>> **You don't have insurance coverage for psychotherapy.** Some insurance companies don't cover psychological services. We hope this will change, but if your insurance covers only medication, and you can't afford therapy, finances may dictate that you go the medication route for defeating your depression.

For many people, medication is a good option. They have minor or few side effects and medication alone helps them get through a difficult time. The following example illustrates a successful trial of antidepressants.

"Doc, I feel terrible," **Bryce** complains. "I can't stand to be around my family, and I get irritated by the smallest things. I'm having trouble sleeping; I wake up at 4 a.m. and usually toss and turn the rest of the night. I feel restless inside; it's hard to describe. I feel pain, but I can't tell you where. All I can tell you is that it hurts. I don't know what's wrong with me. Maybe I have a brain tumor."

After a complete physical and more discussion, Bryce's doctor concludes that he suffers from major depression. His doctor prescribes an antidepressant and explains to Bryce that he has a "chemical imbalance." Slightly puzzled as to how his brain chemicals got out of whack but willing to try out the medication, Bryce agrees to fill the prescription.

At the drugstore, the pharmacist encourages Bryce to look over the literature about the popular antidepressant his doctor prescribed. When Bryce starts to read about possible side effects, he worries. Headaches, dry mouth, dizziness, stomach upsets, and oh no — sexual dysfunction. He wonders whether or not he should just pitch the drugs and tough his depression out. After some pondering, Bryce decides to give the medication a try because his depression feels so awful. Besides, he reasons that if he experiences bad side effects, perhaps the doc will know of a different medication that won't affect him in that way. Bryce made a good decision; his depression began to lift within a couple of weeks.

But what we don't know is whether Bryce's depression will return when he stops taking his medication or will the medication continue to work for him. That's why we generally recommend that people whose depression returns consider psycho-therapy to learn new skills that can help prevent relapse.

Many of you may choose to take medication. Don't worry that you're taking the easy way out. If you have an infection, you take an antibiotic. If you have depres-sion, taking an antidepressant often makes sense.

Taking medication the right way

Antidepressant medications are powerful drugs. They affect the body in numerous ways. That's why they're not sold over the counter. Therefore, keep these tips for taking antidepressant medications the right way in mind should you decide to give antidepressant medication a try.

>> **Tell your doctor about any other physical conditions you have.** Discuss all your current health concerns with your doctor, especially liver disease, hepatitis, diabetes, high blood pressure, or kidney disease.

>> **If you think you may be pregnant, intend to try to get pregnant, or are breastfeeding, let your doctor know.** Certain medications may not be safe.

>> **Tell your doctor what other medications you're taking.** Antidepressants may interfere with other medications, or other medications may interfere with antidepressants. Be sure to include non-prescription medications in your discussion, including over-the-counter allergy, sleeping pills, or pain relievers.

>> **Tell you doctor about any herbs or supplements you take.** Again, there may be interactions with antidepressants. For more about herbs and supple-ments, please see Chapter 18.

>> **Hang in there.** Antidepressant medication usually takes at least two weeks to begin working and may take as long as six weeks for a maximum benefit to occur. And you may not respond to the first attempt. Give your doctor a chance to help you. You may have to go through months of experimentation to find the right drug or drug combination. The good news is that after you

find what works, that drug will likely keep working to alleviate your depression.

>> **Talk to your doctor about side effects.** Although many of the bothersome side effects go away after a couple of weeks, don't suffer in silence. Your doctor may be able to help you manage the side effects with either a change in the dose or by adding another drug to the mix.

>> **Talk to your doctor about *all* side effects.** Okay, one of the most common and somewhat embarrassing side effects of antidepressant medication is a decrease in sexual pleasure. Some experience a decrease in desire. Others may undergo a frustrating inability to achieve orgasm. Tell your doctor. Treatments for this side effect are available.

>> **Don't drink alcohol when you take antidepressants.** Drinking alcohol can boost the mood temporarily, but its overall effect is that of a depressant. Alcohol may interact with antidepressant medication, increasing fatigue or blocking its effects. An occasional drink is probably harmless.

REMEMBER

Whatever you choose, remember that depression is a highly treatable illness. If the method you choose doesn't work, don't give up hope. Be patient, get help, and try something different.

Opting out of medication

If taking a pill can cure you, why not? You may be one of the lucky people who begin taking antidepressant medication, enjoy a reduction of symptoms, have few side effects, and go merrily on with your life.

Why then doesn't everyone fill up at the drugstore? For starters, you should know that cognitive behavioral therapy can give you essentially the same benefits of medications while only rarely encountering side effects and generally preventing relapse. In addition, medication drawbacks include:

>> **Side effects can be very bothersome.** More than a third of people prescribed antidepressant medication discontinue taking their medications. Most stop because of side effects. Side effects can include nausea, headaches, insomnia, dry mouth, weight gain, feelings of apathy, and sexual dysfunction.

>> **Not generally safe for pregnant or breastfeeding women.** Research about the effects of antidepressant medication on the fetus or infant comes from animal studies or case examples. What woman would risk the health of her baby to participate in a drug trial? Not enough information is available to judge the safety of most antidepressant medications. So, talk to your doctor if

WARNING

you're planning on getting pregnant, might be pregnant, or are nursing a baby. In most cases, psychotherapy is a better choice than medication.

Depression after the birth of a baby is a common problem that can become serious if left untreated. Please get help if you experience more than a couple of days of baby blues. (See Chapter 2 for more on postpartum depression.)

>> **Worry about long-term effects.** If you have one bout of depression, your risk of relapse or recurrence increases. If you have more than one major depressive episode, if depression was severe or long-lasting, or your depression never completely lifted, your physician may recommend lifelong medication. Although long-term treatment appears to have little risk, some experts have expressed concern regarding the lack of knowledge about lifelong use of antidepressant medication. And medications only work as long as you keep taking them.

>> **Withdrawal symptoms.** Discontinuing antidepressants can be surprisingly difficult. Anxiety, insomnia, weird dreams, headaches, dizziness, irritability, and fatigue are often reported. In addition, some people feel chills and body aches similar to flu. Others report what have been described as "brain zaps," sensations similar to mild electric shocks. Withdrawal effects can be mitigated somewhat by slowly decreasing the dose over a few weeks or even longer. These symptoms can last for weeks or months and can be confused with the return of the original depression.

>> **Just say no.** Some people don't want to take medication, for religious or philosophical reasons. If you choose this path, please get help for your depression through cognitive-behavioral or interpersonal therapy techniques. Depression requires treatment. If your mood doesn't improve or if your depression feels very deep, please find a mental health professional for assistance. (See Chapter 5 for information on finding professional help).

Working with Your Doctor to Find the Correct Medication

REMEMBER

A positive, collaborative relationship with your prescribing health care practitioner (your primary care physician, psychiatrist, or another practitioner such as a physicians assistant) may be the most important ingredient for successful treatment of depression. You and your health care provider must openly discuss your unique symptoms of depression, your response to the medication, and any side effects you may experience.

Unfortunately, science hasn't yet figured out which particular antidepressant medication is likely to work for any one individual. Some people respond to the first drug prescribed; others will make changes in their medications. The drug your doctor chooses depends on several factors:

>> **Depressive symptoms:** Your doctor will want to know all about your symptoms before choosing a medication. The doctor may want to know the answers to the following questions. Do you sleep too much, or too little? Have you gained or lost weight? Do you have aches and pains? Do you feel anxious as well as depressed? Do you find yourself unable to concentrate?

>> **Side effects:** For most people, the first choice in medication is the drug with the fewest side effects. But side effects of a drug can sometimes be used advantageously. For example, people with sleep problems may do better with a medication that has a side effect of sedation. Again, no one knows how bothered you will be by side effects. Sometimes a change in medication, or a change in the dose, or even the addition of another drug is used to manage side effects.

>> **History of depression:** If you have had previous depressive episodes and have been successfully treated with a particular antidepressant, the same one will likely be used again. And, the doctor may well decide to continue the medication for a much longer period of time.

>> **Family response to antidepressant medication:** Although the evidence is scant that genetics affect how different antidepressant medications will work, if a member of your family had a favorable response to a specific antidepressant medication, let your provider know. Depending on many factors, that antidepressant may be a good first choice.

TIP

Your healthcare provider will attempt to match your particular symptoms with an antidepressant medication. However, be aware that current science hasn't developed a precise way of predicting which symptoms will be best ameliorated by which medications. So, much of the prescribing of antidepressants is based more on the experiences and biases of the provider than a science-based decision.

WARNING

Less than a quarter of people treated with medication for depression get adequate treatment. That means that they don't receive a reasonable number of psychotherapy sessions with treatments found to be effective for depression or take an adequate dose of medications for a sufficient length of time. About 10 percent of people with prescriptions for antidepressants fill the prescription but stop taking their medication within the first week! Many more stop the minute they feel a little better. If you choose to be treated for depression with medication, follow through. Your risk of having a relapse grows when you don't get completely better.

The Seductive Myth of Chemical Imbalance

Despite the fact that there is *absolutely no evidence* that chemical imbalances in the brain cause depression, this myth is pervasive among the pubic as well as too many professionals who should know better by now. One possible reason for this belief is the constant deluge of advertisements that suggest mental illness is a disease caused by some insufficiency in the availability of chemical messengers in the brain. Furthermore, many people feel there's less stigma related to having a physical disease such as a chemical imbalance as opposed to a psychological problem. However, today we know that so-called mental illnesses, including depression, are caused by a multitude of problems including genetic, environmental, and biological factors.

Although pharmaceutical companies spend billions of dollars searching for the next hot treatment for depression, interestingly, no one really knows exactly how antidepressant medication works. Nonetheless, most people believe that antidepressant medications somehow increase one or more of the neurotransmitters in the brain and that doing so improves communication among neurons and ultimately reduces depression.

The relationship between the various neurotransmitters and depression isn't completely understood. However, the three neurotransmitters that are targeted by most antidepressants may have different symptoms associated with them.

>> **Serotonin:** Problems with serotonin are associated with depressed mood, anxiety, insomnia, obsessive compulsive disorder, seasonal affective disorder, and even violence.

>> **Dopamine:** Disruptions in dopamine seem to be related to problems with attention, motivation, alertness, increased apathy, and difficulty in experiencing pleasure.

>> **Norepinephrine:** Disorders in norepinephrine are correlated with lack of energy, decreased alertness, and lethargy.

However, there are major problems with these assumptions concerning specific effects of different neurotransmitters for different symptoms of depression. Once again, that's because scientific data do not support the idea that imbalances in neurotransmitters account for depression. And there is growing evidence that serotonin, dopamine, and norepinephrine have different effects in different people. Here are a few examples the logical and critical problems that the chemical imbalance theory poses:

>> An antidepressant drug used throughout Europe and Asia, Tianeptine, has been found to be effective at treating depression. However, it actually reduces serotonin which contradicts the serotonin depletion hypothesis as a cause of depression.

>> Some patients with depression actually have unusually high levels of norepinephrine and serotonin.

>> Experiments that activated or blocked serotonin receptors have had unpredictable effects on actual depressive symptoms.

>> Some people have very low levels of serotonin and norepinephrine but have never had a history of depression.

>> Many antidepressant drugs quickly increase levels of neurotransmitters yet it still takes weeks to see improvement.

>> Studies that have reduced levels of neurotransmitters failed to produce depression, even though according to the theory, they should.

>> About one third of people with depression do not improve on antidepressants or other psychotropic medications. If the hypothesized chemical imbalance was the cause of depression, then the vast majority of depressed people should improve with appropriate medications.

The bottom line is that the cause of depression, like most emotional disorders, is still unknown. Biological, psychological, and social factors all interact in unknown ways that lead to depression. The chemical imbalance theory is last-century thinking. However, too many ads continue to promote an overly simplified model of causation. For example, headaches are not caused by a lack of aspirin in the brain; however, taking aspirin often cures a headache. The causes of headaches are complicated just as the causes of depression are complex.

REMEMBER

Please realize that we are not suggesting that because the chemical imbalance theory is outdated, that antidepressant drugs have no effect. Some people do feel better and less depressed taking antidepressants. We just don't know how or why they work for some people and not others.

Plunging into Placebos

Placebos are inert treatments or substances such as sugar pills or saline injections. They are often used in experiments to determine the effectiveness and safety of drugs under development. A clinical trial is a design that involves two groups who are getting either an active drug or a placebo. Participants are not told which group they fall into. When the experiment is completed, the groups are compared. If the group given the real drug does significantly better (as determined by statistical methods), then the drug is considered to potentially work. If the groups do the same, or the placebo group does better, then the drug is judged not to work effectively.

However, there is more to the placebo than a fake medical treatment. When given a placebo, the individual receiving it can have what is known as *a placebo effect*. A placebo effect is the reaction people get from receiving treatment purported to be effective. That treatment may be provided in a medical setting (as in a typical drug trial). A placebo effect may also be elicited by undergoing some procedure such as aroma therapy, or by taking a new supplement that promises some benefit. All of these practices involve the instillation of hope and the expectation of feeling better. Hope causes all sorts of positive physiological benefits that increase a sense of well-being.

TECHNICAL STUFF

Placebo effects can also be negative, sometimes called a *nocebo effect*. Some people in clinical trials receiving inert substances (like sugar pills) complain of side effects that are not explained by the placebo but are more likely caused by the participant's expectation of side effects.

So what do placebos and placebo effects have to do with antidepressants? There has been intense controversy about the placebo effect in the treatment of depression. Dr. Irving Kirsch of Harvard Medical School and colleagues have conducted numerous reviews of drug studies sent to the Food and Drug Administration (FDA). These studies were both published and unpublished. Research studies that do not support the efficacy of a particular drug are usually not published. Therefore, by including both published and unpublished studies, this review was quite comprehensive.

These reviews as well as reviews by other scientists have consistently concluded that most of the benefits of antidepressant medication are due to the placebo effect and that there is no clinically significant difference between those taking active drugs and those taking placebo. Dr. Kirsch recommends other treatments for depression that do not have the side effects of antidepressant medication, such as psychotherapy and physical exercise. Psychotherapy and exercise are just as effective as medication and have the added advantage of decreasing the chance of relapse.

TECHNICAL STUFF

There have been criticisms of the conclusions by other authors. Most relate to the differences between clinically different effect sizes. Some argue that antidepressants have a slight, clinically significant better response rate than placebo. These differences are usually measured by small changes on depression measures given before and after treatment.

Others argue that those differences do not make real differences in the lives of the people who are supposedly benefiting from those statistically significant effects. For example, if you scored 100 percent on a test and then lost three points, because of a scoring error, that three points might be statistically significant. However, for you, it wouldn't matter that much because you are still getting an A in the class.

Drugs for Depression

We hope we haven't scared you off from trying medication if that is something you and your healthcare provider think might be beneficial. Just keep in mind, you are engaging in an experiment that may or may not work. Nevertheless, many patients and their doctors report great improvement in depressive symptoms after taking antidepressant medication. How and why those improvements occur is a debate for researchers, not for people with depression and those who are attempting to treat them.

Therefore, in the following sections, we describe the most common prescription drugs used to treat depression. Antidepressant drugs are classified by how they affect one or more of these neurochemicals. We present the most commonly prescribed antidepressants and explain their actions, common uses, problems, and side effects. The following discussion can give you practical information about each class of antidepressant drug. Remember that new antidepressants are constantly being developed.

REMEMBER

We believe that knowledge helps you get the best medical care for your depression. The information we give you below will help you communicate with your healthcare provider. Working together, you can find the right medication or decide on another treatment.

SSRIs

Ever since Prozac came on the market in the late 1980s, *selective serotonin reuptake inhibitors* (SSRIs) have been the most popular antidepressants. One reason for their popularity is that side effects are less severe than older antidepressants and the consequences of overdose are also much less severe.

An SSRI is often the first choice of antidepressant medication. These drugs are used for the treatment of major depressive disorder, persistent depressive disorder, and premenstrual dysphoric disorder. SSRIs are commonly used when depression and anxiety are mixed. These medications are also used for treating other disorders that aren't accompanied by depression, such as anxiety disorders, obsessive compulsive disorder, eating disorders, and some types of chronic pain.

SSRIs ostensibly fight depression by increasing the available levels of serotonin. SSRIs usually take about one to four weeks to become effective. Side effects may include increased anxiety, fatigue, upset stomach, insomnia, apathy, lack of sexual interest, or inability to obtain orgasm. Other side effects include dizziness, sweating, tremors, dry mouth, headache, and weight loss or weight gain. Side effects are worse during the first couple of weeks and generally decrease over time.

WARNING

SSRIs may present some additional complications and problems. Keep these things in mind:

>> If you have bipolar disorder, SSRIs may be dangerous. Occasionally, these drugs activate manic states, which can involve dangerous or risky behaviors.

>> Abrupt discontinuation of SSRIs (or for that matter, any antidepressant medication) can produce flu-like symptoms such as nausea, headache, sweating, fever, and chills. Sudden withdrawal can also cause vivid dreams and problems with sleep. Talk to your doctor if you decide to stop taking SSRIs for advice on how to do so safely.

>> The FDA recently announced that SSRI medications may be associated with an increased risk of self-harm in children, adolescents, and young adults (which could potentially lead to suicidal attempts).

>> Taking SSRIs with another class of antidepressant called MAO inhibititors (discussed more fully later in this chapter) can trigger life-threatening interactions. Other drugs may also interact negatively. Tell your doctor about all of the medications you take.

TIP

Untreated depression often decreases interest in intimacy. And SSRIs can interfere with sexual arousal, pleasure, and interest. If you're in a relationship in which sexual intimacy has already been disrupted, tell your healthcare provider about your concerns.

Other neurotransmitter medications

Antidepressant medication likely works by increasing the amount of certain neurotransmitters in the brain. SSRIs target serotonin, but some antidepressants increase more than one such chemical messenger or act on the neuron and its neurotransmitters in more than one way.

In the following list, we take a look at these medication classes, noting which neurotransmitter system they affect and how it acts on them. You don't need to know the complicated terminology represented by the initials, but we include it in case you run across the terms in other literature.

>> **SNRIs (Serotonin/Norepinephrine Reuptake Inhibitor):** Boosts both serotonin and norepinephrine

>> **NDRIs (Norepinephrine/Dopamine Reuptake Inhibitor):** Boosts both norepinephrine and dopamine

>> **NRIs (Norepinephrine Reuptake Inhibitor):** Selectively boosts norepinephrine

>> **NaSSAs (Noradrenergic/Specific Serotonergic Antidepressants):** Enhances the release of norepinephrine and serotonin while blocking certain serotonin receptors

>> **SARIs (Serotonin-2 Antagonists Reuptake Inhibitors):** Blocks the reuptake of serotonin while also blocking one specific type of serotonin receptor

Other older antidepressants also targeted multiple neurochemicals (Tricyclics, which are covered next). However, these newer versions appear to have fewer side effects and are more specific in their actions on the neurotransmitters than the older tricyclics.

Tricyclics

This class of antidepressant medication was the most widely used for many years. *Tricyclic* medications are thought to have more general effects on neurotransmitters than the newer, more refined medications. The name is based on their chemical structure rather than the way they exert their effects, which vary somewhat from one type of tricyclic medication to another.

The primary reason they're now out of favor is that an overdose can be fatal. The newer antidepressants are much safer. Tricyclics are also associated with a host of side effects. These medications can cause dizziness from *orthostatic hypotension*, a sudden drop in blood pressure upon standing. Therefore, tricyclics are usually not prescribed for people at risk for falling, such as the elderly. Other side effects include weight gain, dry mouth, blurred vision, constipation, sweating, and sexual dysfunction.

Nevertheless, tricyclics are sometimes prescribed when other medications haven't worked or when anxiety mixes with depression.

MAO inhibitors

The first drug to treat depression was discovered in the early 1950s, totally by accident. Scientists were experimenting with a new treatment for tuberculosis. Unfortunately, the drug had no effect on TB, but surprisingly, the patients taking the drug became quite cheerful. Thus, the first antidepressant was born — a *monoamine oxidase inhibitor* (MAO inhibitor).

MAO inhibitors work by zapping a substance that destroys neurotransmitters. Because fewer neurotransmitters are destroyed, this action increases levels of serotonin, norepinephrine, and dopamine. MAO inhibitors are *infrequently* prescribed because of serious side effects when combined with common foods or medications. Side effects can include dangerous spikes in blood pressure that can result in cerebral hemorrhage or death.

WARNING

People taking MAO inhibitors should avoid food with *tyramine* (a natural substance found in the body that also forms as proteins break down as they age) such as sausages, beer, red wine, avocados, aged cheese, and smoked fish. Drug combinations to avoid include any other antidepressant medication, most drugs for colds and asthma, drugs for the treatment of diabetes, blood pressure medication, and some painkillers.

Despite all of the problems with MAO inhibitors, they're still used to treat some forms of resistant depression. When safer medications haven't helped, these drugs can be effective. They're especially useful for the treatment of atypical depression, which often involves overeating, sleeping too much, and irritability.

Looking Beyond Antidepressants

For most people with depression, an antidepressant medication alleviates symptoms. You may have to undergo some initial experimentation, but usually one or more of the drugs we discuss in the "Drugs for Depression" section earlier in the chapter eventually works. However, for some people, another type of medication will need to be tried or added to a mix.

When several different classes of antidepressant medication haven't worked, other types of drugs may be used to augment or enhance the treatment. These pharmacological mixes are usually best prescribed by a *psychiatrist,* a *psychiatric nurse practitioner,* or a *prescribing psychologist,* all specialists trained in the pharmaceutical treatment of mood disorders.

Depression is a deadly disease. Get treatment. If the first trial of medication doesn't work, hang in there with your healthcare professional. Another drug, drug combination, or psychotherapy is likely to help you.

Mood stabilizers

A group of drugs called mood stabilizers don't directly impact serotonin, dopamine, or norepinephrine — the neurotransmitters that antidepressant medications target. No one really knows how mood stabilizers work, but many of these drugs seem to affect two other neurotransmitters, glutamate and gamma-aminobutyric acid (GABA). Usually the first choice in treating bipolar disorder, mood stabilizers are also used in combinations with antidepressants for treating resistant depression.

When taking some mood stabilizers, you'll need to have periodic blood tests to find out the concentration of the medication in your system. These drugs can have serious side effects when levels get too high. Toxic levels can be deadly, so follow your doctor's instructions.

More help for severe depression: Antipsychotics

For people with severe symptoms, a new class of medication called atypical antipsychotics may help. In addition, these medications are sometimes given to those who don't benefit sufficiently from the other antidepressants discussed in this chapter. Antipsychotics may help when individuals suffer from psychosis, paranoia, or delusional thinking. These drugs may also be used when people with depression have problems with controlling their temper, tend to over-react to small frustrations, or swing back and forth from depression to mania.

Antipsychotic medication may cause disturbing side effects. The newer atypical antipsychotic medications have a significantly decreased risk of a long-term side effect known as tardive dyskinesia. *Tardive dyskinesia* involves involuntary movements, often in the face. When tardive dyskinesia appears, it usually does so after long-term treatment. Other serious side effects may include an intense feeling of agitation or restlessness, muscle spasms, muscle stiffness, shuffling gait, sedation, dry mouth, blurred vision, and hypotension. Weight gain is also particularly common and problematic, sometimes leading to diabetes.

A few more for the road

Your physician may prescribe other drugs for the treatment of depression or for the treatment of the side effects of antidepressant drugs. Here are a few examples:

>> **Stimulant medications:** These medications can be used to decrease fatigue, help with sexual drive, and improve attention.

>> **Hormones:** Sometimes hormone therapy is indicated because of abnormalities or as an augmenting agent.

>> **Sedating medications:** These drugs can help calm agitation or help with sleep.

A brief word about ketamine

Ketamine has been used as an anesthetic for over 50 years in operating rooms as well as by medics on battlefields. Recently, the FDA approved a type of ketamine in the form of a nasal spray to be used in conjunction with an oral antidepressant for treatment-resistant depression (that is, those who have failed on multiple trials of other antidepressant treatments). Treatment with ketamine must be closely monitored for side effects such as sedation, problems with attention, judgement, and loss of contact with reality. Therefore the administration of the drug must occur within a clinical setting until the patient is safely ready to leave. The patient is not allowed to drive to or from the ketamine administration sessions.

Ketamine is also given intravenously but under close supervision. Studies in hospital emergency rooms have seen remarkable and quick decreases in agitation and suicidal ideation when ketamine is given through an IV.

Ketamine has much promise as a standard treatment for suicidal crisis and treatment-resistant depression. However, there is a major potential for over-hyping its effectiveness, evidenced by the burgeoning business promoting ketamine clinics for aiding with a variety of maladies such as suicidal ideation, severe depression, pain, migraines, PTSD, bipolar disorder, and life satisfaction enhancement. Because IV-administered ketamine has not been approved by the FDA for these uses, insurance generally will not cover the expenses, which can be considerable. It appears that practitioners may be allowing their enthusiasm to guide their prescribing practices rather than waiting for solid data to establish efficacy for this drug.

One hint that these clinics may skirt the edge of sound, scientifically grounded practice can be found in the fact that some of them are run by providers that may not have appropriate training to treat patients with serious depression as well as other maladies that require specialized expertise. In addition, some providers do not have the experience to manage possible problems that emerge during treatment, such as irregularities in heart rhythm or other complications.

WARNING

Ketamine has interesting properties and possible exciting potential to quickly quell acute suicidal ideation and help those who have treatment-resistant depression. Yet it's too early to endorse this approach broadly to other conditions. Furthermore, it's very important to check out the credentials of the providers in any given clinic. Stay safe.

Chapter **18**

Hype, Help, or Hope? Alternative Treatments for Depression

W hen depression takes over, optimism fades into pessimism, and despair replaces hope. Depression hurts, and getting better seems almost impossible at times. Then you read about a treatment that offers hope in the form of a supplement, pill, new therapy, change in diet, light bulb, or complicated medical procedure. With hope comes a lightening of mood, a little relief, and a small seed of optimism. Hope can be a powerful tonic for depression.

But a general sense of hope in a future free of depression should be tempered with a sense of caution: That "treatment" you've read about may not have been clinically tested and could potentially be dangerous. If you follow a certain course of treatment, you may get a little better because you truly believe that the treatment is going to help you. There is nothing wrong with that — if the treatment is harmless. But, at the same time, we want you to be careful and not get taken advantage of by false promises. That's our purpose for writing this chapter.

Some treatments for depression can be expensive and possibly harmful. The real harm comes from postponing legitimate, evidenced-based treatment. Remember what your mother said: "When something sounds too good to be true, it usually is."

In this chapter, we give you the information you need to decide whether one or more of these alternative treatments may be for you. We present the latest research on treatments you can find at the health food store. Next, we explain what the diet gurus have to say about eating and moods. Finally, we describe electric shock therapy and other advanced medical treatments.

Keeping Your Doc in the Loop

We consider treatments for depression to be *alternative* if they're either not widely accepted as effective by conventional mental health and medical professionals or if these professionals don't use the treatments as first-choice approaches for most cases of major depression.

The *alternative* label certainly doesn't mean they're a secret: A report in the *American Journal of Psychiatry* provided the results of a survey that indicated that well over half of the people with cases of severe depression sought out alternative treatments such as herbs, spiritual healing, vitamins, and special diets. Furthermore, many of the people who used these alternative treatments found them to be helpful.

However, those individuals surveyed also said that they typically didn't inform their doctors about these therapies. That's something of a problem, because certain alternative treatments, such as herbs, may interact badly with some medications. Most of the depressed individuals who sought alternative treatments also used conventional mental health or medical treatment, which is a good thing, because these approaches have the support of a large body of research.

Doctors today are becoming increasingly accepting of alternative treatments. Thus, we urge you to let your healthcare providers in on any alternative treatments you're using for depression. They may be able to tell you whether a particular alternative treatment is known to work, or whether it may interact badly with a medication they're prescribing for you. Either way, this information is important to know.

If you or someone you love suffers from severe depression or has thoughts of suicide, you need to get professional help immediately. Remember, most clerks at health food stores don't qualify as licensed mental health professionals.

Exploring Supplements, Herbs, and Vitamins

Many folks who suffer from depression walk into a health food or supplement store looking for a natural solution to their problems. They walk up to a touch-screen computer, enter the word *depression*, and get five pages of herbs, supplements, and vitamins that promise relief. Some of these promises may pan out, but others won't. And some choices involve significant risks.

WARNING

You may believe that taking herbs, vitamins, and supplements for depression is a relatively harmless and natural alternative. The problem: Most people take these potent pills without medical supervision. Many of these "natural" substances can significantly interact with other medications you're taking and lead to dangerous results. So if you're considering using these alternatives, we strongly recommend that you first consult with your doctor.

If you suffer from moderate to severe depression, taking extra vitamins and minerals isn't likely to cure you. But a lack of certain vitamins and minerals does seem to be related to depression and memory problems. The research seems to clearly show that when people have a deficiency of B vitamins (especially B6, B12, and folic acid), depression is often present. Deficiencies in calcium, magnesium, potassium, iron, selenium, zinc, and sodium also seem to be associated with depression.

REMEMBER

It's important to keep in mind that most people who are depressed don't suffer from deficiencies in these vitamins or minerals. If you have concerns, talk to your primary healthcare provider.

WARNING

Some supplements can be downright dangerous, especially when taken in excessive dosages. Rather than increase your good mood, too many supplements will merely increase your credit card balance.

Herbs and supplements sold in the United States are largely unregulated by the Federal Drug Administration (FDA). Therefore, they are not subject to large-scale safety or efficacy studies. In other words, we just don't know if they work or if they are safe for people to take. Despite the lack of reliable information, the market share of these products is now close to $10 billion in the US.

Nonetheless, millions of people regularly take these supplements and herbs believing that they are working. We have a few caveats:

>> Some of these supplements have been independently tested and found to have dangerous impurities such as lead, other heavy metals, or arsenic.

>> Supplements or ingredients sold in the United States may have been manu-factured in other countries that have less stringent safety standards. You may not be able to determine that from reading the label.

>> Independent testing of products indicates that labeling is sometimes incorrect when a certain amount of a substance or percentage of an ingredient is promised. The potency of the product can be mislabeled.

>> When an adverse reaction occurs following the ingestion of an herb or supplement, there is no accurate tracking of those cases by the healthcare system. This lack of knowledge makes it more difficult to inform patients of potential interactions.

>> Some supplements have negative effects on the functioning of the liver and kidneys without adequate warnings on the label. Other adverse effects are also possible. For example, we love to cook with a variety of herbs and spices. Turmeric is one of our favorites. It is also frequently recommended for inflammation, depression, and pain. Seems pretty innocent. However, when taken prior to surgery, turmeric can cause excessive bleeding. We doubt most people even consider that serious consequence when taking turmeric.

PSYCHEDELICS FOR DEPRESSION?

Back in the 1960s, two Harvard psychology professors experimented with LSD and psilocybin (a hallucinogenic substance found in mushrooms). They had permission to administer their experimental treatment to graduate students. The two professors, Timothy Leary and Richard Alpert, were eventually fired from Harvard. Timothy Leary became an activist leader in the anti-war movement. Richard Alpert went to India and became known as Ram Dass, a spiritual leader. In part due to their association with the anti-establishment, anti-war movement, research on psychedelics was shut down com-pletely by 1974.

In the last few decades, research has been reopened for finding possible beneficial uses of psilocybin. Medium doses of psilocybin produce euphoria, dreamlike states, and per-ceptual changes. People who take high doses report mystical experiences, a sense of beauty, and a sense that love is all important.

Psychedelic-assisted psychotherapy has been provided under close medical supervi-sion. Positive effects have been found on decreasing anxiety at the end of life and reducing depression and anxiety in treatment-resistant patients. These improvements were maintained at 6 and 8 months after the administration. However, much remains to be learned about this promising treatment, but researchers are hopeful.

TIP

Rather than list specific products that advertise benefits for people with depression, we will give you the websites of two sources for information that you can trust. The first is the National Institutes of Health Office of Dietary Supplements. This site offers help in decision-making and fact sheets on vitamins, minerals, and supplements. The web address is www.ods.od.nih.gov. The second site is the National Center for Complementary and Integrative Health. Their website (www.nccih.nih.gov) is packed with information concerning alternative health including research findings and specific complementary approaches to depression.

Happy Foods

Depression can cause a decrease in appetite and lead to weight loss. It can also stir up cravings, which cause weigh gain. In either case, nutrition may suffer. Poor nutrition depletes the body of the nutrients needed for proper brain functioning. When the brain is malfunctioning, the intensity of depression increases. Therefore, when you're depressed, maintaining a healthy diet is especially important. We recommend that you

>> Eat sensible, well-balanced meals.

>> Don't skip meals.

>> Drink alcohol only in moderation, or not at all.

>> Don't beat yourself up if you occasionally indulge in a chocolate chip cookie.

TIP

In addition, you should know about the important role carbohydrates play in regard to moods. Put simply, carbohydrates boost moods. Have you ever craved something sweet when you felt sad or upset? Yum — the smell of fresh baked chocolate chip cookies. This craving for sweets may be your body's way of telling you that it needs a carbohydrate fix. Carbohydrates are broken down and converted to *glucose* (sugar), the fuel that keeps you going.

Two different kinds of carbohydrates exist: simple and complex. The body quickly converts simple carbohydrates (such as white rice, bagels, cookies, crackers, beer, wine, and most pastas) into sugar. The spike in your blood sugar level that results when you eat simple carbohydrates may cause a temporary lifting of spirits.

The problem with simple carbohydrates is that the quick conversion into sugar also signals your body to produce excess insulin. The insulin then causes your blood sugar level to fall. For many, the drop in blood sugar then leads to a lowered mood, irritability, and more cravings for sugar. Doctors believe that these rapid peaks and valleys in insulin levels aren't good for you for numerous reasons, such as a real possibility that they may contribute to the development of diabetes, obesity, and heart disease.

TIP

Complex carbohydrates represent a good alternative method for improving moods. These carbohydrates are found in whole grains, beans, vegetables, roots, and whole fruits. Complex carbohydrates break down into sugar more slowly, allowing your insulin levels to remain more stable. They don't increase cravings or lower moods. Some nutritionists contend that complex carbohydrates also raise serotonin levels. Therefore, consuming complex carbohydrates may be a useful way of improving moods without the peaks and valleys that occur with simple carbohydrates.

If you have depression, what you eat can either make you feel better or worse. Therefore, pay attention to your diet. Make sure it's balanced and contains complex carbohydrates.

Lighting Up the Darkness

If winter consistently brings on the blues, you may suffer from *seasonal affective disorder*, or SAD, a subtype of major depressive disorder. (See Chapter 2 for more information.) Most people feel a little down when the sun rises late and sets early day after day, and the clouds dampen the daylight. However, people with SAD experience symptoms of a major depressive disorder including loss of pleasure and interests, reduced energy, and so on.

SAD can be treated with all the usual treatments for depression that we discuss throughout this book, but light therapy has become a highly popular treatment. With light therapy, a person is exposed to bright light that is from 25 to 100 times more powerful than a standard 100-watt light bulb. Thus, the lighting used with light therapy is much more intense than the lighting you find in a well-lit room.

TIP

Studies generally have shown that the treatment works better than no treatment and placebos. However, the effectiveness of light therapy remains somewhat controversial, and a few studies haven't shown any more improvements than those obtained with a placebo. Many practitioners recommend a daily walk outside during the brightest part of the day as an alternative to light therapy.

Light therapy devices can be purchased online. We checked one popular online source and found hundreds of devices that ranged in price from a low of $17 to one costing close to $500. Many can act as reading lights or lights that gradually brighten and dim to duplicate the sun rising and setting. Please read the reviews before you buy. We suggest that you purchase a well reviewed, relatively inexpensive lamp before spending too much money.

Here are the advantages of light therapy:

>> It often works quite rapidly (sometimes within a week).

>> It has fewer side effects than most medications.

>> After the initial purchase of the equipment, it is inexpensive.

On the other hand, light therapy does have a few, usually mild side effects, which can include headache, nausea, eye strain, jumpiness, sleep disturbance, and agitation. Studies have found that patients who use light therapy for many years don't suffer from any ill effects on the eye. However, the extremely long-term effects of the therapy still remain unknown. And if you suffer from significant eye problems, check with an ophthalmologist prior to using light therapy.

Treating Severe Depression

Unfortunately, some cases of depression are unusually difficult to treat. Medications and psychotherapy occasionally fail to alleviate the pain and suffering of these difficult cases. The following alternative treatments are used specifically for treating especially stubborn depression. We call these treatments alternative largely because they're not used for the vast majority of depressed persons.

Shocking depression

In April 1938, Italian doctors in desperation administered shock to a severely psychotic man. He apparently lived a normal life after receiving the treatment. Thus, *electroconvulsive therapy* (ECT), popularly known as *shock therapy*, was born. The interest in ECT for the treatment of depression blossomed through the 1950s. Soon after, the emergence of antidepressant medication decreased the popularity of ECT. However, ECT is still in use, particularly for treatment-resistant cases of serious depression. In fact, close to a million people still receive ECT each year. That may change due to recent questions about research regarding the efficacy and safety of ECT.

Problems with research on ECT includes the fact that all of the controlled clinical trials occurred more than 35 years ago. There have been relatively few studies, and the ones that do exist had a small number of participants. Methodological quality was also poor.

Recent reviewers published their findings in the journal *Ethical Human Psychology and Psychiatry*. They concluded that evidence does not exist to support using ECT for severely depressed patients, suicidal cases, or treatment-resistant depression. In fact, they recommended that because of the risks of permanent memory loss and death, ECT should be suspended immediately until further, better quality data can be collected.

Once considered the gold standard in the treatment of severe, treatment-resistant depression, there remain some practitioners who continue to recommend ECT to their patients. And there are certainly patients who claim that ECT has helped them. Reviewing researchers counter that these effects are likely due solely to placebos or expectations for positive outcomes and are not worth the risks involved.

TIP

Our take on this controversy is to err on the side of caution and await the collection of more data prior to recommending ECT with its attendant risks. You don't want to lose memories or your life. There are other, less risky alternatives.

Stimulating nerves

Scientists are constantly searching for new treatments for depression. Much of their motivation comes from the fact that a small percentage of people with depression have exceptionally stubborn, treatment-resistant cases. In the past, ECT was one of the few approaches to work for these cases. However, as noted in the previous section, ECT has the potential for serious side effects and is frankly scary to many people.

One of the newer, possibly safer treatments under investigation involves vagus nerve stimulation (VNS). The *vagus nerve* is one of the 12 nerves that run through the head. It controls your heart rate, vocal cords, bronchial constriction, and movements within the digestive tract. Vagus nerve stimulation was first found to be effective in preventing seizures during the 1980s. More recently, it has been applied to the treatment of serious, resistant depression.

The procedure involves implanting a device that intermittently emits a mild electrical impulse to electrodes woven around the vagus nerve in the upper part of the chest. Patients who undergo this procedure report mild side effects, which can include facial muscle weakness, shortness of breath, mild sore throat, and hoarseness or cough.

These side effects are worse while the stimulation is being applied, but they usually decrease over time. Stimulation is typically applied for about a half minute every three to five minutes, 24 hours per day. Patients are given a means for shutting the device off if they find it to be too uncomfortable.

Early evidence suggests that vagus nerve stimulation may result in great improvement in a significant number of patients. And the vast majority of those who improve don't experience early relapse. The treatment takes quite awhile to work. It may also improve in effectiveness the longer it continues. The implanted devices have been approved by the FDA for severe, treatment-resistant depression. However, some insurance companies are reluctant to pay for these devices.

In Europe, there are new VNS devices that don't require surgical implantation. These devices are used to treat depression, pain, and epilepsy. Further research will be required to fully validate their use for treatment-resistant depression. In the United States, the FDA has approved these devices for treating cluster headaches.

Magnetizing depression

We now have several decades of research on a treatment for depression known as *transcranial magnetic stimulation* (TMS). This therapy is safe and noninvasive. It involves placing an electromagnetic coil on the scalp that produces a strong magnetic field. The magnetic pulse stimulates nerve cells in areas of the brain thought to be involved in modulating moods.

TMS is FDA approved for the treatment of severe, chronic depression. It does not require sedation and is essentially pain free. Unlike VNS, TMS does not require surgical implantation, and unlike ECT, it does not require anesthesia or cause seizures. Side effects include headaches, light-headedness, scalp discomfort, and tingling of facial muscles. These side effects tend to go away shortly following sessions.

Originally, TMS was approved for five sessions per week, usually lasting 30 to 40 minutes. These sessions continued for four to six weeks. New devices are intended to allow for shortened treatment times. Patients can drive themselves to and from sessions because no sedation is involved. TMS may not always be covered by insurance, so check your coverage. TMS may prove to be a very effective, simple procedure for severe depression. However, because the approach is relatively new, long-term outcome studies are needed.

WARNING

TMS is not appropriate for people who have implanted electrical or metallic devices. It is also not recommended for patients with brain damage or a history of seizures. Check with your doctor about other potential restrictions.

Searching Further

We searched the literature for additional alternative treatments for depression. Trust us, you don't want to see everything that anyone has ever suggested. However, we will tell you about a small number of other possibilities that may improve an occasional bad mood but can't replace more scientifically validated approaches to treating depression:

>> **Air ionization:** You may have experienced a lift in spirits when standing near a waterfall. That effect may occur because of negative ions in the atmosphere produced by the waterfall. You can purchase machines that produce negative ions, but don't expect major improvements in mood from them. Research has failed to find a positive effect on anxiety, moods, sleep, and relaxation from ionization therapy. However, a small amount of data has indicated that there could be a modest effect on lowering depression scores.

>> **Art and creative therapies:** Activities that allow you to express yourself in creative ways may be effective means to release stress, decrease anxiety, and reduce depressive symptoms. Sessions supervised by an art therapist may be especially beneficial. Research has shown short-term decreases in negative emotions following art therapy. However, we recommend this therapy as an *accompaniment* to standard, empirically validated approaches rather than as a stand-alone treatment.

>> **Massage:** Massage therapy, when delivered by a trained therapist, involves the manipulation of the body's soft tissues. Most people know that a massage can feel pretty good, but can it alleviate depression? Massage can help relieve stress and increase feelings of well-being for a short while. However, it has not shown consistent value as a treatment for major depressive disorders.

>> **Relaxation:** Various techniques exist for teaching people how to relax their muscles. A half dozen or so small, controlled studies suggest that relaxation may be effective for treating mild depression. Once again, however, more research is called for, and studies haven't yet shown whether relaxation training reduces depression over the long run. Nevertheless, relaxation has a very low potential for negative side effects, and it may actually help alleviate depression.

>> **Acupuncture:** This ancient Chinese method ostensibly stimulates the body to correct imbalances in energy flow. Very fine needles are inserted into specific, theoretically relevant body regions. A few studies have suggested that acupuncture effectively decreased depression at three months. It has also been used to treat chronic pain, which is often a risk factor for depression.

TIP

When you are depressed, any activity that brings you temporary relief or good feelings is absolutely fine. We encourage you to try out all sorts of different approaches. However, nothing can substitute for empirically validated treatment. But by all means have as much fun as possible. Just don't spend too much of your hard-earned money or precious time searching for the end of the rainbow.

6

Looking Beyond Depression

IN THIS PART . . .

Prepare a plan for possible relapse.

Understand the relationship between depression and memory, and develop ways to improve memory.

Pour over positive psychology.

IN THIS CHAPTER

» **Understanding the nature and risks of relapse**

» **Protecting yourself against relapse**

» **Handling relapse when it shows up**

Chapter **19**

Reducing the Risk of Relapse

The information in this chapter is especially important after you experience improvement with your depression. If your mood hasn't yet substantially improved, we suggest that you work on your depression before you worry too much about relapse. Parts 1 through 5 of this book may help. If you put in a lot of personal effort, and your depression still hasn't improved much, seek professional help. But if you've seen substantial improvement in your symptoms — or if you don't suffer from depression but you want to find out more about it — keep reading.

Craig took a new position as a high school principal last year. The added responsibility has not been easy for him. He hasn't felt like himself for six months. He feels overwhelmed and yet lacks the drive to solve everyday problems. Craig usually tackles problems head-on, so he makes an appointment with his primary care physician. His doctor prescribes an antidepressant medication. After just six weeks of faithfully taking his prescribed medication, Craig feels on top of the world again. He has no remaining symptoms of depression. Although his doctor recommended continuing the medication for at least six months, Craig chooses to ignore his doctor's advice and stop. Craig "knows" that he'll be alright; after all, he hasn't felt this good in years. Besides, he slowly tapers his medication consumption down so that he can avoid the withdrawal effects that he was warned about. Five weeks later, Craig suffers a relapse and crashes into a bottomless pit, feeling more depressed than he did before he started the medication.

In this chapter, we discuss what is currently known about relapse and depression. *Relapse* refers to a fall or slip back into depression after having largely or completely recovered. We explain how often relapse occurs, and we tell you what you can do to reduce the risk of relapse. We also give you ideas for dealing with relapse in the event that it happens to you.

Risking Relapse with Depression

In writing this book, we choose to shoot straight. That's why our approach to cognitive therapy (see Part 2) recommends that you use objective, evidence-based thinking rather than delude yourself with simplistic positive self-affirmations as a cure-all for your depression. We want you to see yourself and the world as they are, not as a fairy tale. Denial only makes things worse.

So when it comes to the treatment of depression, we give you the good news and the bad. The good news is that, with the wide array of both established and new therapies and medications available today, the majority of people with depression can be successfully treated. By successful treatment, we mean that their depressive symptoms can be eased for at least six months or more. The bad news is that the risk of relapse is distressingly high.

Fortunately, we have more good news — you can do quite a bit to reduce the risk of relapse, and if you should fall back into melancholy, you have a good chance of beating back your depression once again.

Determining what's going on

In Chapter 4, we discuss the fact that, with depression, progress always proceeds in an uneven fashion with many ups and downs along the way. In fact, we can't remember working with anyone who progressed without ever making the slightest slip. Furthermore, everyone has bad moods and rotten days from time to time. So how can you tell if what you're experiencing represents a true relapse?

REMEMBER

When you experience a full-blown relapse of depression, you have clear signs of one of the types of depression we discuss in detail in Chapter 2 following a period of six or more depression-free months. If your symptoms are mild and don't meet the criteria for depression spelled out in Chapter 2, you've encountered one of depression's early warning signs — something to take seriously, but not an actual relapse. To deal with early warning signs, try the suggestions we provide in the "Preparing a Prevention Plan" section later in this chapter. On the other hand, if you're in the middle of a relapse, read the "Reining In Relapse When It Occurs" section, which you can also find later in this chapter.

Evaluating relapse rates

So just how high is the risk of depression relapse? Well, in part, the answer depends on whether your depression was treated with medication or therapy.

If you discontinue medication after your depression lets up, your chances of relapse exceed 50 percent over the next year or two. Your odds appear somewhat better if you received cognitive therapy either alone, or in conjunction with or following antidepressant medication. Interpersonal therapy (we discuss elements of this therapy in Chapters 15 and 16) has also shown promise in reducing relapse. Your odds of reducing the risk of relapse further improve if you also receive behavior therapy, such as problem solving (covered in Chapter 14) or mindfulness techniques (discussed in Chapter 9).

The therapies we chose for this book have been selected in part for their potential to reduce relapse. Combining them gives you particularly robust tools for reducing your risks.

WARNING

Although many treatment avenues lessen the chance of relapse, your risk of relapse is considerably higher if you stop treatment before your symptoms of depression have virtually vanished. In other words, your chances of experiencing a relapse increase if you stop treatment before you are truly back to a full, non-depressed condition. Don't stop treatment until you have months of normal energy, appetite, sleep, and enjoyment of activities.

Rates of depression soared during the 2020 pandemic. Although complete statistics are not currently known, common sense tells us that relapse rates from depression are also high. Social isolation, uncertainty, financial difficulties, and grief are all risk factors.

TIP

If you are suffering depressive symptoms during stressful times and have a history of major depressive disorder, reach out to your healthcare provider for information about getting help.

Getting personal about your risks

In addition to the relapse factors we outline in the "Evaluating relapse rates" section earlier in the chapter, one other intriguing, possible factor is emerging. New evidence suggests a surprising problem that may increase the likelihood of a recurrence of your depression.

TIP

You can take our Relapse Quiz in Table 19-1 to get an idea of whether this risk for relapse pertains to you. For each question, rate your extent of agreement on a scale of 1 to 7. Use 1 if you *completely disagree,* 2 if you mostly disagree, 3 if you disagree a little, 4 if you neither agree nor disagree, 5 if you agree a little, 6 if you mostly agree, and 7 if you *completely agree* with the statement.

TABLE 19-1   ## Relapse Quiz

Statement	Rating of Agreement or Disagreement
I will sacrifice my own needs in order to please other people.	1 2 3 4 5 6 7
I feel I must have the approval of others if I'm going to be happy.	1 2 3 4 5 6 7
I know I can control depression if it strikes.	1 2 3 4 5 6 7
There's nothing I can do to deal with depression.	1 2 3 4 5 6 7
When I feel sad, I'm sure that my view of life is realistic.	1 2 3 4 5 6 7
When I'm depressed, I absolutely know that my thoughts and emotions don't accurately reflect what's going on.	1 2 3 4 5 6 7
I'm the cause of my own depression.	1 2 3 4 5 6 7
I get depressed when I mess up.	1 2 3 4 5 6 7

You score this quiz a little differently than most self-tests. You don't add or subtract any of the scores. Rather, the more items you either *completely agree* or *completely disagree* with, as indicated by a rating of 1 or 7, the higher your odds of relapse.

We know that it sounds strange to hear that your relapse risk rises if you *completely agree* with items such as:

>> I know I can control depression if it strikes.

>> When I'm depressed, I absolutely know that my thoughts and emotions don't accurately reflect what's going on.

And we also know that having an increased risk of relapse sounds strange if you *completely disagree* with items such as:

>> I feel I must have the approval of others if I'm going to be happy.

>> When I feel sad, I'm sure that my view of life is realistic.

Why wouldn't we want you to totally believe that you can control your depression when it strikes? And if you're sad, wouldn't we want you to completely believe that you're viewing life and events unrealistically? Well, sort of, but hold on a moment.

In Part 2, we detail how cognitive therapy helps people to appraise themselves and their world *realistically.* If you've ever experienced a bout of serious depression, absolutely and completely controlling your depression when it strikes probably doesn't sound all that realistic. It may be more reasonable to say that you have *some* confidence in your ability to control your emotions, but not total confidence. You may even be able to say that you have *quite a lot* of confidence, but not *complete* confidence. Stating that you don't believe you need other people's approval to be happy may also be realistic. But isn't it likely that you could have a little doubt?

REMEMBER

Idealistic, overly optimistic thinking just may set you up for relapse. Viewing yourself as superior to other people can put you at risk for disappointment and depression. Similarly, Pollyannaish thinking can do the same.

REMEMBER

Our relapse quiz isn't a scientific test, so don't worry excessively if you respond with quite a few 1s or 7s. However, research does suggest that you want to avoid thinking in absolutist, extreme terms. Also, if you've never been depressed, this quiz has no relevance to whether you may develop depression in the future. Because you've never lived in the pit of depression, it's probably more reasonable for you to have more complete confidence in the views you hold about yourself and the world.

Preparing a Prevention Plan

If you completely ignore the real possibility of your depression returning, relapse may very well lie around the corner ready to jump out and snare you. But you can do a lot to minimize the dangers of a recurrence. We now review the strategies you have available for preventing relapse.

Sustaining success

When depression finally loosens its grip, most people feel like stopping treatment. And we don't blame them for feeling that way. All treatments of depression (including self-help) require time, energy, and at least a little money.

TIP

Given the various challenges that treatment presents, why put in any more effort than you have to — especially when you're feeling good again? Well, we'll tell you: because the risk of relapse is unacceptably high if you stop prematurely, especially when you factor in the debilitating nature of depression.

REMEMBER

Most professionals advocate treating depression until the symptoms completely subside, not just until they're partially resolved. Furthermore, therapists typically recommend continuing treatment for at least a few months following the full remission of depression — a return to normal energy, concentration, appetite, sleep, and enjoyment of life's activities.

The suggestion to continue treatment is based on the idea that attaining a thorough mastery of new skills, behaviors, and ways of thinking is the best approach. Newly acquired, fledgling skills won't hold up in the face of the inevitable adversities of life. The skills you acquire need drill and repetition. In order to hold up under pressure, they need to be "over-learned."

Continue practicing the strategies that first alleviated your depression until you feel you've completely mastered them. In addition, you may want to try something different (such as behavior therapy in Part 3 or relationship therapy in Part 4) and rehearse those new skills. If you haven't yet tackled cognitive therapy (see Part 2), we strongly urge you to do so because thought therapy not only defeats depression, it also helps prevent relapse.

REMEMBER

The more skills you master for handling depression, the less likely you are to experience relapse in the future. Continuing either psychotherapy or medication for some months beyond the alleviation of your depression can help keep relapse at bay.

Even if you choose to treat your depression with medication only, we suggest that you continue taking the medication for at least 6 to 12 months after your depression fully subsides. Doing so will reduce your chances of relapse somewhat, although we highly recommend trying some type of psychotherapy, such as cognitive therapy, in addition to the medication. Alternatively, some folks with a history of recurrent depressions find that continuing to take antidepressant medication for a lifetime provides them with reasonable protection against relapse. (See Chapter 17 for more information about medications.)

Monitoring the signs

In Chapter 2, we review the myriad of ways that depression affects your thoughts, behavior, body, and relationships. If you've worked on beating your depression, you no doubt know what depression looks like for you. We suggest that you observe yourself and the symptoms discussed in the following exercise from time to time.

TIP

Conduct a Depression Review at least once a month. Select a convenient time and pencil your Depression Review in your calendar. We recommend conducting this review for at least a year after the depression lifts. In your Depression Review, ask yourself these questions:

>> Have I been having gloomy, dark thoughts?

>> Have I started avoiding people or situations that make me feel uncomfortable?

>> What is my mood on a 1 (extremely depressed) to 100 (completely happy) point scale? Has my mood dropped from its usual rating by more than 10 points and remained lower for more than a week or so?

>> Am I having any noticeable problems with my appetite, sleep, or energy?

>> Have I been down on myself more than usual?

>> Have I been more irritable than usual?

>> Have I had an increase in guilty feelings?

>> Am I having problems with concentration?

WARNING

If you answer yes to one or more of the questions above, pay attention! This list contains the early warning signs of an impending depression. Of course, anyone can experience a few gloomy thoughts, a little guilt, and difficulty concentrating without sliding into a full-blown depression. However, we recommend taking these warning signs seriously by reinitiating some form of treatment, or possibly self-help efforts if your symptoms are mild.

Using a fire drill

No one knows when a fire will start. That's why school children everywhere periodically engage in fire drills. These drills prepare them for exactly what to do when fire breaks out.

TIP

A Fire Drill for depression involves vividly imagining potential adversities or hardships. Then you ask yourself how you might cope with them. Finally, you imagine yourself coping in a productive manner.

We're guessing that you're not a psychic, so you can't predict which adversities you may encounter in the future or when those hardships may appear. However, you probably do know what types of events have given you trouble in the past, as well as what you fear about the future. Rather than pretend that the entire remainder of your life will be nothing but roses, we suggest that you make up a list of worrisome scenarios.

On your list, include anything that you believe could actually happen to you and that you fear could overwhelm your capacity to cope. A few possibilities include

>> Embarrassment

>> Failing to meet a deadline

>> Financial reversals

>> Illness

>> Injury

>> Isolation caused by a pandemic

>> Losing a loved one

>> Rejection

Next, take your list and select one item. Imagine that event happening and finding a way to cope with the adversity. When you perform a Fire Drill, use the questions in this list to help you come up with ideas on how to cope:

>> How would someone else cope with this situation?

>> Have I dealt with something like this in the past? How did I do it?

>> How much will this event affect my life a year after it occurs?

>> Is this event as awful as I'm making it out to be?

>> Are there any intriguing, creative ways of dealing with this challenge?

TIP

People often dread future possibilities because they assume they'll be unable to cope with them. However, when you face fears head-on, more often than not, you find you can cut them down to size. That's why you should conduct a Fire Drill on each and every item on your list of worrisome scenarios.

Ryan recovered from his bout with depression about a month ago. He feels much better, but he realizes that he needs to consider the issue of relapse seriously. Thus, he monitors his early warning signs of depression and realizes that he's starting to avoid certain people and situations. He knows that, in the past, he's been highly sensitive to embarrassment and rejection.

So he chooses to use the Fire Drill with this issue. He vividly imagines asking Brooke (a girl he's attracted to) out on a date and getting turned down in a hurtful way. Then he answers the coping questions as follows:

● **How would someone else cope with this situation?** "Actually, I bet this happens to people all the time. The key is to accept the rejection, ask myself if there's anything I can learn from it, and move on. It's not like the rejection will be pasted on my forehead for everyone to see."

- **Have I ever dealt with something like this in the past? How did I do it?** "Yeah, I've been turned down before, and I got through it. I didn't like it, but I dealt with it."

- **How much will this event affect my life a year after it occurs?** "If you put in that way, I guess not much at all."

- **Is this event as awful as I'm making it out to be?** "No. I guess I tell myself that it's awful and that it means I'm a total reject, but just having those thoughts doesn't make them true."

- **Are there any intriguing, creative ways of dealing with this challenge?** "Maybe I could try out that new speed-dating service where you meet something like 20 people in an hour. I may meet somebody interesting, and even if I don't, maybe I can learn to deal with rejection better by going straight at it."

Ryan's Fire Drill helps him realize that his ability to cope with feared situations is greater than he has allowed himself to believe. He then imagines getting turned down and dealing with the rejection many times. After he realizes that he can deal with this problem, he asks Brooke out.

TIP

The Fire Drill strategy works best if you first read about cognitive therapy, in Part 2. Cognitive therapy helps you understand how to tackle difficult events with more reasonable ways of thinking. When you perform a Fire Drill, you get extra practice using this type of thinking.

TIP

All too often, people who suffer from depression also struggle with excessive anxiety and worry about future events. And for many, anxiety appears to predate the emergence of depression. If you suffer from anxiety along with your depression, we recommend that you read our other book, *Anxiety For Dummies* (Wiley). Additional work on your anxiety will help you make better use of the Fire Drill technique as well as help insulate you against recurrent depressions.

Reaching for well-being

If you work hard on overcoming depression and search diligently for solutions, the odds greatly favor a positive outcome. In other words, you stand a good chance of defeating your depression. But why stop there? You may no longer feel depressed, but have you achieved a greater sense of well-being?

Tracking your well-being

Some individuals report that they rarely feel a true sense of satisfaction or well-being even when they're not depressed. However, when asked to closely track their well-being, they usually discover that certain types of situations and events do create greater satisfaction than others do. This discovery often inspires them to increase their involvement in gratifying activities.

TIP

Take some time to ponder the activities that feel satisfying to you. Write them down in a notebook or keep a list in your device. Then record the thoughts you have in response to those events as well as how much satisfaction they give you. Rate the intensity of your satisfaction on a scale of 0 to 100. You can use this Satisfaction Tracker to help you discover the activities that improve your sense of well-being. (See Table 19-2 for an example.) Then you can use that information to increase those activities, thereby increasing your overall satisfaction.

Alec no longer feels depressed, but he doesn't feel like he enjoys very many things. His therapist suggests that he use a Satisfaction Tracker to get a better idea of what kinds of situations increase his sense of well-being. Table 19-2 shows what Alec discovers when he records the intensity of the satisfaction he experiences when he participates in specific events.

TABLE 19-2   **Alec's Satisfaction Tracker**

Situation	Satisfying Thoughts	Satisfaction Intensity (On a Scale of 0 to 100)
Taking the dog to the dog park.	I love watching my dog run!	60
Going to a party.	I like talking with a couple of my friends.	40
Showing off my new car to Linda.	I think she might like me.	35
Waxing my new car.	I feel great when I take good care of things.	65
Having lunch with Larry.	I like catching up on things with him.	70
Cleaning out the garage.	It feels good to do things I've been putting off.	65

Alec discovers that a few more things than he thought lead him to feeling satisfied. Clearly, he enjoys taking out his dog and making headway with certain types of chores. He also likes catching up with Larry. He decides to take on at least one satisfying chore, go out to lunch with a friend, and take his dog to the park every week. But Alec also observes that his satisfaction isn't as high as he would have expected on two items — going to a party and showing off his new car. This discovery leads to the next strategy for enhancing your well-being.

Cutting off the well-being interrupters

If you start tracking your satisfying situations as Alec did in Table 19-2, you're likely to discover that some of your satisfactions aren't as terrific as others. When that's the case, take a look at your thoughts regarding the event. First, consider any thoughts you have that involve feeling good about the event. Then ask yourself if you have any thoughts that interrupt that sense of satisfaction. We call those thoughts *satisfaction interrupters* — any thought that takes away from your enjoyment of a positive activity.

For example, **Annette** tracks her satisfying activities as Alec did in Table 19-2. She then chooses a couple of these events that didn't feel as satisfying as she might have expected. Table 19-3 shows the nature of her satisfaction interrupters.

TABLE 19-3   **Annette's Satisfaction Interrupters**

Event	Satisfying Thought	Satisfaction-Interrupting Thoughts
Volunteering at the homeless shelter.	I like contributing something to society.	But then I thought that I really should be working on my school project: I'll never get it done.
Going to a party.	I think Kyle might like me.	Then I thought that he probably has a girlfriend and he's just being polite.

TIP

See how Annette's interrupting thoughts managed to deflate her sense of well-being and satisfaction? If you're not feeling as satisfied by events as you think you should be, try tracking your satisfaction interrupters like Annette did. Then ask yourself the following questions about those deviously disruptive thoughts:

>> What evidence do I have that either supports or refutes my satisfaction-interrupting thoughts?

>> If a friend of mine told me that he or she had this interrupting thought, would I think that it sounded reasonable or merely self-defeating on my friend's part?

>> Do I have experiences in my life that may refute this interrupting thought?

>> Is this interrupting thought distorted in any way?

>> Can I reflect on a satisfaction-interrupting thought that may be more accurate and help me feel better?

When Annette subjects her satisfaction-interrupting thoughts to these questions, she's able to generate a more satisfying alternative. You too will likely discover that subjecting your satisfaction interrupters to scrutiny pays off. When you answer the preceding questions, you'll likely be able to dispute those interrupting thoughts and come up with more satisfying perspectives. We recommend keeping track of this information.

TIP

The strategy of challenging satisfaction-interrupting thoughts may look familiar to you if you read Part 2, which talks about cognitive therapy. In Part 2, you find many more strategies for tackling problematic thinking. The main difference here is that you track *satisfying* events rather than disturbing, depressing ones, and then you record which thoughts *interfere* with that satisfaction.

Changing your lifestyle

A third useful strategy for increasing your overall sense of well-being and decreasing the likelihood of relapse lies in taking a good look at your lifestyle. Ask yourself these Lifestyle Analysis questions:

» Am I spending my time doing things that make me feel good, or do I merely numb myself by doing things like watching excessive television or playing mindless video games?

» Am I working longer hours than necessary?

» Am I obsessing over driven, self-imposed standards of perfectionism that cause unnecessary pressure for me?

» Do I take reasonable vacation times and breaks?

» Do I engage in a reasonable amount of recreation?

» Are there things I have always wanted to do that I haven't gotten around to doing? If so, what are they, and why am I not doing them?

TIP

Take time out to examine your life. Think about whether the way you spend your time reflects your priorities. If it doesn't, consider allocating your time differently. If you feel trapped and unable to make these changes, read Chapters 13 and 14. You may discover a creative way of escaping the trap set by your mind.

Reining In Relapse When It Occurs

Sometimes depression returns despite enormous efforts to fend it off. What do you do in this case? First, you need to know what a true relapse looks like. (Check out the "Determining what's going on" section earlier in this chapter.) Then if you determine that you may be experiencing a relapse, you have to take some steps to deal with it.

The very first step in dealing with relapse is to seek professional help. If you've never seen a therapist or psychiatrist before, make sure that you see one, because self-help alone won't suffice when dealing with recurrent depressions. If you've seen a professional before, don't conclude that a relapse means professional help is useless.

If therapy seemed to help before, then more therapy will likely prove quite beneficial. If you previously tried therapy and it didn't help, you need further treatment — perhaps with a different therapist. (See Chapter 5 for info on finding the right therapist.)

If you haven't tried medication, you may want to consider it. If medication worked before and you stopped, you may want to restart medication or add therapy to your arsenal.

The very worst thing you can do when you experience a relapse is to think of it as a catastrophe and assume that it means you have failed or your condition is uniquely hopeless. You have to understand that depression is a formidable foe with numerous causes, including genetics, trauma, and unknown factors. Professionals don't believe that depression reoccurs because of personal weakness, a lack of moral fiber, or any other fault that resides within a person. Although it may not be pleasant to face this foe again, you can defeat depression.

The vast majority of depression relapses can be treated successfully. You have many treatment avenues to explore.

Chapter **20**

Mending Your Memory

D epression is bad enough. You feel terrible. Your sleep may be disturbed, your appetite may be lousy, and nothing seems like fun anymore. What could be worse? Well, you can add to the mix a significant decline in your ability to remember names, dates, errands, and shopping lists.

But why would we single out memory as a special concern? Mostly because mucked up memory messes up your everyday life. In addition, when you notice memory problems, putting yourself down for having the problem is all too easy. You don't need more sources for negative thinking than depression has already given you.

Depression and memory impairment go hand in hand. Here's the good news: When your depression lifts, your memory will likely improve. But in the meantime, you have many options for aiding and improving your memory, which may in turn improve your mood.

In order to understand how depression damages memory, we first tell you how memory works and then describe the different kinds of memory. Next, we reveal the ways depression depletes and disrupts memory. Some forgetfulness is perfectly normal; we tell you how to know if your problem needs more attention. Finally, we give you sound strategies for dealing with memory problems and boosting your memory skills.

Making Sense of Memory

Think back to when you were a child. What is the earliest memory you can conjure up from childhood? Do you recall where the event took place, who was there, and what you looked like? Good. Now try to remember what you ate for lunch two weeks ago. What? You can remember something that happened years ago, but you can't remember something that happened two weeks ago?

This little exercise demonstrates that memory processes are complex. You don't remember everything that happens to you. We're pretty sure you were awake and paying attention to what you ate two weeks ago. But you probably can't remember the food unless it was unusual, special, or important to you in some way.

Scientists basically agree on how memories are formed. All memory begins with some perception of information or an event by one or more of the senses. Many factors determine the perception that forms a memory and whether or not you're going to recall it. The following sections briefly describe the most important processes involved in memory.

Memory for now: Immediate memory

Think of immediate memory as a photograph or recording of each moment that quickly disintegrates. Right now, you're reading these words, but your senses are also aware of the temperature of the room you're in, the sounds of cars going by, the level of light, and the comfort of your seat. You can turn your attention willfully to any of those sensations, but most of them are never really brought into your awareness.

You use your immediate memory when someone gives you a bit of information such as turn left at the second light or stop at the store and pick up milk and bread. You can remember it for a few minutes and then you forget it entirely. If there are several steps in a set of directions or a grocery list is long, you won't be as likely to recall it even after a couple of minutes.

Your lunch two weeks ago was in your immediate memory for a while. Unless something unusual occurred, such as choking on a chicken bone, the memory of your lunch will probably never move from your immediate memory to long-term memory (which we describe later). Rather, it will be lost forever.

Juggling items in memory: Working memory

When you pay attention to information, your working memory (a temporary holding zone) allows you to use, manipulate, elaborate, or send the information on to long-term storage. Working memory is like a blackboard in your brain that constantly changes. Without working memory, you'd be unable to solve many types of problems that involve thinking about more than one concept at a time. Here's an example: Say all the letters of the alphabet (which you pull from your long-term memory) that rhyme with the word *me*. In order to say these letters, you have to use your working memory to picture all the letters, scan through them, and figure out if they rhyme.

Working memory allows you to consider several aspects of a problem at the same time and come up with solutions. For example, when deciding on whether or not to purchase a new car, your working memory can allow you to think about how nice a new car would look like in your driveway, where you would sell your old car, how much of a hassle it would be to go to a car dealer, and what effect a big car payment would have on your bank balance and lifestyle. People with poor working memory often make impulsive decisions without considering all aspects.

Memory for the long haul: Long-term memory

Most of the information that flows through immediate memory and working memory is quickly forgotten. But when the brain converts a memory into long-term storage, the memory may last a while (maybe even a lifetime). When asked to recall the alphabet, you (hopefully) have no problem remembering the letters. But unless you're a schoolteacher, you probably haven't had to write or recite the letters in order since you were a kid. You can thank your long-term memory for keeping this little nugget of seldom-used info on file. Long-term memory can store huge amounts of information; it's what most people think of when they use the word *memory*.

TECHNICAL STUFF

Long-term memory can be divided into three categories: procedural, semantic, and episodic. Procedural memory involves how to do things. Most people, even with memory problems, can remember how to tie their shoes, brush their teeth, or even ride a bike. Episodic memory is remembering the stories of your lives, like your wedding, a traumatic event, or a favorite trip. Semantic memory is responsible for recalling the meanings of words, geography, and general knowledge.

Bringing back memories: Memory retrieval

You have billions of memories stored in various places in your brain. But sometimes you can't easily find those memories. When you can't remember someone's name and then a couple of hours later it just seems to pop into your brain, you've experienced a retrieval problem. Retrieval (or *recall*) is the process of pulling stored information into conscious awareness.

When all is well, the brain processes, stores, and recalls memories with efficiency and ease. However, memory has many enemies, including neurological injuries or diseases, attentional problems, drugs, alcohol, and emotional disorders. Depression is also a memory antagonist. It disrupts and may even damage the elegant memory system.

Depressing Disruptions on Your Memory

Depression fills your brain with sadness. Your ability to think clearly can be clouded by feelings of hopelessness, helplessness, guilt, and low self-esteem. But depression also affects your ability to think clearly by having a negative influence on all aspects of your memory. In the following list, we describe the ways that depression affects each facet of memory.

Effects on immediate memory

Depression decreases your ability to pay attention to what's going on around you; you may not even notice important information. Things that you normally pay attention to may slip right by.

An overwhelming depression keeps **Aidan** moving slowly through his morning routine. He notices the time and realizes that he'll almost certainly be late for work. Aidan searches frantically for his keys. He tosses papers aside, digs in his brief case, and scurries from room to room. "Damn, damn, damn," he says, as his irritation grows. Suddenly, his hand discovers the keys, in his pocket, where he put them just minutes earlier. "Damn, damn, damn." Everyone probably has something like this happen from time to time, but Aidan is running into this problem almost every day. Aidan's immediate memory is impaired.

Effects on working memory

Depression disrupts your ability to concentrate and hold on to information. Your ability to solve problems plummets.

Throughout her company, folks know **Isabella** as an energetic, kind, and intelligent manager. Lately, she has been experiencing a lack of energy, a poor appetite, and a huge decrease in her usual enthusiasm for her job. Today, she must chair a meeting with six other managers to work on solving a company problem. She begins the meeting by asking the managers to report on their perceptions of the situation. She anticipates finding a solution easily after all the aspects of the problem are exposed. As the meeting progresses, Isabella finds it difficult to listen and hold on to the various ideas in order to compare and contrast them. Her mind floods with negative thoughts. At the end of the presentations, she realizes that she doesn't have a clue about how to approach this problem. Her working memory isn't working very well.

Effects on long-term memory

Depression makes learning new material much harder. Tasks such as studying for an exam can become extremely difficult. Not only is concentrating more difficult, but also the information just doesn't seem to stick.

The cold, slush, and dreary days of winter are especially depressing to **Ethan.** His mood matches the dimming light of the season. But this winter seems worse than past years. Ethan loses his job at an internet company, which deepens his depression. The job market looks terrible, so he decides to get his real estate license. He gathers all the study materials, but when he reads a paragraph, he finds that he can't even remember what he read. He never experienced this kind of problem before. He reads through the book twice, and keeps notes. He takes a practice test and fails miserably. His struggle adds to his depression. Ethan is having trouble getting information to stick in his long-term memory.

Effects on retrieval

Depression makes recalling information like dates or mental shopping lists more difficult. It renders previously learned names, faces, and facts inaccessible. When you're depressed, you're more likely to remember sad and depressing memories, because depression floods your brain with negative memories. You may actually have trouble remembering the periods in your life when you were happy.

"I'll never find a guy," **Emma** complains to her friend Hayley. "Every time I think someone's nice, he turns out to be married, a jerk, or not interested in me. And even the guys who seem interested are only interested in one thing: sex. I've never had a good relationship. They all turn out horrible. I may as well give up."

Hayley is a bit astounded. She remembers plenty of guys who were interested in Emma, and she recalls several long-term, stable relationships that Emma actually broke off. Emma has more dates than anyone in her circle of friends. In fact, Hayley has always been jealous of Emma's ability to attract guys. What gives? Emma is suffering from depression. She really can't remember the good times.

PICTURING THE DEPRESSED BRAIN

TECHNICAL STUFF

Researchers are certain that depressed people have real problems with memory. Exciting brain-imaging techniques are now helping scientists see what depression looks like in the brain. With this knowledge, they're beginning to understand the complicated relationship between mood and memory.

One explanation for poor memory during depression may be found in increased levels of *corticosterone,* a hormone that's released when people experience severe stress. Corticosterone levels increase during depression. Research at the University of California found that high levels of this hormone impaired rats' ability to retrieve information that was previously learned or stored in long-term memory. Another possible explanation for poor memory may be the decreased levels of the brain chemical serotonin found in depressed people. *Serotonin* helps regulate attention as well as the ability to be interested in pleasurable activities.

Research at the Washington University School of Medicine has shown that people who have suffered from depression may have a smaller *hippocampus,* a key region in the brain that is important in learning and memory. According to some speculation, the stress hormone *cortisol* may have toxic effects on the hippocampus.

Worrying about Forgetting

When you experience memory problems as a result of depression, worrying about these problems may deepen your depression, which will no doubt increase your forgetfulness. If you're depressed, don't be too surprised if you forget where you parked, can't remember a word or someone's name, or misplace everyday items. Getting upset about minor problems with your memory can easily make you even more depressed.

TIP

Try to lighten up on yourself and realize that your memory glitches are most likely merely symptoms of depression. These memory problems will likely resolve when your depression lifts. And to take a more active approach in bulking up your memory muscles, use the tips and techniques we provide in the "Boosting Broken Memory" section later in this chapter.

An underlying disease or disorder sometimes causes poor memory. A little forgetfulness is a normal part of aging, too much stress, or depression. But extremely poor memory may be a sign of a more serious problem.

If you notice any of these symptoms, make an appointment for a complete physical:

>> You become confused when performing activities you're very familiar with, such as doing laundry or cooking.

>> You get lost when going to places you routinely visit, such as the post office or grocery store.

>> You get disoriented, unsure about where you are or what you're doing, for more than a brief moment or two.

>> Your memory problems begin to significantly interfere with your everyday work or relationships.

Your doctor may find that a treatable, physical cause is at the heart of these problems. Or she may confirm that your memory problem is due to depression, too much stress, anxiety, or another disease process.

Boosting Broken Memory

So you have some problems with your memory. If you're depressed, you probably don't have lots of enthusiasm for rigorous exercises that can help improve your memory. So we provide *quick, simple* tips and tricks to help you get by until your depression lifts and your memory improves.

TIP

In addition to using the following techniques, practice forgiving yourself for memory lapses. Self-criticism only worsens your memory problems as well as your depression.

Inputting stuff

TIP

The key thing you need to do is admit that you have a problem with your memory, and then compensate for it.

Technology can be very useful for people with memory problems. For example, you can schedule alarms on your smartphone to remind you to check your calendar, take your medication, or perform other daily chores. Or you may find the old-fashioned pen and notepad easier to use.

For most of us, the best thing to do is keep your smartphone handy and use the calendar app to keep track of your schedule. And keep your phone up to date with all of your contacts (both personal and work). Maintain several to-do lists: one for daily chores, one for longer projects, and another for projects you might consider in the future. It's actually kind of satisfying to check things off your to-do lists as you get them done.

Developing routines

Here's the scene: You finally managed to force yourself to do some shopping, and now you're tired. You push your shopping cart out the door and, suddenly, you can't remember where you parked. This situation can happen to anyone, but when you're depressed and distracted, it becomes more likely, it feels horrible, and it gives you one more reason to feel bad about yourself.

TIP

Here's one way to avoid this type of situation: Every time you go to a store, park at the end of a row on either the right or left side of the entrance. If you have a favorite mall or grocery store, pick out a space that is rarely used. Park in that spot even when another space is open right next to the door. Parking in the same spot will not only take care of the problem, but it will also help by making you walk a little more. (See Chapter 12 for information about the benefits of exercise for depression.)

Developing habits and routines for other annoying tasks can also help. For example, find a decorative hook or basket for your keys, and make sure that you put them there every day. Put your mask, purse, or wallet in the same place every day.

Smelling (and touching and seeing) the roses

Most people experience the world through sight, sound, touch, smell, and taste. Memory experts have discovered that when you use more than one sense, your ability to remember something improves. For example, when you listen to several instructions, you're more likely to remember them if you also see them in writing.

TIP

When you need to remember something, try to experience it with as many senses as possible. For example, if you want to remember an address such as 10 Greene Street, you can picture ten people mowing grass alongside a residential street. Use both the image of the green grass and the smell of the grass to plant the address in your memory.

You can also use a familiar tune to help you remember information. You change the lyrics of a song to include the information you want remember. Have you ever noticed how kids learn the alphabet? But don't forget, the best way to remember something is to write it down or input it into your device. Both writing and singing involve more than one sense.

At times, you may find that experiencing something through all the senses doesn't, well, make sense. When you want to remember the names and faces of people you meet, reaching out and tracing the shape of their faces (or other personal places) probably isn't a good idea. And please don't lick anyone you just met. Okay?

Remembering names

Many people complain that they aren't able to remember names. Have you ever forgotten someone's name only seconds after being introduced? It's almost as if the name actually went right through one ear and out the other. It's really hard to recall names when you're introduced to someone in a noisy space with unfamiliar people. You might have been thinking of how awkward you feel or what you might say to continue the conversation. With so many distractions, it's easy to forget names.

If that's a problem for you, try this: Next time you're introduced to someone, use the name at least three times in the conversation. "Hi, Riley, nice to meet you, Riley. So do you live here in town, Riley?"

Try to look directly at the person and take a mental photograph. As you make eye contact, use the name again in conversation. When you turn away, visualize the name, face, and anything interesting you learned about the person. Repeat the name to yourself several more times, and then put the name in your contact list with some descriptive information.

Chunking

Chunking involves grouping or organizing large amounts of information into small units. Doing so facilitates memory. Here's an example of how chunking helps. First, read the following numbers and then close your eyes and try to remember them: 6 3 2 8 9 5 7 4 5.

This exercise may be hard for you to do. One effective technique for remembering strings of unrelated numbers is to put them together in shorter units or chunks. Now read the following numbers and then close your eyes and repeat them: 5 5 4 - 7 5 9 - 8 2 3.

Did you do a little better this time? Your brain can hold on to small amounts of information better than it can hold on to large amounts.

Getting rid of distractions

Do you ever talk on the phone at the same time you answer email? Do you listen to news shows and scroll through your phone simultaneously? The modern world encourages, and sometimes demands, multitasking. However, when you're depressed, your ability to pay attention to multiple things at the same time is compromised. And multitasking takes considerable attention.

TIP

Understand that, during a time of depression, your concentration may not be as good as usual. If you need to remember something or figure out something new, do so in a quiet setting. Concentrate on one thing at a time.

Following through

Do you have several uncompleted projects hanging over your head? The stress of knowing that you have unfinished business may increase your negative mood. When you're having problems with your memory, tracking progress on several different fronts becomes especially difficult.

TIP

When you start something, make sure that you finish it. Don't begin another project until you complete what you start. Alternatively, you can finish a portion of your project and then organize the balance for tackling later. For example, with something as time-consuming as doing your taxes, you may want to tackle it in logical pieces, rather than all at once. And finally, make sure that you plan ahead so that you can devote sufficient time to your project.

Revving up recall

The most annoying memory problem may be forgetting a word or name in the middle of a conversation. You know that you'll remember it tomorrow or in a couple of minutes, but you can't get it out. You feel like kicking yourself. The more you try to remember it, the madder you get.

Stop, take a deep breath, and relax. It happens to us all. Stop trying to remember the word, and think about something else. Then, a little later, take some time to think about associations you may have with that name or word. Most likely, you'll remember it. Don't forget, depression disrupts memory.

Chapter **21**

Pursuing Happiness

P sychologists and therapists in practice spend most of their time with people who have problems. We see people with depression, anxiety, anger, grief, chronic pain, relationship problems, problems with substance abuse, and more. The stories that psychologists hear from their patients are sometimes heartbreaking. And most psychologists carry a bit of that pain in their own hearts.

Yet if you look at lists of the most satisfying careers, you'll almost always find psychology as one of the top-ten professions. When you spend your day with people who are hurting, how can that be so satisfying? Wouldn't it be more fun to be a video game designer or an ice-cream taster?

Ask therapists about what makes their job so satisfying and they are likely to say how wonderful it is to see people feel better, solve their problems, face obstacles, and gain insight. They might explain that learning the challenges of others' lives is a fascinating privilege that allows them to better understand the mysteries of the human mind and behavior. And that making a difference in the lives of other people in positive, meaningful ways is one of the most rewarding gifts of their own lives.

What makes psychology such a gratifying field is the experience of having meaning and purpose from one's work. The field of positive psychology addresses that issue and more. Developed as the 20th century came to an end, the purpose of positive psychology is to go beyond the mere amelioration of misery to help people live an enhanced, full, and satisfying life.

In this chapter, we review key concepts from the field of positive psychology. Hopefully you've reached the point where depression doesn't dominate your life. But we want you to feel better than merely "not depressed." And in discovering how to reach for happiness, we hope that your depression will be less likely to reoccur.

TIP

You'll benefit from this chapter the most if you've already emerged from depression. A number of the ideas contained in this chapter won't seem particularly workable to someone in the throes of a major depression. Please first consider reading other chapters and/or seeking professional help to alleviate your depression prior to seriously looking at achieving true happiness.

The Elusiveness of Happiness

Everyone wants to be happy, right? Not exactly. Some people feel that they don't deserve happiness. Others view happiness as a frivolous pursuit, essentially a waste of time. And finally, some people both desire and pursue happiness, yet fail to find it. We now explain why, for many folks, happiness all too often remains out of reach.

Making the case for being happy

Perhaps you feel that you don't deserve to be happy. If so, you're likely someone who experiences guilt and self-blame rather often. If that description fits you, we suggest reading or rereading Chapters 4, 6, 7, and 8 carefully. You may need further work on certain core change-blocking beliefs or habitual ways of thinking before you embark on a quest for happiness.

On the other hand, maybe you feel as deserving of happiness as anyone else, but you view happiness as flippant foolishness. This perspective is often the result of the messages parents convey to their children. Some children are told that work is the one and only valuable activity in life, and that any other undertaking merely diverts attention from what's important.

REMEMBER

The information gathered from a growing pile of studies stands in stark contradiction to the dreary idea that happiness is irresponsible and wasteful. Today we know that happy people

>> Live longer

>> Are more creative

- » Have lower blood pressure

- » Have more active immune systems

- » Have more empathy for others

- » Make more money

- » Are more productive

So even if work is your primary concern in life, it appears that happiness makes you work more efficiently and productively. Happiness is also good for your health and your overall sense of well-being, and it likely enables you to live longer. It's hard to argue with something so good for you, isn't it?

Looking for happiness in all the wrong places

Many advertisers, booksellers, drug dealers, cult leaders, pornography peddlers, and workshop gurus have something in common. What can it be? To one degree or another, they offer shortcuts and quick-fixes to happiness and well-being. More than a few people must be buying the messages from these quick-fix happiness traffickers. Just take a look at the sales of cars, appliances, clothing, workshop tickets, and even drugs today when compared to 40 or 50 years ago.

A study conducted yearly in the United States asked people to rate themselves on a 1-to-3-point scale of happiness (1 = not too happy; 3 = very happy). The 2019 report (General Social Survey) showed happiness had decreased by more than 50 percent since the 1990s. Poor health appears to predict unhappiness as does excessive social media use, spending time on the internet, and listening to music alone. Those solitary activities typically occur on devices. So in the United States at least, people appear to be less happy than they used to be. Much of the source of this misery may be that more people spend more time engaged in solitary activities as opposed to in-person social connections. The pandemic has no doubt decreased happiness further.

REMEMBER

You may find it hard to believe, but numerous studies have conclusively demonstrated that for most people money fails to substantially improve happiness. If you're not in a state of extreme poverty, money has a low correlation with reported happiness. So you're as likely to be happy if you just have enough money to pay your bills as you are if you have piles of cash you don't know what to do with.

So if money doesn't pave the road toward happiness, what does? According to the *popular* ideas on the subject, the factors that breed happiness include

>> Power

>> Health

>> Education

>> Good looks

>> Youth

>> Good climate

REMEMBER

Guess what? Like money, not one of the issues on the previous list has been found to be a particularly strong predictor of happiness and well-being. Yet many people devote much of their lives in pursuit of these very things, convinced that their quest will lead to happiness. They don't realize that they're chasing highly seductive illusions.

Being healthy doesn't even guarantee happiness. Don't get us wrong; extremely disabling illnesses of long duration do seem to detract from happiness. But studies have shown that, within fairly broad limits, not even less than ideal health hampers happiness.

So if all these rather indisputably desired, sought-after items don't lead to happiness, what does? Though no one knows all the answers, the field of positive psychology is beginning to unearth some interesting possibilities. We devote the remainder of this chapter to some of those possibilities and urge you to consider each of them carefully.

Culture and happiness

The World Happiness Report is an international comparison of levels of happiness across 156 countries. People are asked to rate their life on a scale from one to ten. One would be the worst possible life and ten would represent the best. The five Nordic countries — Finland, Denmark, Norway, Sweden, and Iceland — usually rank among the top ten. What do all of these countries share that appears to be related to happiness? The following factors appear to matter most to people:

>> A well-functioning democracy

>> Reliable and extensive benefits, such as healthcare, childcare, education, income protections

>> Low corruption

>> Freedom and autonomy

>> Social trust toward each other

>> Safe environments

Interestingly, another scale, the Gallup State of Emotions, assesses emotions and positive and negative experiences across 140 countries. A sample of questions from the scale include the following:

>> Did you smile or laugh a lot yesterday?

>> Did you learn or do something interesting yesterday?

>> Did you experience the following feelings during a lot of the day yesterday:

  • Physical pain

  • Worry

  • Sadness

  • Stress

  • Anger

>> Were you treated with respect all day yesterday?

Unlike the World Happiness Report, countries in Latin America represented the most positive feelings and experiences worldwide. Paraguay, Panama, Guatemala, Mexico, and El Salvador took the top-five places in that survey.

The World Happiness Report looks at life satisfaction. The Gallup State of Emotions scale looks at emotions. What is interesting is that life satisfaction does not appear to be highly correlated with positive emotions. They are obviously two widely different measures of well-being. So it is possible that cultural differences in the experience of happiness explain some of the differences across the two measures.

TECHNICAL STUFF

The United States has dropped in happiness rankings three years in a row, recently placing 19th on the World Happiness Report. It is believed by experts that higher levels of anxiety, decreased trust in politicians, and the deadliest drug overdose crisis in history may contribute to this decline.

Language and happiness

The words that we use influence the way we feel. Different languages across the world have culturally inspired specific words to describe feelings or emotions that may not be easily translated or replicated in other languages. For example, the German word *schadenfreude* means the pleasure someone gets at the pain or misfortune of others. It's that feeling you get when a comedian you don't like falls flat on his face, or an unpopular politician stumbles over her words.

English does not have a similar word. Does that mean that people who speak English don't sometimes get a chuckle when someone takes a fall? We don't think so. But because we had no word for the feeling, we either pretend that we don't have that feeling or attribute it to something else.

Words in other languages that refer to different states of happiness reflect cultural differences. Tim Lomas, a lecturer in positive psychology, has studied words across the world for expressions of happiness. Here are a few of the most interesting ones:

» *Wabi sabi* (Japanese): Weathered, imperfect, rustic beauty

» *Fjaka* (Croatian): The sweetness of doing nothing

» *Hygge* (Danish): Being safe, protected, and cared for

» *Morgenfrisk* (Danish): Satisfaction from a good night's sleep

» *Ubuntu* (Zulu): Universal kindness and common humanity

» *Heimlich* (German): Familiar and comfortable

» *Guo yen* (Chinese): Enjoying and satisfying one's cravings

» *Desbundar* (Portuguese): Disinhibited merry making

» *Kefi* (Greek): Frenzied, joyful emotions evoked by social occasions featuring music, dance, and alcohol

» *Charis* (Greek): Kindness, charm, beauty, and nobility

Lomas believes that learning a wider range of words that describe different aspects of happiness and well-being will actually enable people to experience such emotions more frequently and deeply. He further contends that acquiring a broader knowledge of other cultures' expressions will expand our worldview and lead us to new, positive, nuanced interconnections.

Getting on the Right Path to Real Happiness

The steep road to happiness contains no shortcuts. Thus, you may wonder why, in Chapter 13, we advocate indulging in so-called healthy pleasures. Some of our suggestions include short-lived enjoyments such as drinking tea or coffee, eating chocolate, taking a hot bath or shower, playing games, going to a movie, and smelling fresh flowers.

We make those suggestions because people typically avoid anything pleasurable when they become depressed. Temporary, sensory delights don't lead to genuine, long-lasting happiness, but they can kick-start your efforts to climb out of depression. In the following sections, we set aside the tea and chocolate and discuss what may lead to lasting well-being.

Feeling gratitude

Gratitude. We bet that you wouldn't put gratitude at the top of your list if we asked you to compile your ideas about possible foundations for happiness. By *gratitude* we mean an appreciation or thankfulness for the good things that have either happened to you or been bestowed on you by others.

Most of the world's major religions extol the values and virtues of gratitude. And numerous literary references suggest that gratitude may increase a sense of well-being, happiness, and contentment. However, does consciously focusing on feeling grateful lead to happiness?

Studying the effects of gratitude

A colleague of ours volunteered to counsel two different couples who lost their homes and most of their possessions to a terrible forest fire. The first couple focused on the horror of their loss and the magnitude of the work they faced. Insurance claims, government bureaucracies, and rebuilding seemed almost overwhelming. They felt depressed and hopeless.

The other couple had a different take on what happened. They definitely felt a certain amount of sadness and despair, but they also talked about feeling grateful that their family emerged healthy and intact. And they were deeply appreciative of all the help bestowed on them by relatives, friends, neighbors, and even complete strangers.

Both couples received fairly similar acts of kindness and assistance from others. However, the second couple experienced more gratitude. Not surprisingly, they suffered far less emotional pain than the first couple.

We also have some clinical-type proof of the positive effects of gratitude. Researchers, Dr. Robert Emmons and Dr. Michael McCullough, conducted a series of studies that suggest that gratitude does indeed lead to an increased sense of well-being. During these studies, several groups of participants were asked to list items for which they feel *grateful*. These items, which could be large or small, included waking up this morning, performing an act of generosity, or even being able to listen to a favorite musical group. Other groups were asked to list neutral happenings, ways in which they felt others were less fortunate than themselves, and the hassles they experienced during the day.

Overall, the results of the studies were rather striking and impressive. Dr. Emmons and Dr. McCullough found that asking participants to focus on events for which they felt grateful caused a number of interesting changes (when compared to the groups that were asked to track different types of happenings). In general, the groups that focused on gratitude

>> Had more positive feelings

>> Helped other people with their problems more frequently

>> Had less negative feelings (in one study)

>> Slept longer

>> Had better quality sleep

>> Felt more connected to other people

>> Were more optimistic

>> Exercised more, even though no one had asked them to do so (in one study)

>> Reported fewer health complaints (in one study)

These results are particularly amazing given that the groups that focused on gratitude weren't led to expect any particular benefits. Furthermore, these groups tracked their blessings for a relatively short period of time, ranging from a couple of weeks to a couple of months. In addition, people who knew the participants in the gratitude groups reported that they were able to tell that the participants felt better about their lives.

Putting gratitude to work for you

TIP

We recommend that you consider tracking what makes you feel grateful as a way to improve your sense of well-being. We call this strategy the Gratitude Tracker. Perform the following tasks each day for the next month or two:

>> Write down *five* things that make you feel grateful. Review your entire day, and consider both small and large events.

>> Reflect a few moments on how appreciative you feel about each item on your list.

That's it. This exercise only requires about five minutes of your time each day. But we believe that you can use the Gratitude Tracker to start you on the way toward "counting your blessings" as a regular part of your life. The benefits you derive may very well surprise you.

TIP

In down, negative times, you may feel as though you have nothing to feel grateful about. However, even during those negative times, we urge you to ponder and reflect awhile. You'll likely find a few small things to feel grateful about. If, on the other hand, you're so depressed that you find this exercise impossible to do, please work on your depression before going back to this exercise.

Helping others

We believe that a connection exists between *altruism* (unselfish concern for others) and the ability to feel gratitude. Support for this idea can be found in the study we discuss in the "Studying the effects of gratitude" section earlier in this chapter. An increase in gratitude led study participants to help others more often. We suspect that the reverse may hold as well — that an increase in altruism may lead to an increase in gratitude.

TIP

Thus, we suggest that you look for ways to help others. You may wonder how to go about doing this. It isn't that hard after you begin thinking of ideas, but here's a short list to get you started:

>> Find a kid in your neighborhood who needs tutoring, or volunteer to help with a literacy program.

>> Volunteer to read stories to kids at the hospital.

>> Offer to help an elderly neighbor with some chores.

>> Spend a day picking up trash somewhere other than your own neighborhood.

>> Take cans of food to a local food bank.

We won't give you a long list, because we believe that half the fun of performing this exercise is coming up with ideas. You may also want to check out the Random Acts of Kindness Foundation on the internet at www.randomactsofkindness.org.

REMEMBER

If you tend toward cynicism, you may think that people can't truly have unselfish concern for others because, ultimately, the person acting altruistically expects to obtain benefits. Well, we choose not to argue with this idea. We believe that benefits do indeed flow both ways. We're not suggesting that you perform kind acts in anticipation of actual personal gain; that wouldn't be in the spirit of this suggestion. However, we think that you'll derive a considerably more enduring sense of pleasure from altruistic activities than from temporary pleasures such as eating a nice meal or watching your favorite television show. Give altruism a try and see for yourself.

Finding flow

Momentary pleasures won't help you find enduring happiness. Yet it seems that society has gravitated more and more in the direction of cheap, quick-fix approaches to finding happiness. At the same time, we don't recommend that you abandon all small pleasures.

Rather, we suggest searching for engaging challenges. Dr. Mihaly Csikszentmihalyi describes these challenges as something that cause you to feel a sense of what he calls *flow*. When you're in a state of flow, you typically find yourself completely absorbed in the activity you're engaged in (so much so, that you lose a sense of time). These are the activities that you want never to end and that engage you so powerfully that your involvement feels utterly effortless, even if the pursuit is physically strenuous.

You may have to search to find activities that give you this sense of total engagement and flow, but you're likely to discover great value in searching for and finding such completely captivating challenges. Look back on your life and ask yourself what types of activities may have engaged you in the ways we're describing. You'll likely find something if you reflect for awhile. If you don't, search for ideas in hobbies you currently enjoy.

For some people, certain sports like running or tennis do the trick. For others, a particular hobby like painting, gourmet cooking, dancing, or reading a book presents new and stimulating ideas. We sometimes find that writing puts us in a state of flow. Some days we write for hours and barely realize that the clock has moved.

TIP

Activities that stimulate flow require a considerable amount of effort — more than is required by temporary pleasures like watching television, going to movies, or snacking on delightful junk food. Unlike transient delights and amusements, activities that put you in a state of flow require you to hold off gratification for awhile. But at the end of the day, you'll very likely find rich rewards in making the effort.

Most of these fully engaging challenges have the potential to produce failure experiences before and after they become inherently rewarding. In most cases, we think that you'll find these transient failures worth the effort. However, if you're in the throes of a depression, we don't particularly recommend that you start trying to find flow experiences. Recover from your depression first, and then turn your attention to finding activities that produce flow.

Focusing on strengths

We want you to feel better than okay. In order to do that, you'll need to focus on your personal strong points, rather than beat yourself up over your flaws. If you're still in the throes of depression, you'll probably need to work through other parts of this book (especially Part 2) to enable you to let go of your negative focus. But if you have emerged from depression, read on.

Building a definition

What do we mean by strengths? We'll start off by telling you what we don't mean. We don't mean attributes that are largely inherited: Appearance, athletic skill, height, and a great singing voice are features about yourself to appreciate and feel grateful for.

Think about it. You may enjoy hearing a friend sing, but that's not likely why you value that person as a friend. Similarly, you may enjoy watching your children develop as athletes, but we suspect that their athletic skill has little to do with why you love them. When you think about what makes a person invaluable to you, don't you think more about that individual's fundamental human characteristics?

Strengths are really the virtues, attributes, and characteristics that you value in others. Strengths involve a person's core character. The following list provides examples of important strengths, at least some of which you no doubt possess.

Appreciation of beauty/aesthetics	Joy in learning
Compassion	Kindness
Curiosity	Loyalty
Dependability	Listening skills
Empathy	Loving
Generosity	Perseverance
Helpfulness	Sense of humor
Honesty	Trustworthiness

Exercising your strengths

We suggest that you review our list of 16 sample strengths. Ponder which of these strengths capture your personal strong points. Although few people can lay claim to having all these positive attributes in abundance, we also believe that almost no one comes up lacking in all these areas.

TIP

By identifying, appreciating, and building on your strengths, you can find value in yourself and increase your sense of well-being. Start by observing your strengths. Identify the personal strengths you value the most in the previous list, such as honesty, sense of humor, and listening skills. Or perhaps you can think of a few strengths not listed. Then, over the next few weeks, you can work on our Appreciating Strengths Strategy. Get out a notebook and take notes on your strengths.

1. **Notice each time you use one of your personal strengths.**

2. **Notice the type of occasion that allows you to express your strength.**

3. **Observe how you feel when you employ that strength.**

4. **Appreciate how that strength enhances your life.**

5. **Mentally pat yourself on the back for having that strength.**

We hope that, as you try out our Appreciating Strengths Strategy, you'll feel a sense of gratitude for your strengths. Next, we suggest building on your strengths and exercising them often. Look for opportunities to use your strengths at work, home, and play.

> **Anna** cleans houses for a living. She struggles to get through each day and views her work as something she must do to survive, nothing more. Though she's not depressed, her life is dull and lacking in purpose.
>
> By contrast, **Jenna** also cleans houses, but she creates meaning from her work by focusing on ways to express her personal strengths of appreciating aesthetics, kindness, and helpfulness. Jenna approaches her work from the standpoint of how she can "beautify" the homes she works in, not merely clean them. She carefully arranges items in aesthetically pleasing ways; she doesn't just dust them off. She also looks for any opportunity to make her clients' lives easier. Thus, she readily reorganizes pantries and occasionally runs errands without being asked.

Cynics may think that Jenna is merely "sucking up." And indeed she is in far greater demand as a house cleaner than Anna. However, she truly finds joy in expressing her personal strengths through her work. Jenna frequently enters a state of flow, and her work enhances her sense of well-being.

TIP

Given the opportunity, choose work that will maximize your personal strengths. However, no matter what type of work you do, you can find ways to express your strengths and build on them if you try hard enough. And remember that work is just one part of life. Take the opportunity to discover, apply, and build on your strengths in every aspect of your life.

Rejecting the quick fix

Self-restraint, self-discipline, moderation, self-denial, temperance, self-control — these terms don't exactly conjure up images of joy and happiness. In fact, they may even sound downright dreary. Yet the fact remains that self-control will lead you toward happiness more certainly and directly than any quick-fix approach.

Unfortunately, we live in a world that increasingly delivers promises of instant happiness and good feelings. Though we see a role for medications when it comes to treating certain types of depression (see Chapter 17), some advertisements seem to suggest that you should pop pills the moment a bad feeling arises. Other ads condition you to believe that instant happiness will come if you drive the right car or own the best sound equipment available. And instant solutions are offered for every conceivable hassle, from preparing meals to the "horror" of having to wait in line for a rental car.

In addition, books, videotapes, and workshop gurus tell everyone that they should feel good about themselves all the time. And if you don't, they suggest simplistic solutions like merely repeating positive, yet silly self-affirmations over and over every day. Guess what:

>> Quick fixes don't work.

>> No one is happy all the time.

>> The more you expect instant gratification, the more miserable you're going to be.

Psychologists have even found that the ability to exercise self-control and delay gratification is highly predictive of ultimate adjustment and well-being from childhood through adulthood. Although self-control is arguably best figured out in childhood, the good news is that you can increase your self-control at any time.

TIP

Moderation and self-control appear to be valuable for a number of reasons:

>> Many of the most-satisfying goals require considerable patience and work in order to obtain them.

>> When you shower yourself with indulgences, they lose much of their appeal. Psychologists call this phenomena *satiation*. In other words, too much of a good thing ends up feeling less enjoyable.

>> When you have an inflated view of yourself, thinking you're better than others, you may end up causing problems. For example, if you allow yourself to feel superior to other people, others will more likely reject you.

Thus, we advocate moderation as a realistic path toward sustainable happiness. Money, alcohol, drugs, and self-indulgence represent seductive illusions. If you focus your efforts on quick fixes, you'll find yourself disappointed time and time again.

Finding forgiveness

Of all the paths toward happiness, figuring out how to forgive may be the most difficult. When people have been wronged, it can be so tempting to hold a grudge and desperately desire revenge (whether it is ever acted upon or not). And why not? After all, if you did nothing to deserve the injustice, don't you deserve to at least have a *desire* for retribution? Absolutely. You completely deserve to have those feelings!

Unfortunately, those feelings will cost you. Quite a lot, actually. Holding onto feelings of rage and revenge will likely make you feel like a victim. Chapter 4 discusses the harmful effects of feeling like a victim, which include increased anger and a sense of helplessness. We suggest that you read this chapter to discover ideas on how not to feel like a victim.

More importantly, figuring out to forgive is likely to enhance your sense of well-being. Several studies have shown that the more you cling to your resentments and grievances, the less happy and satisfied with life you're likely to be. But how in the world can you find forgiveness if you've been egregiously wronged?

REMEMBER

A few horrific things can happen to people, such as sexual abuse or violence, that you may not be able to forgive. In such cases, it's probably more important to accept one's self and attempt to let go of thoughts of revenge than to actually find forgiveness.

TIP

As we say earlier, finding forgiveness is no easy task. However, you can do it. We recommend the following steps for conducting what we call a Revenge Reanalysis and Forgiveness Technique. See what this process can do for you. We understand that the concept may seem foreign to you at first, but we believe that you're likely to discover surprising benefits after exploring the idea.

1. **Remember the wrong in the most dispassionate, nonjudgmental terms possible. Imagine the happening in your mind and try to avoid feelings of rage, retribution, or sorrow as best you can.**

   Play the tape of your memory many times until your feelings dissipate at least a little.

2. **Search for some understanding of the perpetrator's perspective.**

   This step may be particularly difficult. You may find it useful to realize that people typically hurt others when they feel threatened, fearful, or anxious. Sometimes they perceive a need to defend their honor or self-esteem, even though their perceptions may be misguided. Consider the possibility that many offenders don't understand the hurtfulness of their actions. Some offenders may also feel the need to attack to enhance a self-image that was destroyed by a horrific childhood.

3. **Form an image of yourself in your mind as someone who copes well, rather than as someone who's a victim. Think of yourself as someone with strength and fortitude who can rise above adversity and forgive.**

4. **If thoughts of revenge come into your mind, remind yourself that revenge and retribution will harm you at least as much as the offender, and arguably even more so.**

   Even the thoughts and feelings of revenge inflict damage on your emotional soul — and hurt your body by kicking off a flood of harmful stress hormones that raise blood pressure and may eventually cause damage to your organs.

5. **Dig down deep and forgive.**

   If you can forgive the offender publicly, that's even better. Perhaps you can write a letter of forgiveness. At least write the forgiveness down and then talk about it with others. Give your forgiveness with as much altruism as you can muster, without any regard for yourself.

TIP

When memories of the wrongful act reoccur, go through the forgiveness process again. Don't expect saintly perfection from yourself. Every step you make in the direction of finding forgiveness helps you.

Searching for meaning and purpose

People find meaning and purpose in life in quite diverse ways. Finding meaning and purpose generally involves reaching out and relating to concepts that feel larger, more enduring, and of greater significance than yourself. Of course, religion and spirituality stand as the most prominent methods for finding meaning, and the largest number of people likely employs them.

If you're not very spiritually inclined, you can still infuse meaning into your life. Ask yourself what you want your life to be about. What do you want your legacy to be to the world? Consider the following exercise we call the Eulogy in Advance.

1. **Sit back and relax for a few moments. Take a few slow, deep breaths.**

2. **Reflect on your life for awhile. Don't dwell on past regrets.**

3. **Ask yourself what you want people to say and think of you at your own funeral. What do you want friends, loved ones, or others to remember about your life?**

4. **Consider what you can do with the rest of your life to infuse it with the meaning you want to leave the world.**

Very few people write such a eulogy extolling their appearance, the money they've made, the long hours they worked at the office, or the power they wielded over others. Most people choose to emphasize their strengths of character (such as those listed earlier in this chapter in the section "Focusing on strengths").

TIP

No matter what your age, you can devote at least a portion of your life to enhancing its meaning. These purposes don't need to be monumental. You may choose to

>> Be a kind person.

>> Help others.

>> Advance knowledge in some way.

>> Do something positive for the environment.

>> Be kind to animals.

>> Teach and pass knowledge on to the younger generation.

>> Forgive yourself and others.

>> Express gratitude.

You can fill your life with meaning in any number of ways. All you need to do is connect and contribute to something (almost anything) that feels larger than yourself. Whether you have a day, a year, or decades left on this planet, you *can* make a difference.

7

The Part of Tens

IN THIS PART . . .

Lift yourself out of temporary grumpiness.

Understand how to help kids and teens.

Help friends or lovers cope with dark times.

Chapter **22**

Ten Ways Out of a Bad Mood

Bad mood or depression — what's the difference? Bad moods are typically unpleasant but short emotional states. Depression drags on for weeks, or in some cases, far longer. And after you're over your depression, you'll still encounter occasional bad moods. Nonetheless, realizing that bad moods aren't intolerable and that you can do something about them may help prevent a longer-lasting negative spiral. So, in order to keep your bad moods from spiraling into a depression, this chapter gives you some tips for handling the blues.

REMEMBER

It's totally impossible to feel great all of the time. Negative feelings can alert you that something in your life is not going well and you need to address it. Grief is a normal reaction that takes time to get through. So we are *not* telling you that all bad moods or sadness need to be quelled. Acceptance of negative feelings is a part of life. Nevertheless, the following ideas can be occasional ways of dealing with a fleeting bad mood.

Chomping on Chocolate

Various types of food reputedly affect moods. People probably turn to chocolate as frequently as they do any of the other mood-altering foods. A host of the substances found in chocolate have been cited as responsible for its mood-lifting

CHAPTER 22 **Ten Ways Out of a Bad Mood** 345

effects. However, some researchers believe that chocolate, like most especially palatable foods, alters mood primarily by causing a release of endorphins, the brain's opiates. If you find that chocolate works for you, indulge a little when a bad mood sets in. But if you're a chocoholic and you feel pronounced guilt when you indulge in chocolate, then this isn't the food for you when you feel low. Guilt will only deepen your funk. As with all things, moderation is the key.

Doing Something Nice

Take a page from Chapter 21 on positive psychology. Doing something nice for someone else is one of the best ways we can think of to extricate yourself from a bad mood. It helps you refocus your attention away from what put you in the bad mood and onto other people in a positive way. And your improved mood is likely to last a lot longer than it will with other nice, quick-fix pleasures like chocolate.

Getting a Lift from Exercise

Exercise has the potential to lift you out of a bad mood. Of course, when you're in such a mood, you probably don't *feel* like exercising. But just because you don't feel like exercising, that doesn't mean that you can't do it.

Short-circuit your negative thinking about exercising and just move your body toward doing something active. Getting yourself moving is half the battle. When you get over that hurdle, your momentum will carry you forward.

Take a long walk, jog, lift some weights, take a yoga class, or do whatever form of exercise you prefer. Exercise releases endorphins, improves your health, and helps you feel a sense of accomplishment. For more information about the benefits of exercise, see Chapter 12.

Singing Yourself into a Better Mood

If you like to sing, try it when you feel low. Belt your favorite song out at the top of your lungs. There's something about singing that's almost diametrically opposed to feeling down. Of course, we do recommend an upbeat tune rather than the blues.

Putting your negative thoughts into a whimsical song can also be useful. If you're in a lousy mood, you probably have some negative thinking running through your head. (See Chapters 6, 7, and 8 for more information about this type of thinking.) Listen to those thoughts and write them down. Then use those thoughts as the lyrics to a popular song. Somehow your negative thinking loses some of its meaning when you sing your thoughts in a silly song.

Calling a Long-Lost Friend

If you're like most people, you have friends that you haven't connected with in awhile. If you want to feel good, call one of these friends. Don't wait and talk yourself out of it. Just do it. Besides, research shows that social connections can help with all kinds of ills, including bad moods. So even if you don't have a long-lost friend, call any friend at all. Talking things out may help. And reconnecting feels good.

Dancing to a Different Beat

Do you like to dance? If so, you just may be able to dance your way to a better mood. Dancing, much like exercise, releases endorphins (which is covered in Chapter 12). If you pick the right upbeat song to dance to, the music alone may pull you into a better mood. If you don't have a partner, you can just dance by yourself in the privacy of your home. You can dance in a serious way, or you can create a giddy, whimsical dance (the wilder and crazier the better!).

Soaking the Blues Away

Many people find that a long, hot bath helps soothe the body and mind. A hot tub makes a good alternative. Often, when people end up in a bad mood, doing something soothing doesn't quite "feel" right. Nevertheless, trust us on this idea. Just do it.

Petting Your Way to a Better Mood

If you're in a bad mood, try spending some time with your pet. Don't have one? Consider getting one. Really! Studies are demonstrating that pets actually help people feel better, and they may even improve your health. If we want a good laugh, all we have to do is play with our dogs. Sometimes just looking at them makes us laugh. Pets help you shift the focus from yourself and your problems to something positive — perhaps even something warm and affectionate.

Taking a Hike

Again, we can't exactly say why, but spending time in the outdoors seems to do a much better job of brightening moods than does staying inside. In the winter, it may be the natural light that helps, because the sun emits a far brighter light than you can get inside. And bright light appears to alleviate seasonal affective disorder, or SAD (covered in Chapter 2). However, the outdoors may just lift moods because it puts people into contact with nature. We don't know of specific studies that suggest that nature improves moods, but we do know that almost all our clients report feeling better when they spend time outside of their homes. And there is a bit of research suggesting the benefits of gardening to moods. When you get out there, appreciate what you see.

Mellowing Through Mindfulness

You may be able to get out of a bad mood by accepting that bad moods are an inevitable part of life! Sound confusing? Actually, the idea isn't that complicated. When you can't stand having a bad mood, your mood only gets worse. When you accept bad moods as unpleasant but inevitable, they lose some of their grip on your psyche. If this notion still seems confusing, you may want to read Chapter 9.

TIP

You may also want to consider connecting with the present rather than pondering awful thoughts about the past or future. The following exercise can help you refocus your thoughts on the present.

1. Notice the rhythm of your breathing.

2. Feel the air as it passes through your nostrils and into your lungs.

3. Notice how good the air feels.

4. Notice how your body feels. Focus only on your bodily sensations.

5. Return to the rhythm of your breathing.

6. Feel where your body touches the surface on which you're sitting, standing, or lying.

7. Notice how nice the air feels.

8. Continue noticing these various sensations for five or ten minutes.

When you connect with the present, you let go of negative thoughts about the future or past. The "now" is usually far more tolerable than your mind's worries about the future or concerns with the past.

Chapter **23**

Ten Ways to Help Kids with Depression

D
epression has reached close-to-epidemic levels among our youth. The causes of depression in the young are the same as they are for adults — biology and genetics, trauma, loss, stress, chronic family conflict, and so on. (See Chapter 2 for more about depression's causes.) Of course, the ideal solution is to prevent depression from occurring in the first place.

This chapter provides tips for preventing depression in kids. We also discuss what to do if your child, or a child you care about, becomes depressed, because not all depressions can be prevented, even despite your best efforts.

Finding Fun

Kids flourish when they feel engaged, involved, and interested in what they're doing. Explore activities and hobbies together until your child finds an interest that she can be good at and enjoy. You may have to try many different activities, such as dance, drama, swimming, stamp or coin collecting, tennis, computers, art, soccer, or horseback riding. The goal is to find a hobby that your child both enjoys and feels reasonably competent at performing.

Then make sure that she participates frequently. Getting your child involved in an engaging activity can help prevent depression, because it gives her something to look forward to and helps her develop social support.

TIP

During a pandemic, many children feel lonely and depressed. Get the kids outside. Consider a neighborhood scavenger hunt with painted rocks giving clues to search for hidden treasures. Organize outside activities that can be done while social distancing. In addition, make sure your kids are staying connected with friends and family through technology.

Doling Out Discipline

Many parents are reluctant to discipline their kids. They fear that they'll upset their children and make them feel bad. These parents worry that disciplining their children will turn their kids away from them. They want to be best friends with their children. But parenting isn't about being your child's best friend.

Care enough to discipline your child. Psychologists know that self-control and the ability to tolerate frustration are the two most important skills to learn in childhood. Armed with these skills, kids can face whatever life deals them. Children can't learn self-control unless their parents give them clear rules and consequences. Children need self-control so that they can live up to these rules, and consequences provide an incentive for learning this self-control.

Disciplining children can be hard work. So sometimes it may be tempting to ignore bad behavior. But your children are counting on you. When kids misbehave, take the opportunity to teach an important lesson. Children who learn self-control are far less likely to become depressed.

Giving Feedback

When your child goofs up, criticize the behavior, not your child. Never call a child "stupid" or "bad." Such negative labeling paves the way for the emergence of depression down the road. As an alternative, you can label the behavior "bad." For example, "stealing is bad," or "hitting your sister is wrong." When you apply such labels to your child's entire self, you risk instilling negative self-views that are difficult to alter.

Climbing Every Mountain

Give your child the opportunity to accomplish something difficult. Children learn self-confidence by mastering tough tasks. Help your child enter a race (you can train together), learn how to canoe, or master a piano concerto. During the learning process, your child will no doubt experience frustration and fatigue. Encourage him to persevere.

Life isn't easy. Children who learn how to work hard carry that quality into adulthood. As a result, they're much more likely to be able to bravely tackle life's problems, including depression.

Revving Up Responsibilities

Many parents find it easier to do household chores themselves rather than beg and nag the kids to help out. That's a mistake. Children need to feel connected and useful. Participating in family responsibilities helps kids develop character.

When kids are allowed to take without giving, they begin to feel special — perhaps too special. Laziness at home may work with some moms or dads, but when kids venture out into the real world, others view that sense of specialness and entitlement as simply a case of being spoiled rotten. The resulting rejection may trigger depression.

Talking and Listening

No matter what, you need to make it safe for your children to talk. What do we mean by "make it safe"? First, listen without interrupting. Let your children tell their stories. Next, don't judge or criticize their feelings. The following example illustrates both the wrong way and the right way to listen:

> **Breanna** tells her mother: "No one likes me. Everyone thinks I'm stupid. I feel horrible. I don't want to go to school anymore."
>
> Her mother could respond with, "Don't be ridiculous. You have no reason to feel horrible. You have lots of friends. And don't think for a second that you're going to get away with not going to school!"
>
> But a better response would be, "It sounds like you're feeling down. What happened?"

The better response didn't judge and encouraged more talking. Notice how the first response stopped the conversation cold. Your kids will only talk with you if they feel listened to and understood. Even if you don't agree with what they say, at least let them say what's on their minds.

Recognizing Depression

When children have depression, they experience symptoms that are similar to those experienced by adults. They feel sad, lose interest in things that were previously interesting, have trouble concentrating, and have low self-esteem.

REMEMBER

On the other hand, children may differ from adults in that their moods may vary more over the course of a day. Depressed children are often irritable and moody. The early warning signs of depression in children can include

>> Ditching school

>> Drop in grades

>> Excessive reactions to criticism or rejection

>> Loss of interest in usual activities

>> Risky behavior, such as taking drugs or reckless driving

>> Vague physical complaints, such as headaches and stomachaches

>> Withdrawal from friends

WARNING

Don't ignore such signs of depression in your kids. Depression is a serious problem, and it isn't a normal part of childhood. In fact, suicide is the second leading cause of death in people between the ages of 10 and 24.

Looking Under Rocks

Depression stems from multiple sources. If your child exhibits signs of depression, exploring all possible causes is important. Although depression does have genetic and biological underpinnings, some kind of outside stress often contributes to it.

Many parents blame themselves for their kids' depression. Self-blame and guilt won't help your child. But family life may play a role in depression. Be willing to look at that possibility and get help if you find any indication that your family life is negatively affecting your child.

Children spend much of their lives outside of the home. Some possible causes of depression include

>> Bullying at school

>> Emotional, physical, or sexual abuse (unknown to the family)

>> Social rejection

>> Unidentified academic problems, such as learning disabilities

>> Unidentified health problems

If your child is depressed, carefully explore all possible contributing factors. Treating the depression without understanding the causes may prevent the treatment from working. For example, if your child is depressed due to bullying at school, giving an antidepressant medication won't address the problem.

Getting Help

If you think that your child is depressed, get help. Depression in children can be treated with many of the same tools that help adults — therapy and antidepressant medications. Be prepared to take an active part in the treatment. Don't feel guilty or embarrassed about taking your child for help. If you get treatment early for your child's depression, you may prevent your child from experiencing repeated depressions later in life. See Chapter 5 for advice on how to find the right help.

Loving No Matter What

Part of being a child involves testing the limits. Kids act out, disobey, dress weird, and act out with stupid, childlike behaviors. What would adolescence be without a little rebellion? Some kids go to extremes by shoplifting, using drugs, and shocking their parents with numerous body piercings and tattoos.

Parents typically feel angry and outraged at these excessive behaviors. However, you have to make an important distinction between reacting to unacceptable behavior with feelings and consequences versus total rejection and rage.

REMEMBER

You need to let your kids know that, no matter what, you love them. That doesn't mean that you can't express displeasure or disappointment. Temper condemnation with concern. Care and love walk hand in hand with discipline.

Chapter **24**

Ten Ways to Help a Friend or Lover with Depression

Nothing's much more distressing than seeing someone you love suffer from depression. You care, and you want to help. But most people don't know where to start. This chapter gives you ten ideas for how you can help someone you care about with depression.

Recognizing Depression

You must recognize that your loved one is depressed before you can do anything to help. Of course, you can read the formal diagnosis of depression in Chapter 2 if you want to see an entire list of symptoms. But we don't exactly suggest that you give your friend a diagnosis — that's a task only for professionals.

However, perhaps you've noticed lately that your loved one is acting differently, displaying behaviors such as:

>> Changes in appetite or sleep

>> Disinterest in previously enjoyable activities

>> Increased irritability

>> Lower energy and fatigue

>> Lower mood than usual

>> Problems concentrating or making decisions

>> Self-disparaging talk

If your loved one has more than a couple of these symptoms, she may very well be depressed. As we said, don't make the diagnosis yourself. However, you can gently ask about the possibility of depression, and perhaps urge your partner to check out this possibility with a counselor or the family doctor.

If seeing a counselor or doctor feels too threatening to your loved one, the internet has screening resources. See the Appendix for a list of these and other resources. National Depression Screening Day usually falls in October. You can check out this program at www.mhanational.org. In addition, this site has screening tools you can use at any time of the year.

WARNING

The internet contains an incredible amount of useful information. However, it can't replace professional help. Furthermore, some sites are more reliable than others. We provide you with the web addresses of some high-quality websites in the Appendix.

Referring for Help

One of the more useful actions you can take is to encourage your loved one to get help. You can start by recommending *Depression For Dummies* — just be sure you point out that you're not suggesting that your friend is a dummy in a negative sense! In addition, you can suggest a visit with the family doctor. Finally, if your loved one agrees to see a therapist and doesn't get around to doing so, offer to help find one. Read Chapter 5 for ideas on how to go about finding a good therapist.

REMEMBER

Although you can be helpful to someone you know who has depression, you can't solve the problem. You can't be responsible for the depression or even for insuring that the people you care about get help. You can facilitate help, and that's as far as you can go.

Listening Without Solving

More than anything else, realize that it's truly not up to you to cure your loved one of depression. Even if you're a counselor, physician, or psychologist, you can't treat someone you care deeply about. Friends may not have the necessary objectivity and perspective needed for effective treatment. Your friend needs you to be someone who will listen, not treat or solve the problem.

Therefore, you should provide a sounding board. Listen with empathy and concern. You may want to express that you've had similar feelings at times in the past, if that's truly the case. If you listen carefully, you'll no doubt find yourself tempted to talk your loved one out of the quagmire of depression. Don't give in to that temptation; such attempts will likely be met with resistance and possibly a worsening of symptoms.

REMEMBER

Your loved one needs a sympathetic ear; professionals are the only people who can actually intervene therapeutically.

Taking Care of Yourself

Helping someone you care about who's depressed can drain you of energy and resources. Listening to tales of woe and misery isn't always easy. We advise that you connect, listen, and empathize to the extent that you can. But don't let yourself sink into the throes of depression in the process.

Thus, attending to your own needs is important. Continue to live your life and seek sources of enjoyment. Connect with friends and keep balance in your life. If you invest too much of yourself in helping your loved one, you can easily lose the capacity to help, and you risk falling into your own depression.

Holding Criticism at Bay

If your loved one is depressed, the last thing you need to do is criticize. Nonetheless, you may find yourself tempted to do so when you hear some of the things a person who's depressed may say. For example, your friend may say something like, "I'm no good to anyone anymore."

Upon hearing something like that, you may find yourself blurting out, "That's ridiculous! Why would you ever say something so stupid?"

Try to use empathy instead. Perhaps say, "I know you feel that way. I don't really agree with you, but it must feel awful to have that thought."

In addition, people with depression may bait you to criticize them. Due to the increased irritability, they may criticize you more than usual, and you may feel tempted to defend yourself. Try to resist defending your ego and realize that the criticism is probably due more to depression than anything else.

Depersonalizing Depression

When someone you love is depressed, it's rather easy to think that the depression is the result of something you've done, or that somehow it's your fault. Please realize that depression has many causes — genetics, biological factors, certain diseases or drugs, childhood events, culture, and so on.

That's not to say that your relationship with your loved one has nothing to do with the depression. In fact, it may. Being open to the idea of working on your relationship is a good idea — perhaps through counseling, if that seems appropriate. And consider reading and implementing the ideas presented in Chapter 16. But blaming yourself for your partner's depression won't help. And in most cases, other causes play a far greater role.

Finding Patience

When you're dealing with a case of serious, major depression, you need to understand that treatment takes time. Even antidepressant medication typically requires a few weeks to start working. Furthermore, some depressions require a considerable search for the right medication, which may take many months.

Psychotherapy also takes time to work. An average case may show some improvement within two to three months, but many cases require a longer period of time. As with medications, sometimes the first therapist doesn't work out, and your loved one may need to search for another mental health professional to receive the right type of help. (See Chapter 5 for information about finding help for depression.)

WARNING

Avoid falling into the trap of thinking that your loved one actually *wants* to feel depressed. We truly believe that no one wants to feel depressed. Sometimes a person with depression can act somewhat irrationally or in self-defeating ways, but that doesn't mean that the depression is actually desired.

Try not to lose patience. You may want to consult a therapist yourself if you find the task of getting your loved one to go to a therapist to be too difficult.

Remembering to Care

When people become depressed, they need the care and concern of loved ones more than ever. Unfortunately, people with depression sometimes push others away. Thus, it may seem that they prefer to be alone and isolated.

Don't believe it. Whether your efforts seem appreciated or not, continue to do caring things for someone who's depressed. Send a card or flowers. In addition, look for small caring things you can do. We provide an entire list of nice things you can do for someone in Chapter 16.

Providing Encouragement and Remaining Hopeful

Feeling hopeless isn't unusual for a depressed person. In fact, hopelessness is one of the more common symptoms of depression. Nonetheless, the vast majority of depressed people do manage to improve a great deal.

If you listen too long to what someone with depression says, it can be very easy to start believing in the hopelessness you're hearing. The fact is, many people with depression can present you with an amazing array of evidence concerning the awfulness and hopelessness of their lives. However, you need to understand that depressed minds generate thoughts that are almost always distorted in major ways. Thus, the "evidence" they give you probably isn't accurate. Check out Chapters 6, 7, and 8 for detailed information about how depression inevitably distorts thinking.

When you understand how depressed minds can distort the hopelessness of a situation, it becomes easier to remain encouraging. Your loved one with depression doesn't want you to give up, whether it seems that way or not. Remain hopeful and encouraging.

Exhorting Exercise

As we tell you earlier in this chapter, you can't be a therapist for someone you care about who has depression. That's true without question. Although there is one rather therapeutic thing you can do: Consider encouraging your loved one to find some type of exercise. Ideally, you should also participate. Activity has a positive effect on depression. The more active you are, the better. See Chapter 12 for more about the effects of exercise on depression.

TIP

Although encouraging someone who's depressed to exercise is a good idea, don't push the idea too hard. Some people, especially those with severe depression, simply can't get themselves cranked up to exercise. Pushing hard to get someone to exercise isn't worth harming your relationship.

Appendix

Resources for You

H ere we provide some additional resources for helping you find out more about depression and how to defeat it. In addition, we give you resources for other emotional issues, such as anxiety and relationship problems, that sometimes contribute to depression. Many other excellent books and websites that we have no doubt overlooked are available. In dealing with most any emotional problem, reading more than one book is often a good idea.

Books on Mental Health

Here's a list of books we recommend:

>> *Anxiety For Dummies,* by Charles H. Elliott and Laura L. Smith (Wiley)

>> *Changing For Good: The Revolutionary Program that Explains the Six Stages of Change and Teaches You How to Free Yourself From Bad Habits,* by James O. Prochaska, John C. Norcross, and Carlo C. DiClemente (William Morrow & Co., Inc.)

>> *Changing to Thrive: Using the Stages of Change to Overcome the Top Threats to Your Health and Happiness,* by James O. Prochaska and Janice M. Prochaska (Hazelton Publishing)

>> *Choosing to Live: How to Defeat Suicide Through Cognitive Therapy,* by Thomas E. Ellis and Cory F. Newman (New Harbinger Publications)

>> *Cognitive Therapy of Depression,* by Aaron T. Beck, A. John Rush, Brian F. Shaw, and Gary Emery (Guilford Press)

>> *Don't Believe Everything You Feel: A CBT Workbook to Identify Your Emotional Schemas and Find Freedom from Anxiety and Depression,* by Robert L. Leahy (New Harbinger Publications)

>> *Feeling Great: The Revolutionary New Treatment for Depression & Anxiety,* by David D. Burns (PESI Publishing & Media)

>> *Interpersonal Psychotherapy of Depression,* by Gerald L. Klerman, Myrna M. Weissman, Bruce J. Rounsaville, and Eve S. Chevron (Basic Books)

>> *Love is Never Enough: How Couples Can Overcome Misunderstandings, Resolve Conflicts, and Solve Relationship Problems Through Cognitive Therapy,* by Aaron T. Beck (HarperCollins)

>> *Mind Over Mood: Change How You Feel by Changing The Way You Think,* by Dennis Greenberger and Christine A. Padesky (Guildford Press)

>> *Mindfulness-Based Cognitive Therapy for Depression: A New Approach to Preventing Relapse,* by Zindel V. Segal, J. Mark G. Williams, and John D. Teasdale (Guilford Press)

>> *The Anxiety & Worry Workbook,* by David A. Clark and Aaron Beck (The Guildford Press)

>> *The Seven Principles for Making Marriage Work,* by John M. Gottman and Nan Silverman (Harmony)

>> *Translating Happiness: A Cross-Cultural Lexicon of Well-Being,* by Tim Lomas (The MIT Press)

Resources to Help Children

We recommend the following books for helping your child:

>> *Acceptance and Mindfulness Toolbox for Children & Adolescents,* by Timothy Gordon and Jessica Borushok (PESI Publishing)

>> *Depression: A Teen's Guide to Survive and Thrive,* by Jacqueline Toner and Claire Freeland (Magination Press)

>> *Keys to Parenting Your Anxious Child,* by Katharina Manassis (Barrons Educational Series)

>> *SOS Help for Parents,* by Lynn Clark (Parents Press)

>> *The Optimistic Child: Proven Program to Safeguard Children from Depression and Build Lifelong Resistance,* by Martin E. P. Seligman (Perennial)

>> *Something Bad Happened: A Kid's Guide to Coping with Events in the News,* by Dawn Huebner (Jessica Kingsley Publishing)

Helpful Websites

WARNING

If you type the word *depression* into a search engine, you get access to an endless stream of possible resources. You need to beware, though, because the internet is filled with clever advertisements and gimmicks. Be especially cautious about official sounding organizations that heavily promote expensive materials. And don't believe absurd promises of quick, instant cures for depression.

Many web forums host chat rooms for people who have depression and other related emotional problems. Feel free to access them for support. At the same time, realize that you have no idea who you're talking to when you join a web forum. The other people in the forum may be uneducated about depression or, even worse, try to take advantage of a person in distress.

Here's a list of some legitimate websites that don't sell snake oil but do provide excellent information about depression and related emotional issues:

>> **The American Psychiatric Association** (www.psychiatry.org/patients-families) provides information about depression and other mental disorders.

>> **The American Psychological Association** (www.apa.org/helpcenter) provides information about the treatment of, as well as interesting facts about, depression and other emotional disorders.

>> **The Anxiety Disorders Association of America** (www.adaa.org) lists self-help groups across the United States. It also displays a variety of anxiety screening tools for self-assessment. On their site, you can find an online newsletter and a message board. Because anxiety sometimes accompanies depression, you may want to check this site out.

>> **The Mayo Clinic** (www.mayoclinic.org) gives you a wealth of information on mental and physical health, including medications.

>> **National Alliance for the Mentally Ill** (www.nami.org) is a wonderful organization that serves as an advocate for people and families affected by mental disorders. Information is available about the causes, prevalence, and treatments of mental disorders that affect children and adults.

>> **National Center for Complementary and Alternative Medicine** (www.nccam.nih.gov) is a government-sponsored site designed to provide information about alternative treatments for depression and other disorders. Most of the advice on this site is based upon research (unlike other sites about alternative treatments).

>> **National Foundation for Depressive Illness** (www.depression.org) is a nonprofit group established to provide information about affective disorders.

>> **National Institute of Mental Health** (www.nimh.nih.gov) reports on research about a wide variety of mental health issues. They also have an array of educational materials on depression. They provide resources for researchers and practitioners in the field.

>> **WebMD** (www.webmd.com) provides a vast array of information about both physical and mental health issues, including information about psychological treatments, drug therapy, and prevention.

Index

clinical psychologists, 83

clinical trial, 282–283

cognitive therapy, 15–16, 81, 110

Cognitive Therapy of Depression (Beck, Rush, Shaw and Emery), 362

cognitive-behavioral therapy, 274

communication, relationships and, 267–270

comparisons, critical, 121–122

complex carbohydrates, 296

compliments, giving, 259

connecting

  with experience, 164–169

  losing connections during Covid-19 pandemic, 46

  mindfully, 167–169

  with the present, 166–167

consequences (C), for problem-solving, 230–231

constructive criticism, 258

Consulting the Friend Within strategy, 232

coping, during Covid-19 pandemic, 49–50

corticosteroids, 34

corticosterone, 322

costs, of depression, 12–15

counselors, 83

Covid-19 pandemic

  coping during, 49–50

  depression and, 36, 41, 46–50

  exercise during, 206

  insecurity and, 48

  stress of isolation during, 247–248

  telehealth services during, 50, 85

  working from home, 52

creating

  buffers, 268, 269–270

  Thought Tracker, 128–130

creative therapy, 300

credit, giving yourself, 196–197

critical comparisons, 121–122

criticism

  defusing, 268–270

  holding at bay, 358

crying, 241

Csikdzentmihalyi, Mihaly (doctor), 336

culture, happiness and, 330–331

Cumbay, Traci (author)

  Managing All-In-One For Dummies, 52

D

The Daily News, 261–262

dancing, as a mood lifter, 347

dark depression, 29

Dass, Ram (spiritual leader), 294

dating, for replacing process, 252

debt, paying down, 52

declarations, making, 157

defeating

  defensiveness, 262–266

  demotivating thoughts, 202–204

defensiveness, defeating, 262–266

Defusing technique, 268–270

delusional beliefs, 38

delusions, with postpartum depression, 33

dementia, during Covid-19 pandemic, 47

demotivating thoughts, defeating, 202–204

denial

  about, 99

  as a stage of grief, 243

dependency, managing, 61–63

dependency/inadequacy belief, 61–63

depersonalizing, 264–266, 358

Depressed Behavior Quiz, 23

depression. *see also specific topics*

  about, 7

  adversity and, 12

  behaviors and, 22–23

  biological solutions for, 16–17

  categories of, 8

  causes of, 40–41

  in children, 9–10, 349–354

  costs of, 12–15

  Covid-19 pandemic and, 36, 41, 46–50

  dark, 29

  depersonalizing, 358

  detecting, 19–44

E

eating, mindful, 169

economic change, as a life transition, 246

ECT (electroconvulsive therapy), 297–298

ego, breakups and, 248

electroconvulsive therapy (ECT), 297–298

Elliot, Charles H, (author)

  Anxiety For Dummies, 361

Ellis, Albert (psychologist), 119

Ellis, Thomas E. (author)

  Choosing to Live: How to Defeat Suicide Through Cognitive Therapy, 362

elusiveness, of happiness, 328–332

embracing victimhood, 160

emergency departments, for getting help, 183–184

Emery, Gary (author)

  Cognitive Therapy of Depression, 362

Emmons, Robert (researcher), 334

emotional accounting, 51

emotional reasoning, tracking, 106

emotion-driven behavior, 105–107

emotions

  about, 98

  feelings emerging from your body, 98–100

  feelings guiding behaviors, 101–102

  feelings sprouting from thoughts, 100–101

  handling, 234–236

  therapy and, 89

  thoughts and, 104–105

empathy, expressing, 261

empirical therapy, 81

empty nest, as a life transition, 246

encouragement, providing to friends, 359–360

endorphins, 200–201, 212

entitlement, as a relationship hot button, 266

episodic long-term memory, 319

Ethical Human Psychology and Psychiatry, 297–298

Eulogy in Advance exercise, 342

evaluating

  problem situations (S), 223–226

  relapse rates, 305

events (Thought Tracker), 128–130

everyday routine, introducing nice into your, 261–262

evidence

  checking, 133–137

  dismissing, 113, 117

exaggerating negatives, 256–257

exercise(s). *see also* working out

  mindfulness, 348

  as a mood lifter, 346

  recommending to friends, 360

expecting the worst, 218–220

expenses, cutting your, 52

experience, connecting with, 164–169

expressing empathy, 261

F

facing the worst, 147–149

facts

  feelings compared with, 105–106

  negative thoughts as, 154–155

failure

  expecting, 189

  rewriting stories about, 76–77

family

  breakups and, 248

  discord of, as a suicide risk factor in children/teenagers, 181

  response of, as a factor for antidepressant medications, 280

fatal means, as a risk factor of suicide in adults, 178

FDA (Federal Drug Administration), 293

fear of change, 58–60

Federal Drug Administration (FDA), 293

feedback

  giving, 350

  negative, 257

Feeling Great: The Revolutionary New Treatment for Depression & Anxiety (Burns), 362

feelings

  accepting, 151–169

  avoidance driven by, 106–107

compared with thoughts, 103–104

emerging from your body, 98–100

facts compared with, 105–106

guiding behaviors, 101–102

reflecting on, 224

sprouting from thoughts, 100–101

therapy and, 89

Thought Tracker, 128–130

tracking, 132–133

Feuerstein, Georg (author)

Yoga For Dummies, 208

filtering, 112

finances

breakups and, 248

as a consideration for finding therapists, 84

costs of depression, 13

depression and, 50–52

as risk factor of suicide in adults, 177

finding

adaptive replacement thoughts, 130–141

change-blocking beliefs, 61–71

flow, 336–337

forgiveness, 340–341

guilt, 161

patience, 358–359

replacement thoughts, 137–138

therapists, 84–85

findings, analyzing, 69–71

Fire Drill strategy, 309–311

firearm, suicide by, 173

Firing Your Mind's Faulty Forecaster, 218–220

Fitness For Dummies (Schlosberg and Neporent), 205

flexibility, in goals, 51

floating thoughts, 158

flow, finding, 336–337

following through, 326

foods, happy, 295–296

forgetfulness, 322–323

forgiveness, finding, 340–341

freedoms, loss of during Covid-19 pandemic, 47–48

Freeman, Claire (author)

Depression: A Teens Guide to Survive and Thrive, 362

frequency, of exercise, 205

friends

breakups and, 248

calling, as a mood lifter, 347

death of, 244

giving problems to, 142–143

listening to, 357

providing encouragement to, 359–360

recognizing depression in, 355–356

recommending exercise to, 360

referring for help, 356–357

fun

children and, 349–350

taking it seriously, 209–211

G

GABA (glutamate and gamma-aminobutyric acid), 288

Gallup State of Emotions, 331

gatherings, losing the freedom of, 48

GBD (Global Burden of Disease), 13

geocaching, 213

getting

acceptance, 162–163

help, 182–184

giving

advice, 261

compliments, 259

feedback, 350

Global Burden of Disease (GBD), 13

glutamate and gamma-aminobutyric acid (GABA), 288

goals, flexibility in, 51

good, feeling better than, 17

Gordon, Timothy (author)

Acceptance and Mindfulness Toolbox for Children & Adolescents, 362

Gottman, John M. (author)

The Seven Principles for Making Marriage Work, 362

thinking
   all-or-none, 146–147
   visual, 228
thinking machine, 153
Thought Court, 130–132, 139, 140
thought suppression, 107
thought therapy. *see* cognitive therapy
Thought Tracker
   about, 132–133, 140
   building, 128–130
thought-feeling connection
   about, 97–98
   emotion-driven behavior, 105–107
   emotions, 98–102
   interpreting thoughts, 102–105
   negative thoughts, 107
   pink elephants, 107
thought-repair toolkit, opening, 141–149
thoughts
   about, 127–128
   accepting, 151–169
   building with a Thought Tracker, 128–130
   "can't thoughts," 192–194
   compared with feelings, 103–104
   demotivating, defeating, 202–204
   depression and, 20–22
   emotions and, 104–105
   feelings sprouting from, 100–101
   finding adaptive replacement thoughts, 130–141
   floating, 158
   interpreting, 102–105
   negative, 107
   opening thought-repair toolkit, 141–149
   playing with your, 156–158
   reviewing your, 192–193
   singing, 156
   testing, 144–146
   tracking, 132–133
Thoughts on Trial form, 133–137, 140–141
time
   for exercise, 205
   putting on your side, 143–144

Tip icon, 3
tiredness, 189
TMS (transcranial magnetic stimulation), 299
Toner, Jacqueline (author)
   *Depression: A Teens Guide to Survive and
      Thrive*, 362
touch, 324–325
tracking
   emotional reasoning, 106
   feelings, 132–133
   saboteurs, 72–74
   thoughts, 132–133
   well-being, 312
training, as a consideration for finding therapists,
   84–85
transcranial magnetic stimulation (TMS), 299
*Translating Happiness: A Cross-Cultural Lexicon of
   Well-Being* (Lomas), 362
trauma, as a suicide risk factor in children/
   teenagers, 181
travel, losing the freedom of, 47
treating
   depression, 15–17
   severe depression, 297–299
Trevor Lifeline, 183
tricyclics, 286

U

undeserving outlooks, 63–64
unfairness, 65
unworthiness, as a relationship hot button, 266

V

vagus nerve stimulation (VNS), 298–299
valley, walking in a, 76
veterans, suicide and, 178–179
victim role, 65–68
victimhood, embracing, 160
videos, as resources for self-help, 94
vision, breakups and, 248
visual thinking, 228
vitamins, 293–295

VNS (vagus nerve stimulation), 298–299

volunteer work, for replacing process, 253

vulnerability, as a relationship hot button, 265, 266

W

waiting to be happy, 159

walking, 208

Warning icon, 3

WebMD, 364

websites

American Psychiatric Association, 363

American Psychological Association, 363

Anxiety Disorders Association of America, 363

Cheat Sheet, 4

Mayo Clinic, 364

National Alliance for the Mentally Ill, 364

National Center for Complementary and Alternative Medicine, 364

National Center for Complementary and Integrative Health, 295

National Depression Screening Day, 356

National Domestic Violence Hotline, 55

National Foundation for Depressive Illness, 364

National Institute of Mental Health, 364

National Institutes of Health Office of Dietary Supplements, 295

Random Acts of Kindness Foundation, 336

as resources, 363–364

as resources for self-help, 94

WebMD, 364

Wegner, Daniel (doctor), 107

Weissman, Myrna M. (author)

Interpersonal Psychotherapy of Depression, 362

well-being

about, 311

changing lifestyle, 314

satisfaction interrupters, 313–314

tracking, 312

Wenzlaff, Richard (doctor), 107

Williams, Mark G. (author)

Mindfulness-Based Cognitive Therapy for Depression: A New Approach to Preventing Relapse, 362

withdrawal symptoms, antidepressant medications and, 279

women, depression in, 11

work, losing the freedom of, 47

working memory

about, 319

effect of depression on, 320–321

working out

about, 199–200

defeating demotivating thoughts, 202–204

easing into, 204–205

options for, 206–208

during a pandemic, 206

reasons for, 200–202

World Happiness Report, 330–331

worst

expecting the, 218–220

facing the, 147–149

Y

Yates, Andrea, 38

yoga, 208

Yoga For Dummies (Feuerstein and Payne), 208

yourself

taking care of, 357

talking to, 235–236

Z

zovirax, 34

About the Authors

Drs. Smith and Elliott are clinical psychologists and have worked on numerous publications together. They are coauthors of *Anxiety For Dummies (Wiley)*; *Quitting Smoking & Vaping For Dummies* (Wiley); *Anger Management For Dummies* (Wiley); *Borderline Personality Disorder For Dummies* (Wiley); *Child Psychology & Development For Dummies* (Wiley); *Obsessive Compulsive Disorder For Dummies* (Wiley); *Seasonal Affective Disorder For Dummies* (Wiley); and *Anxiety & Depression Workbook For Dummies* (Wiley). They have committed their professional lives to making the science of psychology relevant and accessible to the public.

Authors' Acknowledgments

We want to thank our outstanding team at Wiley. As usual, their expertise, support, and guidance was of immeasurable help. From the beginning, our acquisition editor, Kelsey Baird, helped us formulate and execute a plan for developing this new edition of *Depression For Dummies*. Tim Gallan, masterful project editor, ensured that our text stayed coherent and on point. We also thank our technical editor, Joe Bush, PhD, for his insightful contributions.

Publisher's Acknowledgments

Acquisitions Editor: Kelsey Baird

Project Editor: Tim Gallan

Technical Reviewer: Joseph P. Bush, PhD

Proofreader: Debbye Butler

Production Editor: Tamilmani Varadharaj

Cover Image: © DNY59/E+/Getty Images